RECENT ADVANCES IN PERIODONTOLOGY
VOLUME II

RECENT ADVANCES IN PERIODONTOLOGY VOLUME II

Proceedings of the fourth International Academy of Periodontology Meeting, Istanbul, 17–20 September, 1990

Editors:

STEVEN I. GOLD
Columbia University
School of Dental and Oral Surgery
New York, N.Y.
U.S.A.

MARSHALL MIDDA
Department of Clinical Periodontology
University of Bristol Dental Hospital
Bristol
U.K.

SERDAR MUTLU
Centre for the Study of Oral Disease
University of Bristol Dental School
Bristol
U.K.

 1991

EXCERPTA MEDICA, AMSTERDAM – NEW YORK – OXFORD

International Congress Series No. 957
ISBN 0 444 81424 8

This book is printed on acid-free paper.

Published by:
Elsevier Science Publishers B.V.
P.O. Box 211
1000 ED Amsterdam
The Netherlands

Sole distributors for the USA and Canada:
Elsevier Science Publishing Company Inc.
655 Avenue of the Americas
New York, NY 10010
USA

Library of Congress Cataloging in Publication Data:

International Academy of Periodontology. Meeting (4th : 1990 :
  Istanbul, Turkey)
    Recent advances in periodontology : volume II : proceedings of the
  Fourth International Academy of Periodontology Meeting, Istanbul,
  17–20 September 1990 / editors, Steven I. Gold, Marshall Midda,
  Serda Mutlu.
        p. cm. -- (International congress series : no. 957)
  Includes index.
  ISBN 0-444-81424-8 (alk. paper)
  1. Periodontics--Congresses. I. Gold, Steven I. II. Midda,
  Marshall. III. Mutlu, Serdar. IV. Title. V. Series.
  [DNLM: 1. Periodontal Diseases--congresses. 2. Periodontics-
  -trends--congresses. W3 EX89 no. 957 / WU 240 I597 1990r]
  RK361.A2R43   1990
  617.6'32--dc20
  DNLM/DLC
  for Library of Congress   91–24889
                                               CIP

Printed in The Netherlands

INTRODUCTION

The fourth meeting of the International Academy of Periodontology provided an opportunity to bring together more than a thousand dental professionals, who are involved in treating and investigating periodontal diseases in man, from around the world. The main symposium themes included recent advances in the diagnosis and treatment of periodontal diseases, chemical plaque control of gingivitis and periodontal disease, reappraisal of longitudinal studies, new surgical approaches to the regeneration of periodontal tissues and the periodontal application of dental implants.

As is the custom of the International Academy of Periodontology, speakers were drawn from more than 30 countries and from all continents. The most current advanced work being done aroud the globe was presented and freely discussed in a collegial atmosphere. This open exchange of information and opinion is the foundation of good science and good international relations, and both were features of this unique gathering in Istanbul. It is a tribute to Professor Sandalli, and his hard working committee, that the warm and friendly gathering of dental professionals was both productive and rewarding.

These proceedings record the symposia and lectures of researchers who were essential to the process of bringing a clear picture of the changing patterns of the diagnosis and treatment of periodontal diseases to colleagues from around the world.

In addition to the opportunity for professional growth, the exciting venue of Istanbul provided the perfect environment for the social events that enhance an international congress of this calibre. The Turkish hosts and IAP officers created a series of events that took full advantage of the three thousand year history of the metropolis of Istanbul, with its sites commemorating the contributions of Greek, Roman, Byzantine and Ottoman culture to human civilization. This blend of ancient and modern was an ideal forum for consideration of the coming developments in dental practice as the International Academy of Periodontology honoree, Professor Harald Löe noted in his keynote address 'The Changing Face of Dentistry'. In the past 40 years caries has declined and periodontal diseases, as well as other oral diseases, have become proportionately more important to dental practitioners. The training and research of the 21st century will have to reflect these changes.

In reviewing the papers presented at this Congress the reader will note a thread of an increasing awareness of the potential for regeneration of periodontal tissues. This has been an elusive goal in the last quarter century. Current approaches draw upon chemotherapeutic and biological concepts which have emerged in the last decade. Other papers record the precision of increasingly sensitive ultrastructural and histochemical probes of disease activity. The subject of the periodontal implantology was a popular topic, emphasising the increasing role of the periodontists in this developing discipline.

The editors are grateful for the opportunity to share with its readership the Proceedings of the 4th Meeting of the International Academy of Periodontology with the hope that it will contribute to continued improvement in the development of periodontology and continued development of internationalism among dental professionals.

On behalf of the IAP and the local organising committee we would like to express our gratitude to our major commercial sponsors without whom this meeting would not have been possible. For the publication of these proceedings we particularly thank Colgate–Palmolive, Sunstar Inc., The Lion Foundation for Dental Research and Unilever.

Steven I Gold, A.B., D.D.S.
Marshall Midda, B.D.S., F.D.S., F.F.D.
Serdar Mutlu, B.D.S., M.Sc.

CONTENTS

SYMPOSIA

FREE PAPERS

POSTER PRESENTATIONS

LECTURES

© 1991 Elsevier Science Publishers B.V.
Recent advances in periodontology Vol. II,
S.I. Gold, M. Midda and S. Mutlu, eds.

THE CHANGING FACE OF DENTISTRY

HARALD LÖE

Director, National Institute of Dental Research, National
Institutes of Health, Building 31, Room 2C39, Bethesda, MD
(United States)

We are living at a remarkable time in human civilization. I
believe this period will be remembered as a turning point in
history, one that is changing the world of politics,
communications and science. The movement towards democracy that
has swept across Eastern Europe from Poland and Czechoslovakia to
Hungary, the Baltic nations and Russia itself is nothing short of
a tidal wave that has not crested yet. And it is all happening
simultaneously and literally before our eyes.

Today the Middle East is the focus of world attention,
reminding us of the pivotal role this region has played in human
history. Indeed, civilization as we know it began in the valley
of the Rivers Tigris and Euphrates flowing out of Turkey to
nourish the ancient kingdoms of Mesopotamia and Babylon.

Over the centuries Turkey's command over the eastern end of
the Mediterranean made it the crossroads of East and West; the
seat of the Byzantine and Ottoman Empires; and the magnet for
trade and travel for the peoples of the Levant and beyond.
Everywhere around us are the natural beauties of landscape and
harbor and the cultural monuments that make Istanbul the Jewel of
the Bosphorus.

But we are not here to celebrate past glories. It is a
tribute to the sponsors of this Fourth Meeting of the
International Academy of Periodontology and the 21st Annual
Meeting of the Turkish Society of Periodontology that we are
meeting here in modern Istanbul to talk about modern science.

For surely the remarkable changes we are seeing in the political face of Europe and the Middle East, the abundant developments in computer science and communications that are making the world truly a global village, are more than matched by what we are seeing in biomedical science. Fundamental advances and discoveries are changing the way we live today and the way our children will live tomorrow.

From our own perspective, the past decades of dental research--of periodontal disease research in particular--are cause for celebration. Indeed, what has happened in the past quarter of a century has changed the face of dentistry--for all time.

I mean that literally. We know from surveys in America and in other industrialized countries, that oral health has improved significantly over the last 25 years. And it shows no sign of stopping. With regard to children, the NIDR conducted a survey in 1986-87 in which we examined some 40,000 schoolchildren between the ages of 5 and 17 representing America's 44 million school-children. Primarily, we wanted to see if the declines in dental caries in children we had documented earlier were levelling off. They were not. Caries prevalence among schoolchildren is continuing to decline. Fifty percent of the children in America are now caries free; never had a cavity, never had a filling. So we are seeing a continued change in the face of youngsters for the better.

Also, I should add--those who still have caries have much fewer and smaller lesions than just 10-15 years ago.

For the first time we were able also to mount a national assessment of juvenile periodontitis in America. (For all I know, this may have been the first national survey ever and anywhere on early onset periodontal disease.) At any rate, we examined 11,007 youngsters aged 13 to 17 years old for their patterns of periodontal destruction.

Approximately 0.53 percent of American children between 13-17 were found to have localized juvenile periodontitis; 0.13 percent to have generalized juvenile periodontitis, and 0.47 percent to have incidental loss of attachment--for a total of 1.13 percent. These percentages are not high, but the actual number of children affected is not trivial. Close to 150,000 children below 18 years in the United States are estimated to have some form of early onset periodontitis.

With regard to adults, the NIDR conducted a major national survey of caries and periodontal diseases in 1985-86. Over 15,000 employed adults 18 to 65 years old were examined at their workplaces and over 5,000 Americans 65 to 103 years old were seen at senior citizen centers. When we looked at the data by age groups it was clear that the young-to-middle-aged cohorts are in far better oral health than their forebears. So the face of many adults in America is also changing for the better. A significant indicator of that was the finding that only 4 percent of adults 18 to 65 years old are edentulous.

The situation with respect to the periodontal diseases is also improved. To be sure, the diseases are still highly prevalent and worsen with age. However, overall, the workers are experiencing the milder forms of disease; there are relatively few cases of severe, advanced destructive periodontitis among working individuals in America.

The situation with regard to older Americans is far worse. Forty-two percent of the senior citizens (65 years and older) have lost all their teeth. The older groups have more coronal caries and the prevalence of root caries is three times what was seen in younger adults. The seniors also have more severe and extensive signs of periodontal disease.

I should remind you that the older people studied in this survey were well enough to walk or travel to senior citizen centers. So, the oral health status of the homebound, handicapped, or frail elderly was not represented and is probably worse.

RESEARCH AND ACTION

Concern over the situation in older Americans and of some of the other adult risk groups--combined with a desire to maintain the state of good oral health of younger adults through the retirement years--has become the driving force behind a major initiative at the NIDR called "The Research and Action Program for Improving the Oral Health of Older American and Other Adults at High Risk." Our goals are to eliminate toothlessness in America; to prevent the further deterioration of the oral health of those with compromised dentitions; and to ensure that adults in good oral health maintain that state as they advance to the retirement years.

By any standard, this is an ambitious undertaking. But what is happening here is that NIDR is changing the focus from a preoccupation with primary prevention in children's teeth to a concern for the whole spectrum of oral health problems of children, adults, and old people. We need to look at the oral aspects of normal development, maturation, and aging, including changes in the oral micro-ecology, in the immune system, and in the capacity for tissue repair, as well as research on the various oral conditions and how they affect and are affected by systemic disease and treatments. Most importantly, we need to get on with the job of finding out who is at risk and why.

That means basic molecular research and more analytical epidemiology studies; risk factor analysis and behavioral and social science research. It also means concentrated efforts to develop new and innovative preventive measures appropriate for different individuals and risk groups.

At the same time, we are moving ahead to forge links with public and private agencies and individuals who can conduct the kinds of activities that will shorten the distance from the lab to the chairside and promote information. We want to make sure that the message is heard in the dental schools and is reflected in the education of dental students; we want to see that it reaches the practitioners, the public, the health policy and health-financing organizations, and anyone else who can facilitate the transfer of technology for oral health promotion and disease prevention.

If the past is any guide, there is good reason this program will succeed. The improvements in oral health we are currently seeing have been attributed to a number of factors: improved oral hygiene practices, the use of fluorides, healthier diets, more knowledgeable patients, better trained dental professionals. But the real explanation is that we basically understand the etiology of the major dental diseases. That understanding is the basis for the rational approaches to prevention and treatment that we employ today and is a direct reflection of the power of dental research.

Many of us here today have personal experience of that fact. We have seen an exponential growth in knowledge about the periodontal diseases and in the application of that knowledge in our lifetimes. Thirty-five years ago we in periodontal research banished idle speculation as the major approach to understanding periodontal biology and pathology. Theories of simple mechanical etiologies of periodontal diseases collapsed under the weight of scientific evidence. Basic and clinical studies established the role of supra- and subgingival plaque in the development and progression of periodontal diseases. The new understanding that the periodontal diseases were <u>bacterial infections</u> compounded by <u>host inflammatory processes</u> revolutionized the field, intensifying research to identify the bacteria involved, clarify host-bacteria interactions, and determine the importance of genetic and environmental factors in the natural history of the diseases.

All at once there was an explosion of activity in microbiology and immunology. Animal models like the beagle dog, and, more recently monkey species, were developed. Experimental antiseptic therapies were tried and surgical and non-surgical procedures reevaluated.

But the work was not conducted in a vacuum. By the 1970s, the whole world of biomedical research was becoming molecular and getting computerized. Step by step we are learning the genetic and biochemical rules that govern the functions of cells from birth to maturity to old age.

MOLECULAR BIOLOGY IN PERIODONTAL RESEARCH

At a molecular level we now are beginning to understand the processes by which the normal oral flora becomes established in the mouth. We know that within moments after a tooth has been cleaned that saliva will lay down an "acquired pellicle" that will provide a receptive surface for early colonizers like

<u>Streptococcus sanguis</u>. Other bacteria will find their niches on the tongue, the palate, and other mucosal surfaces. In turn, specific proteins and surface features of the early colonizers permit interactions with other bacteria leading to co-aggregations, creating the complex assemblage that we call plaque. Here is a real potential for the development of a new kind of a molecular anti-plaque attachment agent or rinse which would prevent co-aggregation of bacteria, and thereby halt plaque formation.

Also, new approaches are now available for studying familial forms of periodontal diseases. Immunologists have raised the possibility of a hereditary defect in neutrophils in cases of localized juvenile periodontitis. It is now possible to study samples of DNA from members of large families affected by this disease, and the hope is to find a genetic marker to identify family members at risk for early onset periodontitis. These children are obvious risk groups and have been for a long time. I suggest that now is time for an aggressive approach to deal with their problems.

Molecular technology is also speeding up the process of isolating and identifying periodontal pathogens. We now have an assortment of new genetic probes and monoclonal antibodies that have been produced to detect oral pathogens or the byproducts of disease in crevicular fluid, oral tissues, or plaque samples. Some of these probes are already commercially available in kit form for diagnostic use in the dental office.

These molecular techniques should also help to resolve a key question in periodontal disease research today: the issue of disease activity versus inactivity. In turn, those findings could lead to better diagnosis and prognostications, but also

could lead to more selective therapy: the use of "narrow
spectrum" antibacterial agents specifically directed against the
bacterial species identified.

Finally, I should mention one of the most exciting and
celebrated directions that periodontal disease research has taken
in the past few years. That is the work on regeneration of the
periodontium. The concept of guided tissue regeneration is based
on the hypothesis that periodontal ligament cells have the
potential of developing new connective tissue attachment and bone
in areas or sites affected by advanced periodontitis. Both the
concept and the techniques have shown great promise in clinical
studies and represent an entirely new and innovative approach to
treatment of periodontal disease.

All these examples reflect some of the exciting areas of
contemporary periodontal disease research. Clearly, in a
relatively short time, we have progressed from ignorance to
understanding and from impotence to power in diagnosing,
preventing, and treating periodontal diseases.

MOLECULAR BIOLOGY IN CARIES RESEARCH

And the same could be said for dental caries. Whereas
fluoride programs of various kinds continue to be the mainstay of
caries prevention and most likely are the explanation for the
dramatic reduction of caries in children and young adults, we
should not forget that there are billions of people who today--
for one reason or another--do not benefit from this technology.
For them, the possibility now exists that caries can be prevented
by an anti-caries vaccine. Yes, indeed, we now think this long
dream of research could become a distinct reality. In the past,
crude extracts of <u>Streptococcus mutans</u> or killed or weakened

strains were used as the immunizing agent. These materials were often effective in evoking an immune response, but there were always concerns that the antibodies raised might cross-react with healthy tissue.

The new approach takes advantage of an understanding of the molecular genetics of the bacteria. Microbiologists have now identified specific virulence factors on the cell surface of _S. mutans_. The genes coding for these proteins have been cloned and introduced into a harmless strain of bacteria that normally inhabits the intestine. The idea is to use these genetically engineered bacteria as an oral vaccine. Once swallowed, the bacteria would settle in the intestine, express the S. mutans proteins, and stimulate lymphoid tissue lining the intestine. The activated lymph cells would generate anti-caries antibodies which then would be released in the mouth via salivary secretions.

A number of laboratories are conducting this research with the potential of developing polyvalent vaccines: a vaccine that might combine caries protection with protection against oral herpes--which has also been the target for recombinant DNA vaccine research. In turn, protection against these oral diseases might be combined in a vaccine against polio, measles, influenza, or other serious disease--all in a single easy-to-swallow dose. Such an approach might be the preventive method of choice in individuals at high risk for disease or in areas where the availability of health services and trained health professionals is problematic.

IMPLICATIONS FOR THE FUTURE

Probably the ultimate measure of how well we in science and practice are doing in our efforts to control oral disease is the extent of toothlessness. However, tooth loss is not only a function of disease. It also reflects socioeconomic conditions, individual and cultural differences, and the dental delivery system. These factors include a person's perception of the need, of self-care practices, and of the cost of dental services as well as their availability and utilization.

Earlier, I mentioned the impressive gains in oral health among the working population of America, including evidence that very few do experience extensive and severe periodontal disease. These findings have revised our thinking. We no longer believe that the periodontal diseases are the major cause of tooth loss in adults in the U.S. As a matter of fact we have data to show that even in the adult population, caries and its sequelae-- restorations, recurrent caries, pulpal disease--are the major contributors to tooth mortality over the lifetime.

Over the last 150 years dentistry in industrialized societies has evolved in three phases: First, there was a preoccupation with relieving pain and extracting teeth. Second, we developed technologies that enabled us to save teeth by filling cavities. Third is the phase that Western dentistry is entering in full force: prevention. We are now able to take advantage of what research has taught us about the cause of oral diseases and to get on with the job of prevention in all its complexity--from the development of vaccines to the behavioral strategies aimed at getting people to adopt sound life styles and abandon destructive habits.

Furthermore, the growth and expansion of dental science have resulted in an increasing investment in activities going beyond the traditional dental disorders to include all the diseases and disorders affecting the orofacial tissues.

We continue to explore the genetic and environmental factors that can result in cleft lip, cleft palate, and other serious craniofacial defects. In some cases we understand, at the molecular level, when and how the damage can occur.

Soft tissue lesions, salivary gland research, bone disease, research on acute and chronic pain--all have grown to become major fields of oral and dental science in the past quarter of a century, defining the expanding scope of the future dental practitioner and the future curricula of our dental schools.

These are exciting developments in the history of dentistry. Progress in understanding the transition from health to disease and from disease to health has gained enormously as we have passed from the level of the organism, the tissue, the cell and now the molecule. But the reverse journey is equally important. Once we have a handle on the cell and molecular derangements in disease processes, we must go up the scale to engage the whole organism in the healing process. And beyond the whole organism there is society itself--and the community of societies that constitutes the world today.

We come together at this conference as representatives of those separate societies united by common interests in periodontology as a basic clinical discipline in comprehensive oral health care. But more than that, we are united by the common ground of our humanity and our concerns for the health of all people. It is in this context that I look forward to a productive meeting, one that can take us one step farther toward our goal of modern dentistry: The complete control of the two major oral diseases and the preservation of the natural dentition for a lifetime.

© 1991 Elsevier Science Publishers B.V.
Recent advances in periodontology Vol. II,
S.I. Gold, M. Midda and S. Mutlu, eds.

PERIODONTOSIS (JUVENILE PERIODONTITIS) UPDATE

Paul N. Baer, Professor and Chairman, Department of Periodontics, School of Dental Medicine, Stony Brook, NY 11790

All patients with periodontosis (J.P.) may appear to be similar clinically. However, the disease may have different etiologies in different patients. In some, the genetic factors may play the dominant role, in others it may be the microflora, where the predominant cultivable microorganism is the actinobacillus actinomycetemcomitans (A.A.) while in still others, it may be a combination of factors. This would explain why in some patients the A.A. cannot be found, why in others there is no familial background and why in still others, one finds both a familial background and the Actinobacillus actinomycetemcomitans to be the predominant microorganism present. An interesting aspect of the ongoing reasearch in this disease has recently been reported. Investigators have found a strong assoiciation between the presence of <u>Actinobacillus actinomycetyemcomitans</u> (A.A.) as well as a greater prevalance of antibody of this microorganism among subjects with juvenile periodontitis (J.P.) than in subjects with either no periodontitis or other forms of periodontitis. Yet none of the investigators who reported on these findings mentioned that the majority of their subjects with juvenile periodontits (J.P.) were black while their non-periodontal disease controls were white. Gunsolley noting this omission recently repeated

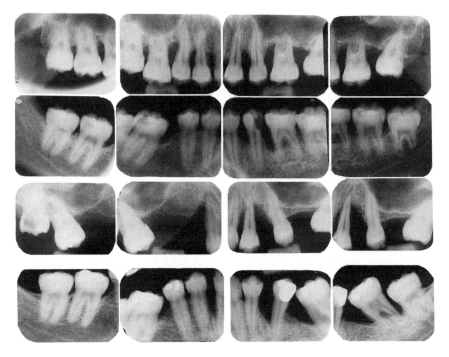

Figure 1   An example of a rapidly progressive generalized juvenile periodontitis or periodontosis.
TOP--Radiographs of patient at age 16
BOTTOM--Radiographs of patient at age 21

these studies using race-matched controls (1). The results: while some differences might still exist, these investigators felt that the results obtained by others were largely the result of the racial composition of their groups. Once race-matched controls were used, these differences were greatly reduced.

In regards to etiology, I have observed the localized and generalized forms occurring in siblings born of the same parents. This suggests that the localized and generalized forms have similar etiologies and differ only in the severity of their clinincal manifistations. Furthermore, these are two distinct clinical

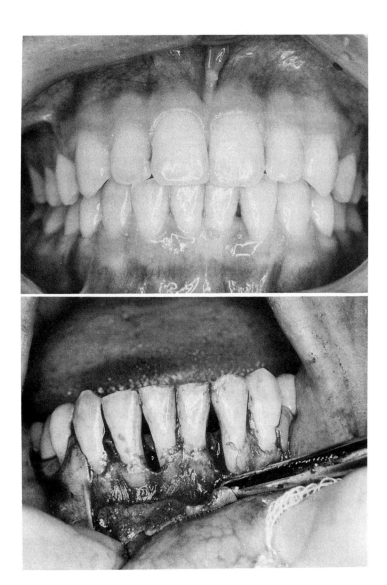

Figure 2   Patient with a chronic slowly progressive generalized
                periodontosis or juvenile periodontitis.
                TOP--Appearance of patient at age 19
                BOTTOM--Bony defects at time of surgery, age 19

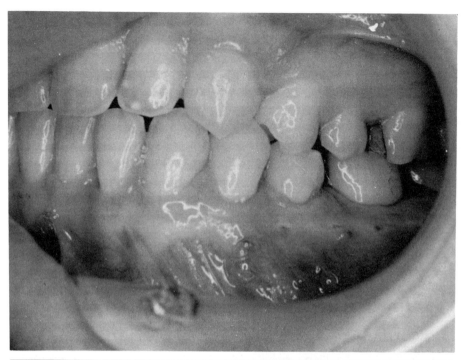

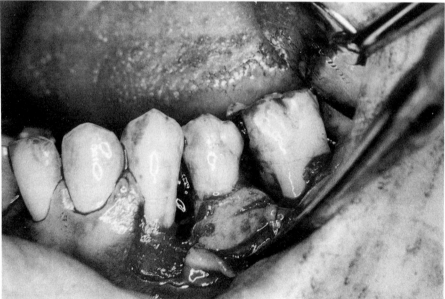

Figure 3   TOP--Patient at age 19 (same patient as Fig. 2)
                 BOTTOM--Bony defects present at time of surgery, age 19

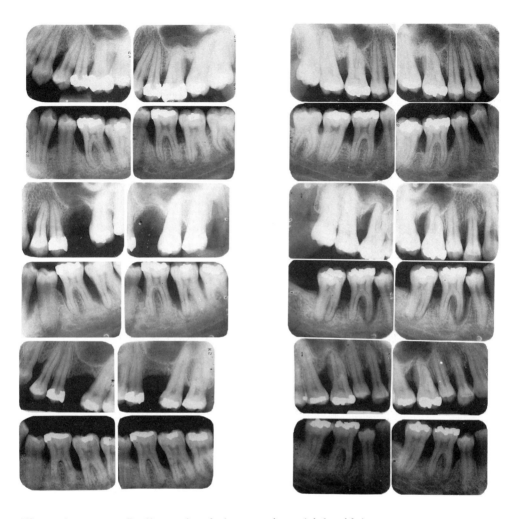

Figure 4   Radiographs of above patient, (right side).
                TOP--age 19
                MIDDLE--age 27
                BOTTOM--age 40

Figure 5   Radiographs of above patient, (left side).
                TOP--age 19
                MIDDLE--age 27
                BOTTOM--age 40

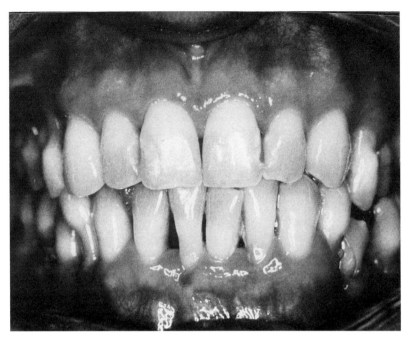

Figure 6   Appearance of patient today. Compare with figure 2.

manifestations of the generalized form. An acute disseminated type which is rapidly progressive, Figure 1, and a chronic slowly progressive type figures 2-6. While the chronic generalized disease has the more favorable prognosis, nevertheless, even the acute type, which frequently results in loss of all the maxillary teeth, tends to spare many of the mandibular teeth. I have never observed a case where patients with this disease following therapy have become completely edentulous in the mandible. In regards to therapy, I recommend that antibiotics be used as adjuncts to surgical treatment in both the acute and chronic forms of this disease.

REFERENCES

1. Gunsolley, J. C. et all (1988) J. Periodont Res: 23:303-307

Recent advances in periodontology Vol. II,
S.I. Gold, M. Midda and S. Mutlu, eds.

MECHANISMS AND CONTROL OF ALVEOLAR BONE LOSS IN PERIODONTAL DISEASE

JOHN E. HORTON AND LAURIE K. MCCAULEY

Department of Periodontology, The Ohio State University College of Dentistry, Columbus, Ohio, 43210. U.S.A.

INTRODUCTION

The pathogenesis of alveolar bone loss in periodontal diseases (PD) is complex due to direct and indirect effects on tissues by bacterial deposits and host defense mechanisms. This loss appears to exist independent of a generalized skeletal response or disruption in systemic mineral metabolism to suggest that specific biologic molecules exist at the local site to control cellular responses (1). Justification for such a local regulation of osteoclastic activity is further exemplified in the growth and development of long bones, fracture repair, and rheumatoid arthritis. Consequently, recent studies utilizing immunologic and tissue culture assays have revealed that specific biologic molecules operative in localized reactions of osseous tissue do exist. While incomplete, such knowledge has formed the basis for suggestion of chemotherapeutic agents to intercept the activity of some of these biologic molecules. However, a clear treatment approach which incorporates knowledge of bone cell activities with clinical responses remains to be elucidated. This review will center on these issues with information from basic studies and recent clinical studies using chemotherapeutics on alveolar bone loss in PD.

THE OSTEOCLAST AND BONE RESORPTION

Walker originally revealed the osteoclast was derived from a hematopoietic precursor rather than from the historical belief of a stromal cell lineage (2). While intense efforts sought to identify the monocytic macrophage as the direct osteoclast precursor based upon several similarities between the two (3), the more current revelation of many other differences between the two rule out the role of the monocytic macrophage as the precursor to the osteoclast (4-7). Currently it is believed that a granulocyte-macrophage progenitor cell is formed from a multipotential hematopoietic stem cell and is the precursor to the osteoclast and monocyte (8-11). Specific regulatory molecules, colony stimulating factors (CSF's), are believed to influence the progenitor cells to form either pre-osteoclasts or monocytic macrophages via irreversible pathways. Those reported to influence the formation of osteoclast-like cells in vitro include interleukin-3 (IL-3), granulocyte-macrophage CSF (GM-CSF), and macrophage CSF (M-CSF) (12-14).

The resorption of mineralized tissue such as calcified cartilage, dentin, cementum, and bone is long recognized as the function of osteoclasts for differences between chondroclasts and odontoclasts are unknown (15). Non-calcified osteoid and cartilage are believed ignored by osteoclasts, although some degradation of osteoid adjacent to active osteoclasts has been reported (16,17). Early concepts suggested the osteoclast possessed all cellular functions needed to resorb both the mineral and collagenous organic matrices of bone (18). However, at present little evidence exists for collagenase production or collagen phagocytosis by osteoclasts (19). Further, current concepts suggest that the bone surface lining of osteoblast cells and non-mineralized osteoid are two interposed barriers covering the bone which prevent the osteoclast from gaining access to and contact with the mineralized tissue (20).

BONE RESORBING STIMULANTS AND REGULATORS

In the regulation of bone resorption, the classic systemic hormones, parathyroid hormone and 1,25 (OH_2) vitamin D_3, are prominent in the regulation of calcium flux from bone calcium stores. Recent studies utilizing immunologic and tissue culture methodologies have expanded the knowledge of cellular mechanisms and interactions to identify and characterize specific local factors operative in resorptive bone pathophysiology.

Prostaglandins (PGs) are unsaturated, oxygenated fatty acids synthesized from arachidonic acid. They are produced locally by many cells and rapidly degrade. PGs stimulate at corresponding concentrations both bone resorption and formation via effects on osteoclasts and osteoblasts, but in high concentrations are reported inhibitory (21).

The concept that the immune system plays a significant role in bone resorption was strengthened by the detection of the first cytokine with bone resorbing activity termed osteoclast activating factor, now identified as IL-1ß (22,23). Interleukin 1 has been shown to be a potent stimulator of bone resorption both in vitro and in vivo (24). Other cytokines, tumor necrosis factor alpha and beta (TNFα, TNFß) and transforming growth factor alpha (TGFα) stimulate bone resorption while TGFß also stimulates bone growth (25,26). CSFs, as previously indicated, may determine the osteoclast lineage. In addition, recent studies indicate lymphocytes possess receptors for bone resorbing agents such as PTH (27,28). Furthermore, studies evaluating parameters of bone turnover in immune deficient animals indicate the role of the immune system may be of greater significance in pathologic bone resorption than physiologic bone metabolism (29,30). While regulatory interactions between systemic and local factors undoubtedly exist, in localized bone disorders exogenous agents disrupt this interaction with deleterious effects at specific sites of assault.

OSTEOBLASTIC CONTROL OF OSTEOCLASTIC ACTIVITY

The osteoblast was traditionally believed responsible only for bone deposition. Recent studies indicate it also may possess the key to the control of bone resorption by potentially mediating osteoclast activation (31). Bone cell receptors to PTH and vitamin D_3 exist only on osteoblasts and in response to PTH osteoblasts change shape, flatten and detach from the bone surface (32,33). Osteoblasts are potential sources for PGs, IL-1, GM-CSF, M-CSF, differentiation inducing factor, and platelet derived growth factor (34-40). Further, osteoblasts may be responsible for the digestion of osteoid and the collagenous matrix since they synthesize collagenase in response to bone resorbing agents (41,42). Sakamoto proposed that bone resorbing stimulants induce the osteoblastic bone lining cells to synthesize and release collagenase which would then digest osteoid and the organic bone matrix. The osteoblasts would also retract from the external bone surface to expose the underlying surface of mineralized bone to recruited osteoclasts which then dislodge and engulf bone mineral (43). The reversible inhibition of osteoclastic activity by anti-collagenases lends support to this concept (44-46).

PERIODONTAL DISEASES AND BONE RESORPTION

Bacterial plaque colonizing at the dento-gingival junction induces host inflammatory reactions and immunologic reactions in the periodontal tissues (47). Initially the predominant organisms are gram-positive non-motile aerobes; however, with pocket development gram-negative motile anaerobes establish and increase in numbers (48).

Cell wall components from gram-positive bacteria (lipoteichoic acid; LTA) and from gram-negative bacteria (lipopolysaccharides; LPS) have been shown to stimulate osteoclastic bone resorption, with the lipid-A portion or free fatty acid comprising the active component (49). Plaque material also was found to stimulate the immune system resulting in the production of IL-1 by activated leukocytes (23,50).

IL-1 is also known to be produced by macrophages and epithelial cells, significant cellular components of the periodontal tissues. IL-1 has been found in gingival crevicular fluid, and its presence has been identified in the lamina propria of gingival biopsies (51,52). Purified LPS from B. gingivalis and extracts from A. actinomycetemcomitans and C. ochracea, putative periodontal pathogens, have been reported to induce bone resorption and IL-1 and TNF production in murine and human monocytes and macrophages (53-55).

In diseased versus healthy gingival tissues, and in crevicular fluid from diseased versus healthy periodontal tissue sites, PGEs are reported present in higher concentrations (56,57). Additionally LPS preparations from suspected periodontal pathogens are capable of stimulating PGE_2 release from human monocytes (58).

CLINICAL STUDIES ON ALVEOLAR BONE LOSS IN PERIODONTAL DISEASE

Knowledge from basic bone cell studies has led to attempts to intercept alveolar bone loss with non-steroidal anti-inflammatory drugs (NSAIDS). The basis for this treatment stems from the fact that the production of PGs is promoted by many factors and results in osteoclastic activation via the osteoblast. High levels of PGs are found in cultured gingiva and many studies attribute alveolar bone loss in PD to arachidonic acid metabolites (56,57). Caution interpreting these studies is imperative since PGs stimulate both bone resorption and formation and in the high concentrations found in gingival tissues inhibit bone resorption (21); consequently their role is unclear.

Indomethacin, flurbiprofen, ibuprofen, and naproxen have been studied for their ability to reduce bone loss in PD (59-62). These NSAIDS act by blocking the action of cyclooxygenase which catalyzes PGs formation from membrane derived arachidonic acid. Results of these studies indicate a reduction in the rate of alveolar bone loss when matched with untreated controls. However, an "escape" phenomenon has been found with fluribroprofen whereby at 24 months the rate of bone loss in treated and control sites was equal to baseline (63). Therefore, blocking

PGs synthesis by NSAIDS may affect some cellular responses but may not affect other bone resorbing agents such as IL-1 and TNF (64-66).

While the present efficacy for treating PD with NSAIDS is debatable, future studies may combine this therapy with other treatments. One possibility could be with the use of a specific anti-collagenase which would prevent the osteoblastic collagenase from digesting osteoid and the organic bone matrix, thereby inhibiting osteoclastic access to the mineralized portion of bone. Another exciting avenue could be to prevent the osteoblast from secreting a putative osteoclast activating agent. Once identified, chemotherapeutic intervention at this level could prove to have a striking impact on the prevention and treatment of PD.

SUMMARY

Exogenous agents which invoke the inflammatory and immune responses induce the production of cytokines and growth factors to stimulate and regulate cellular and inter-cellular activities. Such mechanisms are of major significance when considering the origin and function of the osteoclast operative in the localized loss of alveolar bone as well as skeletal homeostasis and other systemic and localized bone disorders. While progress in elucidating the cellular interactions of such mediators has been made with resultant information enabling the initial development and testing of interceptive and/or therapeutic agents, the complete role played by these molecules is still incompletely defined.

In periodontitis, the loss of alveolar bone is a well-recognized result of the inflammatory and immune responses to products of exogenous bacterial plaque. Yet, the concept that many of these mechanisms are operative in gingivitis which does not convert to periodontitis nor cause bone loss is still enigmatic.

REFERENCES

1.   Horton JE, Tarpley TM and Davis WF (1978) (eds). Mechanisms of Localized Bone Loss. Information Retrieval Inc., Washington, D.C. and London

2.   Walker DG (1975) J. Exp. Med. 142:651

3.   Teitelbaum SL, Kahn SJ (1980) Miner. Electrolyte Metab. 3:2

4.   Schneider GB, Byrnes JE (1983) Exp. Cell. Biol. 51:44

5.   Chambers TJ, Magnus CJ (1982) J. Pathol. 136:27

6.   Hogg N, Shapiro IM, Jones SJ, Slusarenko M, Boyde A (1980) Cell. Tiss.Res. 212:509

7.   Horton MA, Rimmer EF, Moore A, Chambers TJ (1985) Calcif. Tiss. Intl. 37:46

8.   Burger EH, VanderMeer JWM, Vande Gevel JS, Gribnau JC, Thesingh CW, VanFurth R (1982) J. Exp. Med. 156:1604

9.   Ibbotson KJ, Roodman GD, McManus LM, Mundy GR (1987) J. Cell. Biol. 99:471

10.   Nijweide PJ, Burger EH, Feyen JHM (1986) Physiol. Rev. 66:855

11.   Thesingh CW (1986) Dev. Biol. 117:127

12.   McDonald BR, Mundy GR, Clark S, Wang EA, Kuehl TJ, Stanley ER, Roodman GD (1986) J. Bone Min. Res. 1:227

13.   Metcalf D (1985) Science 229:16

14.   Scheven BAA, Visser JWM, Nijweide PJ (1986) Nature 321:79

15.   Boyde A, Jones SJ (1987) Scan. Microscop. 1:369

16.   Chambers TJ, Thomson BM, Fuller K (1984) J. Cell. Sci. 70:61

17.   Reid SA (1986) Anat. Embryol. 174:225

18.   Vaes G (1968) J. Cell. Biol. 39:676

19.   Wirl G (1984) Cancer Metastasis Revs. 3:237

20.   Zambonin-Zallone A, Teti A, Primavera MV (1984) Cell. Tissue Res. 235:561

21.   Nefussi JR, Baron R (1985) Anat Rec 211:9

22.   Horton JE, Raisz LG, Simmons HA, Oppenheim JJ, Mergenhagen SE (1972) Science 177:793

23.   Dewhirst FE, Stashenko P, Mole JE, Tsurumachi T (1985) J. Immunol. 135:2562

24.   McCauley LK, Rosol TJ, PC Stromberg, Capen CC (1990) Toxicologic Pathology (in review)

25.   Ibbotson KJ, Harrod J, Gowen M, D'Souza S, Smith DD, Winkler ME, Derynck R, Mundy GR (1986) Proc Natl Acad Sci USA 83:2228

26.   Centrella M, McCarthy TL, Canalis E (1988) FASEB J 2:3066

27. Yamamoto I, Bringhurst FR, Potts JT, Segre GV (1988) J. Bone and Min. Res. 3:289

28. McCauley LK, Rosol TJ, Capen CC (1990) J. Bone and Min. Res. 5:S194 (Abs)

29. McCauley LK, Rosol TJ, Capen CC, Horton JE (1989) Bone 10:29

30. McCauley LK, Rosol TJ, Capen CC, Horton JE, Shanfeld J (1989) Bone 10:389

31. Jilka RL (1986) Bone and Mineral 1:261

32. Jones SJ, Boyde A, Shapiro IM (1981) Metabol. Bone Dis. Rel. Res. 2:335

33. Jones SJ Boyde A (1976) Cell. Tiss. Res. 169:449

34. Rodan SB, Rodan GA, Simmons HA, Walenga RW, Feinstein MB, Raisz LG (1981) Biochem. Biophys. Res. Commun. 102:1358

35. Hanagawa S, Ohmori Y, Amano S, Myoshi T, Kumegawa M, Kitano S (1985) Biochem. Biophys. Res. Commun. 131:774

36. Robey PG, Young MF, Flanders KC, Roche NS, Kondaiah P, Reddi AH, Termine JD, Sporn MB, Roberts AB (1987) J. Cell. Biol. 105:457

37. Valentin-Opran A, Delgado R, Valente T, Mundy GR, Graves DT (1987) J. Bone Min. Res. 2:254 (Abs)

38. Shiina-Ishimi Y, Abe E, Tanaka H, Suda T (1986) Biochem. Biophys. Res. Commun. 134:400

39. Horowitz M, Colman D, Kupper TS, Jilka R (1987) J. Bone Min. Res. 2:234 (Abs)

40. Elford PR, Felix R, Cerchini M, Treschel U, Fleisch H (1987) Calcif. Tissue Intl. 41:151

41. Heath JK, Atkinson SJ, Meikle MC, Reynolds JJ (1984) Biochem. Biophys. Acta. 802:151

42. Sakamoto M, Sakamoto S (1984) Biomed. Res. 5:29

43. Sakamoto S, Sakamoto M (1986) In: Peck WA (ed) Bone and Mineral Research 4. Elsevier, Amsterdam, pp 49-102

44. Horton JE, Wezeman FH, Kuettner KE (1978) In: Horton JE, Tarpley TM, Davis WF (Eds). Mechanisms of Localized Bone Loss. Information Retrieval Inc. Washington D.C. and London, pp 127-150

45. Wezeman FH, Kuettner KE, Horton JE (1979) Anat. Rec. 194:311

46. Horton JE, Harper E (1980) Biochim. Biophys. ACTA 630:459

47. Horton JE, Oppenheim JJ, Mergenhagen SE (1974) J. Periodont. 45:351

48. Listgarten MA Hellden L (1978) J. Clin. Periodont. 5:115

49. Hausmann E, Raisz LG, Miller WA (1970) Science 168:862

50. Horton JE, Oppenheim JJ, Mergenhagen SE, Raisz (1974) J. Immunol. 113:1278

51. Charon JA, Luger TA, Mergenhagen SE, Oppenheim JJ (1982) Infect. Immun. 38:1190

52. Jandinski JJ, Leung C, Macedo B, Rynar J, Deasey M (1987) J. Leukocyte Biol. 42:601

53. Hanazawa S, Nakada IK, Ohmoiri Y (1985) Infect. Immunol. 50:262

54. Lundemann RA, Economou JS (1988) J. Periodontol. 59:728

55. Bottenbley CJ, Shurin SB, Jenkins SD, Socransky SS, Horton JE (1982) J Dent Res 61:338

56. El Attar TMA, Lui HS (1981) J Periodontol 52:16

57. Offenbacher S, Odle BM, Gray RC, Van Dyke TE (1984) J Periodont Res 19:1

58. Garrison SW, Holt SC, Nichols FC (1988) J. Periodontol. 59:684

59. Lasfargus JJ, Saffer JL (1988) J. Periodont. Res. 18:110

60. Williams RC, Jeffcoat MK, Kaplan ML (1987) J Periodont Res 22:403

61. Williams RC, Jeffcoat MK, Howell TH (1988) J Periodont Res 23:166

62. Williams RC, Jeffcoat MK, Howell TH (1989) J Dent Res 68:243 (Abs)

63. Williams RC, Jeffcoat MK, Howell TH (1989) J Periodontol 60:485

64. Gowen M, Wood DD, Mundy GR, Russell RGG (1985) Prog. Leukocyte Biol. 2:85

65. Yocum DE, Esparza L, Dubrey S, Benjamin JB, Volz R, Scuderi P (1989) Cellular Immunology 122:131

66. Stashenko P, Dewhirst FE, Peros WJ, Kent RL, Ago JM (1987) J. Immunol. 138:1468

© 1991 Elsevier Science Publishers B.V.
Recent advances in periodontology Vol. II,
S.I. Gold, M. Midda and S. Mutlu, eds.

Longitudinal Studies of Various Periodontal Therapies - A Reappraisal

Raul G. Caffesse

Professor and Chairman

During the last 25 years a significant body of information has been produced in several clinical research centers evaluating the therapeutic responses of the periodontal tissues to different modalities of therapy.

These studies which started in the early sixties at the University of Michigan, provided an objective, unbiased evaluation of the results achieved. In essence, they compared the outcome of treatment after several years of maintenance when periodontitis was treated with different therapeutic approaches, such as, scaling and root planing, Modified Widman flap, subgingival curettage, or apically positioned flap with and without osseous resection. The clinical results were mainly evaluated in terms of changes in probing pocket depth and clinical attachment levels.[1] Other studies evaluated primarily the effects of maintenance on the results achieved. Several reports from the University of Gothenburg, Minnesota, Washington, Nebraska, as well as the Royal Dental College were published during the past two decades together with new reports from Michigan.

Long-term studies

The first Michigan studies[2-6] basically compared subgingival curettage, Modified Widman flap and pocket elimination using a split mouth design where each subject was randomly treated by two of the three modalities tested. These subjects were seen on a 3 month maintenance regimen, and 8 years results have been reported.[6]

Another Michigan study[7-9] compared scaling and root planing, subgingival curettage, Modified Widman flap and pocket elimination with random quadrant assignment. Parameters were also recorded after completion of the hygienic phase of therapy. Again, 3 month recall maintenance was provided. The report covered 5 years follow-up.[9]

Coming from Sweden,[10-13] studies performed at Gothenburg evaluated the response of patients treated with several surgical approaches including: apically positioned flap with and without osseous resection, Modified Widman flap with and without osseous resection and gingivectomy.   After treatment subjects were divided in 2 groups according to maintenance: test subjects were followed with an ideal recall regimen, i.e. professional tooth cleaning every two weeks, while controls received professional tooth cleaning at 6 or 12 months intervals.   Two years results were reported.

The Minnesota study[14-15] compared in a split mouth design the results of scaling and root planing and Modified Widman flap followed by 3-4 month professional maintenance.   Six and one half years results have been reported.

The Washington study used also a split mouth design to compare the results of osseous resection with those achieved with open flap curettage.   Maintenance was provided at 3-6 month intervals.   Five years results were published.[16]

The Nebraska study[17-18] is an on-going evaluation of four approaches to therapy, randomly assigned to quadrants: scaling and root planing, Modified Widman flap, osseous resection and coronal polishing.   Two years results have been reported, after a 3 month maintenance schedule.

The Danish study,[19] from the Royal Dental College in Aarhus reported also a 5 year study on the effects of scaling and root planing and Modified Widman flap on patients that were maintained on a 3 month recall regimen.

Results

All studies have shown the long time benefits of periodontal therapy for moderate and advanced periodontitis.[1]   The following are general statements which summarize the results of the above mentioned studies.

It has been shown that <u>probing pocket depth</u> gets reduced after treatment. However, the reduction in probing depth depends on the severity of the disease treated. Pockets 1-3 mm show initially minimal reduction which disappears over time; moderate disease, 4-6 mm in depth, reduces probing depth in around 2 mm, while pockets $\geq$ 7 mm show a 4 mm reduction. These results remain stable over time if proper maintenance is instituted. Minimal variations, of no clinical significance, have been reported when different treatment modalities were evaluated. In general, scaling and root planing reduces pockets the least together with subgingival curettage, followed by Modified Widman flap and with osseous resection reducing pockets the most. Although some studies have reported statistical significance among those differences, over time they become insignificant.

When changes in <u>clinical attachment levels</u> are evaluated the studies show different results for different severities of disease. Shallow pocket depth areas, 1-3 mm, show a loss of clinical attachment with all procedures tested, which does not repair over time. Moderate disease areas, with 4-6 mm pockets, gain around 1 mm of clinical attachment, however, according with certain studies over time this clinical gain becomes insignificant when compared to baseline recordings. Deep pockets, $\geq$, 7 mm in depth do get an initial gain of attachment of around 2 mm. This gain also reduces with time, producing changes from baseline which are insignificant. When different modalities are compared scaling and root planing and gingival curettage provide the greatest gain in clinical attachment, followed by Modified Widman flap, and osseous resection which gains the least. However, as with probing depth changes, over time the existing differences among techniques become insignificant. Frequency distributions have shown similar number of sites gaining or loosing attachment for each procedure, with those loosing attachment generally concentrated in a reduced number of subjects.

Those studies which here evaluated <u>maintenance regimens</u> here clearly demonstrated that, professional maintenance is paramount to maintain stable results after treatment. The least the recall interval the better the maintenance results as far as probing depth reduction and changes in clinical attachment levels is concern. Although biweekly maintenance seems ideal, 3 month recalls seem effective in stabilizing results, while 6 month maintenance does not seem to be effective in achieving such goal. Under these circumstances probing depths increase and clinical attachment is lost. All modalities have shown similar deterioration with improper maintenance.

<u>Plaque accumulation</u> gets reduced after therapy and is maintained reduced with proper maintenance. Similarly, <u>gingival inflammation</u> gets reduced and is maintained reduced under those circumstances. The reductions achieved are highly significant when compared to baseline values. No differences have been reported between the techniques tested as far as reduction of plaque accumulation or control of gingival inflammation. No single study has shown the superiority of a particular technique in maximizing plaque control or facilitating maintenance.

In summary, all studies performed have reported results to substantiate the beneficial effects of periodontal treatment in controlling the progression of the disease. Furthermore, they have failed to show significant differences between treatment modalities, whether surgical or non-surgical, as far as probing depth reductions and changes in clinical attachment levels. Proper maintenance seems imperative to maintain stable results. Under these circumstances all techniques reduce plaque accumulation and gingival inflammation in a similar manner.

The Tucson Study

In 1984 a longitudinal study was started which was unique in several aspects.[20] First, it was planned by the close cooperation of academicians and periodontists in private practice; second, it was performed in a private practice setting with the subjects selected from the patient population of a private periodontal practice and with the maintenance protocol used in that office; third the treatment modalities were provided by experienced periodontists with high expertise in the particular technique performed. In this fashion, we tried to address several of the criticisms raised by the previous studies.

Sixteen subjects were selected for the study. They suffered from moderate to severe periodontitis, which by the criteria of two of the investigators could be amenable to treatment either by Modified Widman flap or osseous resection surgery. After the hygiene phase procedures by a hygienist which took no more than four sessions of 1 1/2 hours each, periodontal procedures were performed. The same day one periodontist performed on one posterior sextant osseous resection while another performed Modified flap on the contralateral sextant. The sextant selection was accomplished by the toss of a coin. An opposite sextant was consequently scaled and root planed under anesthesia by a periodontist. A 3 month maintenance schedule was followed. Results up to 5 years have been reported.[20-23]

The results of this study confirm all the findings reviewed previously. All three therapeutic techniques, scaling and root planing, osseous resection and Modified Widman flap, are equally effective in controlling plaque accumulation and in reducing gingival inflammation. They also showed similar performance as far as probing pocket depth and clinical attachment changes. Shallow pockets lost clinical attachment, while moderate and severe disease sites showed probing depth reductions and changes in clinical attachment of similar amount for all modalities. After one year the initial differences seen between procedures disappeared.

The lack of differences among the three procedures tested was found both when mean differences and frequency distributions of sites were statistically analyzed.

In essence, the results of the Tucson study confirmed those reported by the university based studies previously reviewed.

Conclusions

After reviewing all the long term clinical studies performed to evaluate the behavior of different therapeutic approaches, as well as the extensive literature available to assess the wound healing mechanisms associated with these techniques, the following conclusion can be drawn regarding the potentials and effects of different treatment modalities in the control of periodontitis:

1. Surgical approaches should be avoided in the treatment of shallow pockets (1-3 mm).

2. Moderate pockets can be treated by different therapeutic approaches, since all provide similar long-term results.

3. Judicious osseous surgery can be used in the treatment of shallow craters in moderate disease at the discretion of the therapist. However, it needs to be emphasized that this is not mandatory to achieve long-term results.

4. Severe pockets (≥ 7 mm) can be treated by several modes of therapy which have shown effective in restoring health on a long term basis. A more conservative approach allows the maintenance of seriously involved teeth which otherwise would have to be extracted.

5. Subgingival curettage does not offer any advantage over scaling and root planing, since it does not provide any additional accessibility for root instrumentation.

6. Osteoplasty can be safely performed to reduce ledges, and to allow for better flap adaption.

7. The apically positioned flap represents the treatment of choice when maximum pocket reduction is the primary objective.

8. Ostectomy could be used with an apically positioned flap for crown lengthening procedures. However, the effects of bone removal in neighboring teeth must be considered.

9. Leaving radicular bone exposed should be avoided, whenever possible.

10. Although pocket reduction is a desirable objective, it is not mandatory for the success of therapy.

REFERENCES

1. Caffesse, R.G.: Longitudinal evaluation of Periodontal Therapy. Den Clin N Amer 24:(4) 751, 1980.

2. Ramfjord, S., Nissle, R., Shick, R., and Cooper, Jr., H.: Subgingival curettage versus surgical elimination of periodontal pockets. J Periodontol 39: 167, 1968.

3. Ramfjord, S., Knowles, J., Nissle, R., et al.: Longitudinal study of periodontal therapy. J Periodontol 44: 66, 1973.

4. Ramfjord, S., Knowles, J., Nissle, R., et al.: Results following three modalities of periodontal therapy. J Periodontol 46: 522, 1975.

5. Knowles, J., Burgett, F., Nissle, R., et al.: Results of periodontal treatment related to pocket depth and attachment level. Eights years. J Periodontol 50: 225, 1979.

6. Knowles, J., Burgett, E., Morrison, R., et al.: Comparison of results following three modalities of periodontal therapy related to tooth type and initial pocket depth. J Clin Periodontol 7: 32, 1980.

7. Hill, R., Ramfjord, S., Morrison, E., et al.: Four type of periodontal treatment compared over two years, J Periodontol 52: 655, 1981.

8. Ramfjord, S., Caffesse, R.G., and Morrison, E.: Four modalities of periodontal treatment compared over five years. J Periodont Res 22: 222, 1987.

9. Ramfjord, S., Caffesse, R.G., Morrison, E., et al: 4 modalities of periodontal treatment compared over 5 years. J Clin Periodontol 14: 445, 1987.

10. Nyman, S., Rosling, B., and Lindhe, J.: Effect of professional tooth cleaning on healing after periodontal surgery. J. Clin Periodontol 2: 80, 1975.

11. Rosling, B., Nyman, S., and Lindhe, J.: The effect of systematic plaque control on bone regeneration in infrabony pockets. J Clin Periodontol 3: 38, 1976.

12. Rosling, B., Nyman, S., Lindhe, J., and Jern, B.: The healing potential of the periodontal tissues following different techniques of periodontal surgery in plaque-free dentitions. J Clin Periodontol 3: 233, 1976.

38

13. Nyman, S., Lindhe, J., and Rosling, B.: Periodontal surgery in plaque-infected dentitions. J Clin Periodontol 4: 240, 1977.

14. Pihlstrom, B., Ortiz-Campos, C., and McHugh, R.: A randomized four-year study of periodontal therapy. J Periodontol 52: 227, 1981.

15. Pihlstrom, B., McHugh, R., Oliphant, T., and Ortiz-Campos, C.: Comparison of surgical and nonsurgical treatment of periodontal disease. J Clin Periodontol 10: 524, 1983.

16. Olsen, C., Ammons, W., and van Belle, G.: A longitudinal study comparing apically repositioned flaps, with and without osseous surgery. Int J Periodontics Restorative Dent 3: 10, 1984.

17. Kaldahl, W., Kalkwarf, K., Patil, K., et al.: Evaluation of four modalities of periodontal therapy, J Periodontol 59: 783, 1988.

18. Kalkwarf, K., Kaldahl, W., and Patil, K.: Evaluation of furcation region response to periodontal therapy. J Periodontol 59: 794, 1988.

19. Isidor, F. and Karring, T.: Long-term effect of surgical and nonsurgical periodontal treatment. A 5 year clinical study. J Periodont Res 21:462, 1986.

20. Becker, W., Becker, B.E., Ochsenbein, C., Kerry, G., Caffesse, R.G., Morrison, E.C., and Prichard, J.A. : A longitudinal study comparing scaling, osseous surgery and modified Widman procedures. J Periodontol 59: 351-365, 1988.

21. Becker, B., Kerry, G., Becker, W., Ochsenbein, C., Caffesse, R.G., and Morrison, E.C.: Changes after three modalities of periodontal therapy - 3 year follow-up. J Dent Res 67: 272, 1988.

22. Becker, B.E., Becker, W., Caffesse, R.G., Kerry, G.J., Ochsenbein, C., and Morrison, E.C.: Three modalities of Periodontal Therapy - 5-Year Final Results. II. J Dent Res 69: 219, 1990. (Abst)

23. Kerry, G.J., Becker, W., Morrison, E.C., Ochsenbein, C., Becker, B.E., and Caffesse, R.G.: Three Modalities of Periodontal Therapy - 5-Year Final Results. I. J Dent Res 69: 246, 1990. (Abst)

© 1991 Elsevier Science Publishers B.V.
Recent advances in periodontology Vol. II,
S.I. Gold, M. Midda and S. Mutlu, eds.

LONGITUDINAL FOLLOW-UP OF PERIODONTAL TREATMENT AND ITS
EVALUATION USING STANDARDIZED RADIOGRAPHIC TECHNIQUE

HITOSHI KAWASAKI   D.D.S.   D.D.Sc.
KAWASAKI INSTITUTE OF PERIODONTICS, Minato-ku, Tokyo   107   JAPAN

In order ot assess the effects of periodontal treatments
various means are used clinically. Commonly used are measurements
of tooth mobility and pocket depth, plaque charts, various
indices such as gingival index, and radiography. Furthermore,
as a means to prove the post-operative bone regeneration,
re-entry is also employed. This is certainly most accurate and
objective means of assessing bone regeneration. The most dis-
advantageous of this method, however, is that it needs patient's
consent, and then the patient must undergo the same painful
experience as the operation itself, and that the consent may not
be obtained sometimes.

In 1962, I reported standardized radiographic technique as a
means to evaluate periodontal treatment. I have observed post-
treatment changes of bone objectively, using this technique.
    This technique is much better than conventional radiography
in its objectivity which is realized by standardization.

The purpose of this report is to explain the technique of
standardization and to present some case reports which show how
bone is regenerated with this assessing technique.

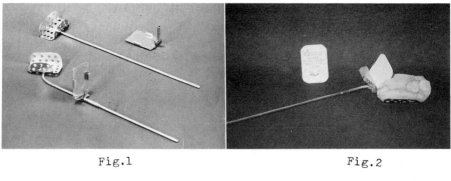

Fig.1   Fig.2

Anchor Part   Self Curing Resin
                     Film Holder
Aluminum Step
                     Hook
Guide Wire
                     Dental Film

                     Extension Cone

Fig.3   Fig.4

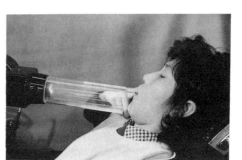

Fig. 1 shows the half-finished device used for this technique, which is manufactured and distributed by Yama-ura Manufacturing Co. (Tokyo, Japan).

This device is consisted of three parts: 1. anchor part, 2. film holder, 3. direction guide wire (Figs.1,2 and 3).

In order to set this device on the plaster cast of a patient adjusting to the site to be radiographed, first bend the guide wire so that the film holder is properly positioned toward the tooth to be radiographed. Then solder the film holder to the guide wire. Next pour autocuring acrylic resin into the setting part and press down on the dentition of the cast while it's soft,

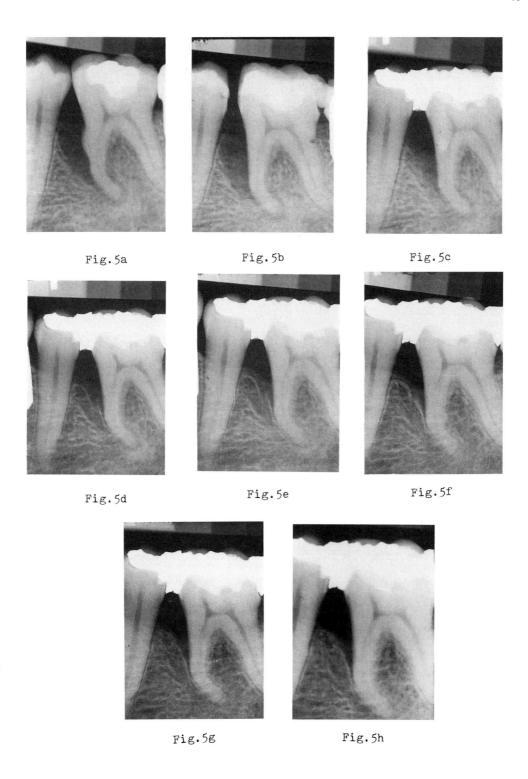

Fig.5a Fig.5b Fig.5c

Fig.5d Fig.5e Fig.5f

Fig.5g Fig.5h

and wait for curing. When cured, take out the device, polish
the resin to be finished (Figs. 2 and 3). The finished device
should be stored for many years and be used as many times as
necessary (Fig.4).

Next, changes of alveolar bone after periodontal treatment,
as observed using this standardized radiographic technique, are
shown.

Fig.5 shows a case in which a pocket of 8 mm of depth and a
two wall bone defect are seen on the medial side of the first
mandibular molar. In this case, flap operation was performed
after usual initial preparation.

Fig.5a, taken before the treatment, shows the vertical bone defect,
calculus on the root surface and bone resorption in the furcation
area.

Fig.5b shows post-operative condition.

Fig.5c that of one month later.

Fig.5d, 2 months later, shows slight change in the bone defect.

Fig.5e shows the condition 3 months after the operation.

Fig.5f and Fig.5e, those of 6 mons. and 10 mons. later respectively,
show gradual changes in the bone.

Fig.5h, one year later, shows that almost all of the defect are
filled with new bone. Lamina dura is also seen along the root
surface, and the furcation lesion has disappeared.

Fig. 6a shows the flap operation (F.Op.) for a 2 wall infrabony
pocket on the medial side of the first mandibular molar.

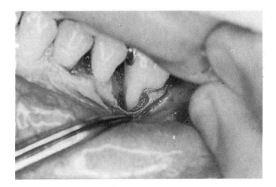

Fig.6a

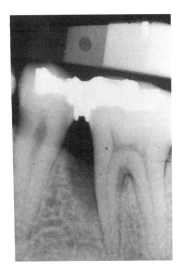
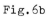

Fig.6b

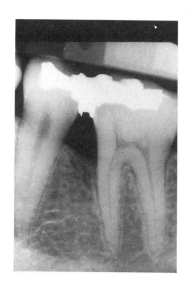

Fig.6c

Fig.6b is the preoperative standardized radiograph.

Fig.6c, one year later, shows the bone defect is filled with

new bone almost completely. Lamina dura (L.D.) is also seen.

44

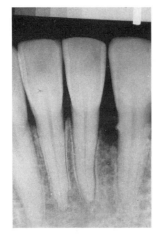

Fig.7a

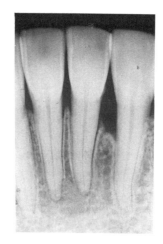

Fig.7b

REPAIR OF BONE DEFECT

After Operation	1M	2M	3M	6M	10M	12M	18M
Increase of Bone Height No. of Improved Cases / Total No. of Cases	41/71	64/71	71/71	71/71	71/71	55/55	40/40
0.1 - 1.0	41	56	58	43	33	24	16
1.0 - 2.0	0	7	10	21	26	21	17
2.0 - 3.0	0	1	3	6	9	8	5
3.0 - 4.0	0	0	0	1	2	2	2
4.0 - 5.0	0	0	0	0	1	0	0
Maximum (mm)	1.0	2.4	3.0	3.7	4.5	4.0	3.5
Average (mm)	0.2	0.5	0.8	1.1	1.4	1.5	1.4
Appearance of Lamina Dura No. of Improved Cases / Total No. of Cases	0/71	1/71	5/71	26/71	38/71	43/55	36/40

Table 1

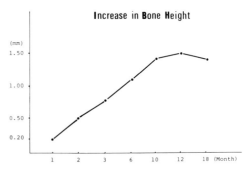

Increase in Bone Height

Fig.8

Is regeneration of bone possible with only initial preparation (I.P.)?   Fig.7a is pre-treatment radiograph.
Fig.7b is 10 months after I.P. Bone regeneration is seen just as
in the case where F.Op. was performed. L.D. is also clearly seen.
Table 1 shows the results of a study done in 1962. In this
study, changes of the bone after F.Op. in 71 cases were observed
for 18 months.   The results were: changes in bone were ob-

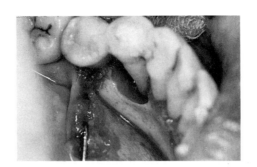

Fig.9a

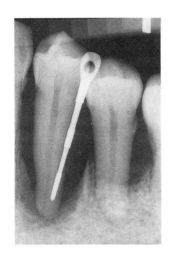

Fig.9b

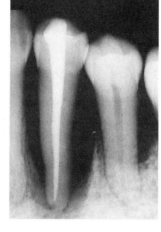

Fig.9c

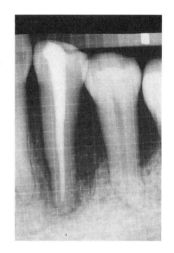

Fig.9d

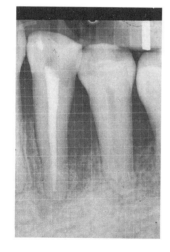

Fig.9e

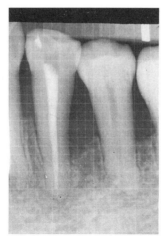

Fig.9f

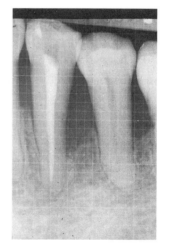

Fig.9g

served in 41 cases one month after F.Op., and in almost all cases those were seen 3 months after F.Op. L.D. appeared a little later than those bone changes.

Fig. 8 shows the increase in bone height. Up to the 10th month after F.Op. the increase is recognizable in the radiograph. In 10 to 12 months it reaches the maximum height and becomes stable.

Fig.9a: 42 year old female. Chief complaint: mobility and bleeding of the left first mandibular premolar. She had a pocket of 8 - 10 mm of depth. The photo shows F.Op., which was performed after I.P. A large 4 wall bone defect was found.
Fig.9b: preoperative stadardized radiograph. The probe is in the pocket.
Fig.9c: condition immediately after F.Op.
Figs. 9 d, e, f and g: taken one month, 4 months, 6 and 12 mons. later respectively. Bone regeneration is already seen one month later. That is more clearly seen 4 mons. later. In 6 to 12 mons. the bone defect is filled with new bone.

As seen in the above, by standardizing the radiographs the observation of change and the highly objective evaluation becomes possible. And I believe this technique is very effective for evaluation of treatment results.

© 1991 Elsevier Science Publishers B.V.
Recent advances in periodontology Vol. II,
S.I. Gold, M. Midda and S. Mutlu, eds.

THE VALUE OF THE COMMUNITY PERIODONTAL INDEX OF TREATMENT NEEDS
(CPITN) IN PERIODONTICS

T. W. CUTRESS

Dental Research Unit, Medical Research Council, P.O.Box 27007,
Wellington (New Zealand)

INTRODUCTION

Periodontal disease appears to have affected mankind
throughout recorded history[1-3]. We know that it is a consequence of
ubiquitous commensal bacteria of the gingival crevice[4-5] but
explanations of the incompatibility between dental plaque and
healthy gingival tissues remain obscure.

Despite an incomplete understanding of the initiation and
progression of destructive periodontal diseases, prevention and
control are feasible in most individuals[6-8]. It appears that the
high prevalence of disease in most populations[9,10] reflects not only
the low priority given to oral hygiene by an unaware public but
also an apparent lack of concern for periodontal care by the
private and public sectors of dentistry[11-13]. Implementation of
known, effective methods of controlling periodontal diseases is an
increasing challenge to dentistry as public awareness of 'gum
disease' increases and tooth loss due to caries decreases[14].
Accountability for periodontal care requires a practical procedure
for documenting periodontal needs, monitoring outcomes and
assessing effectiveness of periodontal treatment and self-care.

In the absence of other standardised screening procedures,
compatible with everyday clinical practice, the basic periodontal
examination known as the CPITN offers advantages to general dental
practice, periodontology and public health dentistry. Also the
brief documentation required appears to satisfy ethical
responsibilities.

Comprehension of the initiation, progression and pathology of
periodontal diseases has changed significantly in the past 20
years. The value of CPITN is that it offers guidance to clinicians
on chair-side management and treatment decisions and is helpful in
the promotion of periodontal health. This is particularly
important during an era of changing concepts in periodontology.

CHANGING CONCEPTS OF PERIODONTAL DISEASES

Destructive periodontal disease does not necessarily follow

the traditionally accepted concept of a slow, continuous,
progressive destructive condition commencing as gingivitis and
extending to advanced disease and tooth loss[15]. Increasingly,
clinical and epidemiological evidence reveals that much disease is
confined as simple, marginal chronic gingivitis or early chronic
periodontitis[5,16,17]. The rate of disease progression reflects a
balance between 'bursts' of destructive activity and periods of
repair and quiescence[5,15,16]. This is substantiated by
epidemiological findings in many populations of a high prevalence
of gingivitis, calculus and early periodontitis but a low
prevalence of advanced disease[9,10,17,18] and tooth loss[19-21].

Recent important developments in our understanding of the
natural history of the diseases have led to a re-evaluation of
their traditional signs and symptoms and their relevance to the
progression and destructiveness of disease and hence risk to tooth
function and retention. However the move away from traditional
concepts of periodontology has probably created more rather than
less confusion in diagnosis, prognosis and treatment. For example,
the traditional concept offered predictability on the progression
of the disease whereas current concepts are more conservative on
disease progression. Terms such as, specific periodontal
pathogens, active and inactive disease, 'burst ' theory of
progression, etc. define the sophistication of recent research but
add little to the practical armamentarium of clinicians and public
health planners.

Classification and diagnosis of periodontal diseases is, in
most instances, not a critical issue. Marginal chronic gingivitis
alone or together with chronic periodontitis are the dominant
disease forms. Variability in disease patterns and progression can
be explained as the balance between the common initiating factor of
bacterial plaque and variation in the host immunological and
cellular defence systems. Recourse to complex classifications of
disease types appears unnecessary. A modest classification[5] of
disease entities such as pre-pubertal, juvenile periodontitis,
rapidly progressive, and adult onset periodontitis appears is
realistic. However 'Adult onset' periodontitis is, by far, the
predominant disease pattern. Hence diagnostic problems are
essentially concerned with assessing the severity of this disease
type and whether it is precocious for age. Nowadays practitioners
can expect that most disease observed will be the common diseases
of 'simple' gingivitis and adult onset periodontitis. The severity

and extent can be appraised and the appropriate level of treatment intervention assessed by relatively unsophisticated procedures.

How dental plaque initiates disease and the mechanism of disease progression remain obscure. Explanations in terms of specific bacterial types, endotoxins, bacterial invasion of tissues, immunopathology and systemic factors each have their protagonists. From a practical viewpoint we are faced with accepting that variations in disease prevalence and severity represent a balance between the pathogenicity of a complex microbial plaque and numerous host defence factors. Dental plaque is the primary determinant in disease progression: absence of plaque means absence of disease.

While the improved knowledge in periodontology promises great advances in future care and treatment its immediate application to the practitioner, patients, treatment prescription or patient motivation is limited. Of more immediate value to dental practitioners and public health services would be guidance on the routine management of periodontal disease within the existing framework of proven prevention and treatment procedures. It is important that the periodontal 'at risk' potential of individuals and communities be assessed using realistic criteria that are translatable into action by the patient and clinician. Screening, 'diagnostic' or assessing procedures which encourage the inclusion of periodontal assessment into routine dental care are of value to private dental practice as well as public health dentistry.

SCOPE AND PURPOSE OF CPITN

A basic periodontal examination, to become known as the CPITN, was introduced originally as a epidemiological survey procedure for gross screening of the magnitude of the need for periodontal care of groups or communities and the requirements for oral health personnel [22,23]. The Index has the potential to integrate dental professional, patient and community endeavour in reducing the prevalence of chronic periodontal diseases and tooth loss. The CPITN is compatible with current concepts of disease progression and control. It confines clinical observations to those criteria most relevant to periodontal treatment needs, that is, periodontal pockets, gingival inflammation (identified by bleeding on gentle probing), and dental calculus and other plaque retentive factors. Assessment of past and present deviations from health, such as gingival recession, tooth mobility and loss of periodontal attachment, are considered irrelevant to improving periodontal health[4], although not, of course, irrelevant to research.

The major advantages of CPITN are seen as its simplicity, speed of use and international uniformity. Primarily it is a screening index for periodontal disease both at the community and individual level. Appropriate oral care services can then be planned for populations and for individuals although social, economic, personnel and other factors will influence decisions on priorities[6,19,24,25].

Despite its simplicity the CPITN procedure appears to satisfy a need as a basic periodontal examination for clinicians and their patients. Consequently with some modifications the CPITN has achieved some relevance to every day dentistry. The label Community Periodontal Index of Treatment Needs is now becoming a misnomer as it functions in a wider role as a basic (preliminary) periodontal examination(BPE). Various debates have ensued over the value of CPITN both in its original (epidemiological and Public Health) and general dentistry roles. Criticisms include use of index teeth, non differentiation of sub and supra calculus, limited pocket depth discrimination and no measurement of total attachment loss. Nevertheless the basic examination does appear to be useful in assigning of patients to basic care modalities and identifies the magnitude of essential treatments. Also it lends itself to patient involvement, and monitoring. 'Treatment Needs' should be interpreted as guide to the level of care that would be required to improve periodontal health; it is not intended as prescription for treatment.

THE CPITN PROCEDURE

Full details of procedures are available in several publications[22,23,26].

For epidemiological and dental practice the objectives are to assess the severity and extent of periodontal needs, and appropriate treatment intervention.

The basic periodontal examination (BPE):
The highest score in each sextant is determined after examination of all teeth in the sextant (for epidemiological purposes only selected index teeth are scored). Scores are based on the presence of calculus, pocket depth and bleeding of inflamed tissues. Only six scores are recorded which give some guidance on the severity and extent of disease for each patient.

The average time for a CPITN assessment is 3-4 minutes.

Categories Periodontal Treatments:

The value of the basic periodontal examination is as an initial indicator of the magnitude of likely care or treatment required by a patient. The actual specific individual treatment modality prescribed will depend on the extent and severity of the disease, the age and oral condition of the individual. This will usually be decided following a more detailed and confirming diagnostic examination when resources are available for individual care. When resources are very limited priorities of care will need to determined - usually meaning that early prevention rather than 'late treatment' will dictate the actions taken.

The CPITN spectrum of treatment needs recognises four general levels of care: (1) No care required - no gingivitis, calculus or pocketing present; (2) Improved oral hygiene -inflammation present but no calculus or pocketing - This is considered as primary prevention not requiring the direct assistance of dental personnel; (3) Improved oral hygiene and calculus removal - calculus and/or shallow pockets present (4-5 mm). This is considered secondary prevention requiring some level of professional assistance:(4) Complex periodontal care. This is considered as tertiary prevention, to prevent progression of advanced disease and tooth loss. It requires particular clinical skills and may involve pocket eradication plus scaling and oral hygiene.

Another important objective of the CPITN screening procedure is to stream individuals to the appropriate source of care, that is, self-care, dental auxiliary, practitioner or specialist.

IMPLEMENTATION

CPITN has been adopted by WHO and many public health services promoting awareness of periodontal disease on a mass scale. Well-organized promotions of periodontal health are reported in various countries including the U.K., USA (Indian Health Service), Finland, Sri Lanka, New Zealand, Italy, Portugal and Columbia[27].

In the United Kingdom and New Zealand periodontal awareness programmes include a 'Gum Health Plan' which includes self-assessment, a self-help guide, and free educational and promotional material. In the U.K. a pilot study revealed a most favourable response from more than 80 percent of general practitioners. Because detailed periodontal examinations are impractical on a mass scale the British Society of Periodontology encourages the use of

CPITN in promoting a greater awareness of periodontal disease, its prevention and treatment[28].

A trial of CPITN screening by practitioners compared favourably with more detailed diagnosis of treatment needs by periodontists.

More recently the American Academy of Periodontology recognized the value of CPITN as a basic periodontal examination which fulfils a practical and effective screening role.

The value of CPITN or similar procedures is primarily in coordinating a realistic approach to an oral health affection which has largely been ignored, and yet can be prevented or controlled sufficiently for most people to retain a functional natural dentition for life.

REFERENCES

1. Ruffer MA (1921) Studies in the Paleopathology of Ancient Egypt. Chicago: University of Chicago Press

2. Sagnes S, Olsson G (1977) Studies of periodontal status of a medieval population. Dentomaxillofac Radiol 1977; 6:46-52

3. Wilkinson FC, Adamson KT, Knight F (1929) A study of the incidence of dental disease in the Aborigines. Aust Dent J 33:109

4. WHO: (1978) Epidemiology, etiology, and prevention of periodontal diseases   Technical Report Series No. 621, Geneva

5. Page RC, Schroeder HE (1982) Periodontitis in Man and Other Animals: A Comparative Review. Basel: S. Karger

6. Birkeland JM, Axelsson P (1976) Preventive programs for children and teenagers with special reference to oral hygiene. In Preventive Dentistry in Practice. Fransden A. (Ed). Copenhagen: Munksgaard

7. Horowitz HS (1980) Established methods of prevention. Brit Dent J 149:311-318

8. Soderholm G, Attstrom R (1984) Longitudinal data on practice based preventive periodontal care. In Public Health Aspects of Periodontal Disease. Frandsen A. (Ed). Quintessence Publ. Co.

9. Pilot T, Barmes DE, Leclercq MH, McCombie BJ, Sardo Infirri J (1986) Periodontal conditions in adults 35-44 years of age: an overview of CPITN data in the WHO Global Oral Data Bank. Community Dent & Oral Epidemiol 14:310-312

10. Pilot T, Barmes DE, Leclercq MH, McCombie BJ, Sardo Infirri J (1987) Periodontal conditions in adolescents 15-19 years of age: an overview of CPITN data in the WHO Global Oral Data Bank. Community Dent & Oral Epidemiol 1987; 15: 336-338

11. Flores-de-Jacoby L, Jacoby R (1984) Experiences in periodontal care under an insurance scheme in West Germany. In: Public Health Aspects of Periodontal Disease. Frandsen A. (Ed). Quintessence Publ. Co.

12. Brown L (1988) Factors influencing the provision of periodontal services by general dental practitioners. Thesis, University of Melbourne

13. Bader JD, Kaplan AL (1984) Treatment distributions in dental practice. J Dent Ed 47:142-148

14. Renson CE (1985) Changing patterns of oral health and implications for oral health manpower: Part 1. Int Dent J 35:235-248

15. Genco RJ (1984) Pathogenesis of periodontal disease: New concepts. J Canad Dent Assn 50:391-395

16. Goodson JM (1984) Acute exacerbation in chronic periodontal disease. J Canad Dent Ass 50:380-387

17. Cutress TW (1988) Can treatment needs be defined on the basis of epidemiological studies? In: Periodontology Today. Int. Congr., Zurich, pp 77-85

18. Barmes DE (1984) Prevalence of periodontal disease. In Public Health Aspects of Periodontal Disease. Frandsen A. (Ed). Quintessence Publ. Co.

19. Corbet EF, Davies WIR (1986) Reasons for extraction of teeth in Hong Kong. J Dent Res Abstr. 607. 65:793

20. Schaub RMH, Jansen J, Pilot T (1979) The prevalence of periodontal disease in an adult Dutch population. J Dent Res 58: Spec.Issue D. 57

21. Bailit HL, Braun R, Maryniuk GA, Camp P (1987) "Is periodontal disease the primary cause of tooth extraction in adults?" J Am Dent Assoc 114:40-45

22. Ainamo J, Barmes DE, Beagrie G, Cutress TW, Martin J, Sardo Infirri J (1982) Development of the WHO Community Periodontal Index of Treatment Needs. Int Dent J 32:281-291

23. Cutress TW, Ainamo J, Sardo Infirri J (1987) The CPITN procedure for identifying periodontal treatment needs in individuals and populations. Int Dent J 37:222-233

24. Pilot T (1984) Implementation of preventive periodontal programs at the community level. In Public Health Aspects of Periodontal Disease. Frandsen A. (Ed). Quintessence Publ. Co. Ltd.

25. Listgarten MA (1979) Prevention of periodontal disease in the future. In Prevention of Major Dental Disorders. Symposium Proceedings, Marabou, Sweden.

26. Ainamo J (1984) Assessment of Periodontal Treatment Needs. In Public Health Aspects of Periodontal Disease. Frandsen, A. (Ed) Quintessence Publ. Co.27.

54

27. FDI (1987-1988) Newsletters Nos. 152-156

28. Smales EC, Mosdale RF, Floyd PM (1987) Policy for Periodontal
    Care. Brit Dent J 167-169

© 1991 Elsevier Science Publishers B.V.
Recent advances in periodontology Vol. II,
S.I. Gold, M. Midda and S. Mutlu, eds.

IS REGENERATION OF THE PERIODONTIUM POSSIBLE?

BERNARD S. MOSKOW, D.D.S., M.Sc.D.

Clinical Professor of Dentistry, Center for Clinical Research in Dentistry,
Columbia University, School of Dental and Oral Surgery, New York, N.Y. 10032

The restoration of periodontal structures lost as a result of periodontitis
has occupied the interest of the dental profession for more than a century.
(Marshall 1883), yet it continues to remain an elusive challenge to those individuals who treat periodontal disease. The early literature is replete with
clinical case reports claiming "reattachment" or "regeneration" and in several
instances, histologic documentation was provided by surgically retrieved block
sections of treated lesions. Many of these reports provided attractive and con-
vincing evidence that regeneration or repair of the periodontium was a distinct
possibility, but in general, this material has not gained the hallmark of
acceptance, since the results were generally unpredictable and the reports in
many ways were anecdotal.

While the term "regeneration" in the context of periodontal lesions is bandied
about glibbly, it should be pointed out, that in most instances, it is a totally
inaccurate description of what is achieved even under unusual circumstances.
Melcher has pointed out that regeneration implies the complete restoration of a
structure in so far as form and function are concerned to the state that existed
prior to the outset of the disease. It, therefore, would be more accurate to
refer to most healed lesions following treatment for periodontitis as a form of
repair - even in instances where the clinical result is exemplary and dramatic.
Repair then is "the biologic process in which the continuity of the destroyed
tissues is restored by new tissues which do not totally replicate the structure
and function of the lost tissues".

With the world wide interest in this approach to periodontal therapy, it is
important to reflect on and assess carefully the aims and objectives of so called
"regenerative therapy" to attempt to achieve a more rational perspective. Indeed,
interest in bone grafts to achieve this end has occupied the interest of periodontists for years and, more recently the concept of "guided tissue regeneration (GTR)" has garnered a great deal of appeal and interest. To be sure, in
1990, it could be considered a growth industry as more and more commercial interests are becoming involved in the manufacturing of membranes to be employed
in GTR.

While there is an abundance of literature on the subject of regeneration,
there remains considerable doubt as to whether either one of these techniques
truly are capable of replicating the entire periodontium. The concept that

various types of bone and bone substitutes placed in a periodontal defect can
induce the formation of a functional periodontal ligament, new cementum formation and new alveolar bone must still be questioned from a biological point of
view. Surely, there is no question that new bone can form around particles of
bone grafts placed in a periodontal lesion, but the idea that bone has the capability of inducing the formation of a new periodontium lacks good scientific documentation. Those who in fact have published reports showing the formation of
new periodontal tissues following bone graft therapy, are quick to defend their
published material, but there are adequate arguments that can be put forth to
question their conclusions. Similarly, the philosophy of GTR, is innovative and
interesting indeed and microscopic demonstrations in animals of its potential
for restoring lost periodontium are intriquing and impressive. Unfortunately,
to date, there is no good histologic evidence in humans that indicates the technique is capable of inducing the formation of new alveolar bone, although new
connective tissue attachment to roots denuded by periodontitis has been adequately
documented. Based on past knowledge relating to the dynamics and biology of the
periodontal structures, one would expect that the formation of a new connective
tissue attachment to the root would carry with it the potential for new bone
to form, however the best clinical material presented to date and what little
human histology that is available does not give the impression that new alveolar
bone is formed.

In any form of treatment rendered to a patient, the cost benefit ratio must be
evaluated, not only in terms of money spent, but more important whether the
procedures performed actually provide sufficient long term benefits to the patient to warrant their usage. There is no data available that demonstrates that
periodontal lesions treated by so called "regenerative techniques" enhance the
chances of tooth survival or have a clinical behavior more efficient than other
clinical techniques available. These are important rhetorical questions to be
posed, given the complicated, often costly and lenghty operations required. Once
more, there is an increasing body of literature suggesting that there is a
potential for spontaneous repair of periodontal lesions following conventional
forms of periodontal therapy beyond what has been traditionally thought.

Over the last two decades, there has been a tremendous amount of scientific
data made available regarding the microbiologic implications in various forms
of human periodontitis. Given the greater understanding of the organisms involved
in the etiology of periodontitis and the associated immunologic and host factors
operative in the diseases, there is a tendency in 1990 to think more about directing our therapeutic measures to the potential bacterial causes of the disease.
Antibacterial agents, including certain antibiotics are playing a useful and
important role in periodontal therapy. Once more, there is increasing evidence

that tetracyclines which are effective against gram-negative anaerobes, important pathogens in periodontitis, appear to inhance the potential for repair and
regeneration of periodontal tissues (Moskow 1983, Mattout, Moskow & Fourel 1990,
Moskow and Tennenbaum 1991). Golub and co-workers have shown that, in addition
to their antibacterial properties, tetracyclines have the additional property
of inhibiting the production of collagenases, endogenous enzymes which have the
capability of destroying collagen, the main component of periodontal tissues
(Golub et al, 1984, 1985). This anticollagenytic property of tetracycline suggests
a definite role for these drugs in the treatment of periodontitis, but they are
also being used to advantage in other diseases characterized by collagen breakdown, such as corneal ulcers, dystrophic epidermolysis, rheumatoid arthritis
and diabetes.

There is always the argument that periodontal defects which heal spontaneously
following conventional periodontal therapies such as scaling and curettage or
open debridement of osseous defects should be open to the same scrutiny as bone
grafting or GTR in so far has histologic evidence for "regeneration" of all components of the periodontium are concerned. While clinical and radiographic evidence
of dramatic reconstruction of periodontal structures can be consistently shown,
the exact nature of the healed tissues needs further documentation. From a biologic point of view, it seems more rational to anticipate formation of new periodontal ligament, cementum and alveolar bone in a healing of a normal periodontal
wound, then one in which artificial substitutes such as bone grafts have been
inserted. There is histologic evidence to show that junctional epithelium tends
to grow down inbetween the root surface and the bone in this type of wound, but
there is reasonable histologic and experimental evidence to postulate that this
situation would gradually change and that the dynamic nature of the periodontal
structures would ultimately result in a normal functioning attachment apparatus.
There is more than adequate documentation that such naturally healing periodontal wounds can remain free of disease and be resistant to periodontal breakdown
after extended periods of time.

Infraosseous lesions, particularly those where multiple bony walls enclose the
defect are particularly amenable to "fill" when treated by simple debridement.
While there is no doubt that new bone is filling into these lesions, there is
the connotation that in periodontal jargon, the word "fill" implies that the
other structures of the periodontium, namely periodontal ligament and cementum
are also part of the healing process. Moskow has demonstrated predictable and
dramatic repair of "craters" (1977) and other confined oseous lesions such as
the "interproximal channel" (1978).

While the prospect of extensive repair and (?) regeneration following periodontal therapy can be an exciting and dramatic outcome of periodontal therapy, it

58

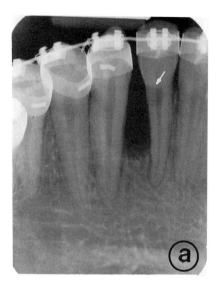 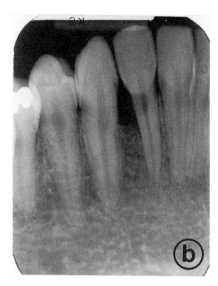

Fig. 1A. Deep interproximal crater in 16 year old male patient at the end of orthodontic treatment. Arrow denotes resorptive lesion in tooth at level of cemento-enamel junction.

B. Healing of crater 11 months following open flap and debridment.

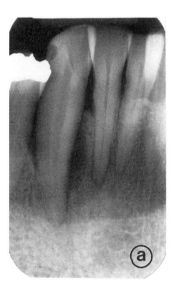 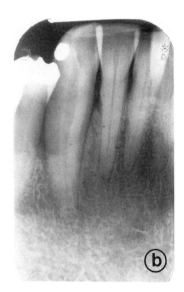

Fig. 2A. Interproximal channeling lesion on mesial and lingual aspect of mandibular cuspid.

B. 3 years after flap and debridment. There is extensive healing on the proximal and lingual aspect of defect.

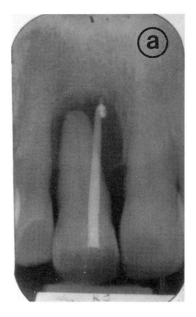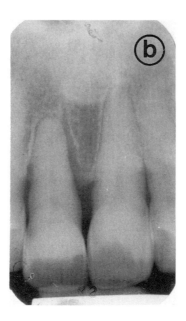

Fig. 3A. Central incisor with extensive loss of periodontal structures encompassing all surfaces of the root. The tooth was given a hopeless prognosis.
  B. Dramatic repair of lesion after administration of 1 gram of tetracyline per day for 3 weeks. Radiograph taken 9 years later.

can tend to overshow the true purpose of treating periodontal disease. That is, to arrest the disease process and maintain the periodontal tissues in a state of health and function over an extended period of time. There is evidence in carefully carried out clinical studies that a number of approaches to treating periodontal disease, some very simple, can accomplish this if routine and careful maintenance programs are carried out (Lindhe & Nyman 1987). There is a tremendous amount of priority given to this area of "repair and regeneration" and one can question its real importance in tackling the monumental, ubiquitous and endemic problem of periodontitis in the world.

ABBREVIATED REFERENCE LIST

1. Marshall JS (1883) A remarkable case of pyorrhea alveolaris, with reproduction of bone occurring in the practice of Dr. Allport, Chicago, Ill. Journal of American Medical Association 1, 641-643

2. Melcher AH (1976) On the repair potential of periodontal tissues. Journal of Periodontology 47, 256-260

3. Moskow BS (1977) Healing potential in periodontal lesions: The interdental crater. Journal of Periodontology 48, 754-767

4. Moskow BS (1978) Repair potential in periodontal disease: The interproximal channel. Journal of Periodontology 49, 55-59

5. Moskow BS (1983) Repair of an extensive periodontal defect after tetracycline administration. Journal of Periodontology 57, 29-34

6. Golub LM, Ramamurthy NS, Mc Namara TF, et al (1984) Tetracyclines inhibit tissue collagenase activity: A new mechanism in the treatment of periodontal disease. Journal Periodontal Research 19, 651-566

7. Golub LM, Goodson JM, Lee HM, et al (1985) Locally and low-dose systemically administrated tetracycline inhibit tissue collagenase activity: Potential new approaches in the treatment of periodontal disease. Journal Periodontology 56, 93-97 (special issue)

8. Mattout P, Moskow BS, Fourel J (1990) Repair potential in Localized Juvenile Periodontitis. Journal Clinical Periodontology - in press

9. Moskow BS, Tannenbaum P (1991) Enhanced repair and regeneration of periodontal lesions in tetracycline treated cases. Journal of Periodontology - submitted for publication

© 1991 Elsevier Science Publishers B.V.
Recent advances in periodontology Vol. II,
S.I. Gold, M. Midda and S. Mutlu, eds.

TREATMENT OF PERIODONTAL DISEASES BY LOCAL DRUG DELIVERY

J. MAX GOODSON

Forsyth Dental Center, 140 Fenway, Boston, MA 02115

The end of the 20th century will mark the introduction of localized drug delivery systems for treating periodontal diseases. It is appropriate to consider their development, which has been an international occurrence, at an international conference. This paper will review the concepts underlying the technology involved and discuss some principles found to be important in using local drug delivery systems to treat periodontally diseased patients.

Intrapocket Delivery Systems. Delivery systems investigated for the intrapocket delivery of drugs to treat periodontal diseases can be classified into three general categories: fibers, films or inserts, and gels or semisolids. The first delivery devices placed within the periodontal pocket for therapy were hollow fibers, initially reported 11 years ago[1]. They were small diameter dialysis tubing that could be loaded easily with any pharmacologic agent and placed into the pocket to test the drug's effects. This system failed to provide therapeutic levels for longer than 24 hours because of its primary delivery from the cut ends of the fiber. The delivery profile was exponential, with a half–time of 1 to 2 hours. Technical difficulty in sealing the ends of fibers precluded development of this approach for practical application in sustained drug delivery. Nevertheless, this system provided investigators [1-6] with evidence of the effects of drugs delivered from a system placed within the periodontal pocket and targeted directly to the site of disease activity.

The monolithic drug delivery system, introduced in 1983 [7], is a soft tetracycline (TC) loaded fiber retained in the pocket by application of an overlying adhesive. The term monolithic served to indicate the uniform composition of the fiber (versus a layered or membrane–encapsulated structure) and to differentiate it from the hollow fibers previously tested.

Soon after study of monolithic fibers had started, other systems were reported, including ethyl cellulose films [8-12] and methacrylate inserts [13-18]. Like monolithic fibers, these systems are nonbiodegradable. Unlike the monolithic fibers, however, these polymers are stiff, requiring their application as preformed films or inserts. Retention in the pocket was by physical shape and intrinsic adhesion.

Reports on biodegradable intrapocket delivery systems also began to appear in 1983 [19]. Hydroxypropyl cellulose films [20-22], collagen films [23,24], polyactide films [25], and novel two–polymer biodegradable delivery systems have been described [22]. In addition, semisolid preparations have been tested for local delivery of drugs to the periodontal environment [26-29].

This brief overview of research on local delivery of drugs for periodontal therapy serves to indicate the widespread interest in studies in this area. Most of the delivery systems described have been shown to affect periodontal microbiota. In pilot studies, some have demonstrated beneficial effects on pocket depth, attachment level, bleeding, and bone loss. Except for the TC fiber system, however, scant detail is available from published data to characterize any of these delivery systems adequately. Therefore, I will concentrate on the TC fiber system, for which considerable data are available, and will try to identify the characteristics that contribute substantially to its efficacy and safety.

THE TETRACYCLINE FIBER DELIVERY SYSTEM

Characteristics. The TC fiber delivery system (Actisite® (tetracycline HCl) Periodontal Fiber, ALZA Corporation, Palo Alto, CA) has only two components: tetracycline and ethylene vinyl acetate (EVA) copolymer. This copolymer is soft, flexible, and biologically compatible, but nondegradable. It is extruded as a 0.5 mm diameter fiber loaded 25% with tetracycline HCl crystals which are distributed uniformly throughout the copolymer matrix. The fiber will be supplied in packages, 9 inches per package, containing a total of 12.7 mg tetracycline. On average, one package should suffice to treat 1 or 2 teeth with 6–10 mm pockets.

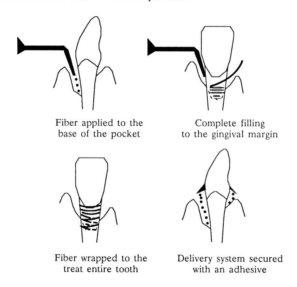

<table>
<tr><td>Fiber applied to the
base of the pocket</td><td>Complete filling
to the gingival margin</td></tr>
<tr><td>Fiber wrapped to the
treat entire tooth</td><td>Delivery system secured
with an adhesive</td></tr>
</table>

Fig. 1. Application of the TC fiber delivery system.

Application. The system is applied (Fig. 1) by filling the deepest sites first. This appears important to give the delivery system direct access to the advancing disease front and to compensate for the flushing action of the gingival fluid. As the fiber is soft and flexible, it can be closely adapted to the irregular contours of the periodontal pocket. Next, successive layers are applied until the entire circumference of the periodontium of a tooth is exposed to the delivery system. Clearly, the periodontium of a tooth is potentially a contiguous environment. Eradication of all pathogen reservoirs in this environment is the aim. Fiber application is completed when no more fiber can be placed. Excess is trimmed to the gingival margin, and a thin coat of adhesive is applied to maintain the delivery system. The adhesive currently preferred, based on its simplicity of application and functionality, is a cyanoacrylate. It is recommended that the fibers be retained in the pocket for a week to 10 days. If applied for shorter periods, their full beneficial effect may not be realized. At the end of therapy the fibers, being nonbiodegradable, must be removed which takes only a few minutes.

The average fiber length to treat a 6–10 mm pocket is 5 inches. The rule, however, is to use whatever amount is necessary to treat the entire tooth and completely fill the pocket. The average time to apply fibers is 5–15 minutes, depending on the location of the tooth and the operator's experience. As this is a new technique, there is a learning curve; proficiency is usually achievable after 10 or fewer applications. The technique is similar to that used to apply gingival retraction cord. The average dose/tooth delivered over 7 to 10 days is approximately 2 mg. Anesthesia is generally not required. 95% of subjects treated with TC fibers have found the procedure not at all uncomfortable or only slightly so. In one study, 19% of 113 subjects found application mildly uncomfortable. Usually over 90% of those treated state that they would definitely or probably have the therapy again if needed, indicating a high level of patient acceptance. Compliance requirements are simple. Patients are advised not to brush the treated area, not to chew on the side of fiber application, and not to eat crusty foods. These actions would tend to break the cyanoacrylate, which could result in premature fiber loss.

Design Strategy. The underlying strategy adopted in developing this delivery system is to maximize drug effectiveness and minimize side effects. To maximize effectiveness, drug application is targeted to the disease site and confined to the treated area. Targeting is achieved by placing the delivery system directly into the periodontal pocket. Confinement to that area is accomplished by applying the adhesive, which minimizes drug loss from the pocket and washout by saliva. As a result of this design, the delivery system rapidly establishes a high antibiotic concentration within the pocket, sufficient to inhibit growth of all oral bacteria. Equally important is the ability to maintain high TC concentration for sufficient time to allow the optimal drug effect to occur, as all drugs require time to act. Indeed, inadequate duration of drug presence is a common reason for therapeutic failure. Finally, to minimize low–level drug effects that might encourage development of drug resistance, the system is designed to terminate rapidly, which is an advantage of a removable, non–biodegradable system.

Therapeutic Effects. Since 1983, controlled clinical trials based on examination of more than 500 subjects have been conducted to explore therapeutic effects of the TC fiber system under a variety of conditions. Results indicate that this delivery system reduces pocket depth [30-33], produces attachment gain [30,32,33], reduces bleeding on probing [30-33], reduces darkfield counts [34], and numbers of probable periodontal pathogens [31,35]. Effects on suppuration [32] and tooth mobility [32] have also been reported. In addition,

64

studies have reported additive or cooperative effects with scaling and root planing [31] and with chlorhexidine mouth rinses [36].

Biphasic Release and Reserve Delivery Capacity. Two important characteristics of the TC fiber delivery system are biphasic release and reserve delivery capacity (Fig. 2). The *in vitro* profile of drug release by this system is by an initial burst of approximately 40–60 µg/cm/h from surface exposed drug, followed by sustained release of 1–2 µg/cm/h over several days. The initial burst provides a loading of nonspecific drug binding sites while the sustained release component replenishes TC lost by gingival fluid washout (ca. 30 µg/h/tooth).

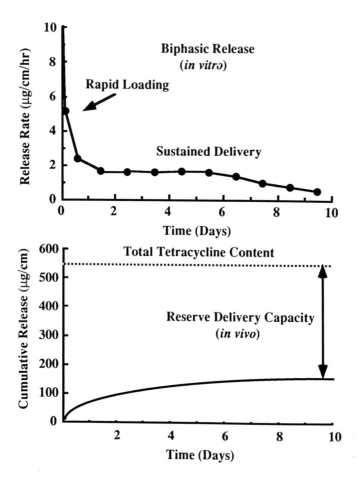

Fig. 2. Biphasic release characteristics and reserve delivery capacity.

The reserve delivery capacity of the fiber is necessary to maintain controlled TC release. Systems that severely deplete their reserve capacity cannot sustain delivery. After 10 days of *in vivo* release, approximately 75% of the drug remains in the fiber [30] to provide the driving force necessary to maintain controlled release. In clinical application, an average of 5 inches of fiber may be placed in a 6 mm pocket. The volume distention of the pocket is approximately 50–fold, increasing from an initial value [37] of approximately 0.5 μl to 25 μl after fiber application. This results in a total reservoir capacity of approximately 7 mg, of which approximately 2 mg is released *in vivo* over a 10 day period.

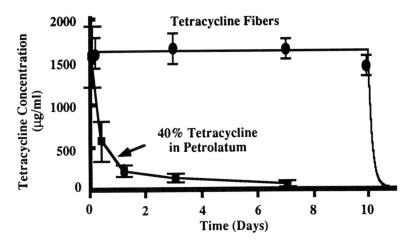

Fig. 3. Concentration of tetracycline in gingival fluid following TC fiber placement [38] or 40% TC in petrolatum [28].

Effect of Sustained Concentration. Placement of the TC fiber delivery system into the periodontal pocket results in a concentration of greater than 0.13% TC (1300 μg/ml) which is maintained for 10 days (Fig. 3). By comparison, Eckles *et al.* [28] demonstrated that administration of 40% TC in petrolatum maintained high concentrations of TC only for the first day. Although antibacterial levels persisted for 7 days, clinical responses to TC in this study appeared minimal. In this study, pocket depth reduction at 56 days by scaling was 1.6 mm. In a study of TC fiber application [33], supragingival scaling produced 1.2 mm pocket depth reduction and subgingival scaling produced an additional 0.7 mm reduction at 60 days resulting in 1.9 mm overall pocket depth reduction. These data suggest that the scaling response in these two studies were comparable. However, application of 40% TC in petrolatum resulted in 0.7 mm less pocket depth reduction than scaling, whereas with application of TC fibers, a 0.3 mm improvement relative to scaling was reported. Further, application of 40% TC in petrolatum failed to provide significant attachment level gain, whereas significant attachment level gain was observed following TC fiber application [33].

These data suggest that a sustained high level of TC may be important and that maintenance of low antibacterial levels is not sufficient for optimal effectiveness. One explanation of this observation is that concentration is the driving force to penetrate poorly accessible microenvironments from which residual pathogenic bacteria can recolonize. Several relatively protected environments for bacteria have been identified, including dentinal tubules [39], surrounding diseased soft tissue [40], dense bacterial plaques, and tooth irregularities such as furcations and accessory canals.

Many antibacterial agents have been tested for intrapocket delivery, including tetracycline [13,17,19-21,23-26,28-38], doxycycline [26], chlorhexidine [8-10,12,13,16-18,20,21,25,26], metronidazole [11,13-17], ofloxacin [22], and sanguinarine [25,26]. Considering the high drug levels attainable by intrapocket drug delivery, it is not clear that any of these agents has a preferred role. However, several nonantibiotic effects of TC such as collagenase inhibition [41], anti-inflammatory activity [42], inhibition of neutrophil chemotaxis [43], and possible function as a root conditioning agent [44] may materially contribute to therapeutic response of this drug in periodontal disease.

EVA is a soft and flexible copolymer that allows adaptation of the delivery system to the irregular contour of the periodontal pocket. Many other delivery systems are inflexible and not as adaptable. In addition, EVA provides sufficient bulk to maintain its position within the periodontal pocket despite gingival fluid flow. Some of the other intrapocket delivery systems are rapidly displaced. Another useful characteristic of EVA is that high drug loading (i.e., 25%) can be obtained without substantial alteration of polymer characteristics. Some delivery systems must limit their load to much lower (ca. 2-3%) drug levels thereby limiting their reservoir capacity.

Intrinsic Safety. An important feature of the TC fiber system is its intrinsic safety. Low systemic drug dosage (ca. 2 mg/tooth) results in negligible systemic effects. Application of high concentrations for a short duration minimizes the probability of developing bacterial resistance. Tetracycline itself has long history of safe topical usage (eg. in acne) and it is no longer considered crucial for treatment of life-threatening diseases. EVA, as a delivery matrix, is nontoxic, biocompatible, and nonbiodegradable; thus, no toxic degradation products are formed. EVA has a long safe history as a platform for drug delivery.

Precautions. Experience in the use of TC fibers has revealed few precautions, except allergy to any of its components:

1. Severely abscessed teeth cannot be tightly packed with the TC fibers without risk of forming a lateral drainage canal. In this case, light packing without adhesive application is recommended until the abscess subsides.

2. It has been noted in patients with existing candidiasis, or a propensity to develop candidiasis, that TC fiber application can lead to an exacerbation in clinical symptomatology. This can be treated by prior or concomitant antifungal therapy.

3. Although fiber application is largely painless, it may cause pain on insertion at a few sites in some patients. Such pain, rapidly subsides and does not constitute a reason for discontinuation of therapy.

4. Premature fiber loss occurs in approximately 20% of patients and requires replacement. However, this principally represents an inconvenience.

SUMMARY

The TC fiber delivery system represents a safe and effective means to assist in the treatment of periodontal diseases. As other systems are developed and introduced, evaluation of their ability to achieve the more important performance characteristics embodied in the TC fiber delivery system will become critical to understand their strengths, weaknesses, and potential utility.

REFERENCES

1. Goodson JM, Haffajee AD, Socransky SS (1979) J Clin Periodontol 6:83–92

2. Lindhe J, Heijl L, Goodson JM, Socransky SS (1979) J Clin Periodontol 6:141–149

3. Coventry J, Newman HN (1982) J Clin Periodontol 9:129

4. wan Yusof WZA, Newman HN, Strahan JD, Coventry JF (1984) J Clin Periodontol 11:166

5. Newman HN, Yeung FIS, wan Yusof WZA, Addy M (1984) J Clin Periodontol 11:576

6. Hoerman KC, Lang RL, Klapper L, Beery J (1985) Quintessence Int 2:161

7. Goodson JM, Holborow D, Dunn RL, Hogan P, Dunham S (1983) J Periodontol 54:435

8. Soskolne WA, Friedman M, Golomb G, Sela M (1982) J Dent Res 61:273

9. Friedman M, Golomb G (1982) J Periodont Res 17:323

10. Soskolne A, Golomb G, Friedman M, Sela MN (1983) J Periodont Res 18:330

11. Golomb G, Friedman M, Soskolne A, Sela MN (1984) J Dent Res 63(9):1149

12. Stabholz A, Sela MN, Friedman M, Golomb G, Soskolne A (1986) J Clin Periodontol 13(8):783

13. Addy M, Rawle L, Handley R, Newman HN, Coventry JF (1982) J Periodontol 53:693

14. Addy M, Alam L, Rawle L (1984) J Clin Periodontol 11(7):467

15. Newman HN, Yeung FIS, wan Yusof WZAB, Addy M (1984) J Clin Periodontol 11:576

16. Addy M, Langeroudi M (1984) J Clin Periodontol 11:379

17. Addy M, Langeroudi M, Hassan H (1985) Int Dent J 35(2):124

18. Brook IM, Douglas CWI, van Noort R (1986) Biomaterials 7:292

19. Dunn RL, Perkins BH, Goodson JM (1983) J Dent Res 62:289 Abstr 1084

20. Noguchi T, Izumizawa K, Fukuda M, Kitamura S, Suzuki Y, Ikura H (1984) Bull Tokyo Med Dent Univ 31:145

21. Noguchi T, Fukuda M, Kitamura S, Kobayashi M, Umeda M, Ishikawa I, Suzuki Y (1986) Nippon Shishubyo Gakkai Kaishi 28(2):737

22. Higashi K, Morisaki K, Hayashi S, Kitamura M, Fujimoto N, Kimura S, Ebisu S, Okada H (1990) J Periodont Res 25:1

23. Minabe M, Uematsu A, Nishijima K, Tomomatsu E, Tamura T, Hori T, Umenoto T, Hino T (1989) J Periodontol 60:113

24. Minabe M, Takeuchi K, Tomomatsu E, Hori T, Umemoto T (1989) J Clin Periodontol 16(5):291

25. Harkrader R, Rogers J, Godowski K, Dunn, R (1989) J Dent Res 68:322 Abstr 1127

26. Dunn RL, Southard GL, Tipton AJ, Yewey GL, Reinhart PC, Menardi EM, Rogers JA (1990) J Dent Res 69:245 Abstr 1095

27. Williams RC, Jeffcoat MK, Howell TH, Reddy MS, Johnson HG, Hall CM, Goldhaber P (1988) J Periodont Res 23(4):225

28. Eckles TA, Reinhardt RA, Dyer JK, Tussing GJ, Szydlowski WM, DuBois LM (1990) J Clin Periodontol 17:454

29. Tokumoto K, Tsuchida K, Kawamura M, Nakamura M, Hasegawa K, Iwamoto Y (1985) Nippon Shishubyo Gakkai Kaishi 27(4):923

30. Goodson JM, Hogan PE, Dunham SL (1985) J Periodontol 56:81

31. Heijl L, Dahlen G, Sundin Y, Goodson JM (1990) J Clin Periodontol (in press)

32. Goodson JM, Cugini MA (1988) Compend Cont Educ Dent, Suppl No 12:S418

33. Cugini MA, Goodson JM (1989) J Dent Res 68:197 Abstr 123

34. Goodson JM, Offenbacher S, Farr DH, Hogan PE (1985) J Periodontol 56:265

35. Tanner A, McArdle S, Goodson JM (1989) J Dent Res 68:197 Abstr 124

36. Holborow D, Niederman R, Tonetti M, Cugini MA, Goodson JM (1990) J Dent Res 69:277 Abstr 1346

37. Goodson JM (1989) J Dent Res 68:1625

38. Tonetti M, Cugini MA, Goodson JM (1990) J Periodont Res 25:243

39. Adriaens PA, DeBoever JA, Loesche WJ (1988) J Periodontol 59(4):222

40. Christersson LA, Wikesjo UME, Albini B, Zanbon JJ, Genco RJ (1987) J Periodontol 58:540

41. Golub LM, Goodson JM, Lee HM, Vidal AM, McNamara TF, Ramamurthy NS (1985) J Periodontol 56:93

42. Plewig G, Schopf E (1975) J Invest Dermatol 65:532

43. Martin RR, Warr GA, Couch RB, Yeager H, Knight V (1974) J Infect Dis 129:110

44. Wikesjo UME, Baker PJ, Christersson LA, Genco RJ, Lyall RM, Hic S, DiFlorio RM, Terranova VP (1986) J Periodont Res 21:322

© 1991 Elsevier Science Publishers B.V.
Recent advances in periodontology Vol. II,
S.I. Gold, M. Midda and S. Mutlu, eds.

HYDROXYAPATITE IMPLANTATION IN PERIODONTAL OSSEOUS SURGERY

YOSHITAKA HARA

Department of Periodontology, Nagasaki University School of Dentistry, Sakamoto-machi 7-1, Nagasaki 852 (Japan)

INTRODUCTION

Recently hydroxyapatite has been used as a bone graft material in periodontal osseous surgery. This paper reports the basic characteristics of hydroxyapatite and their significance in clinical application.

BASIC CHARACTERISTICS OF HYDROXYAPATITE

Biocompatibility and stabilization

When we implanted hydroxyapatite granules into the jaws of dogs, no subsequent encapsulation by connective tissues, phagocytosis by foreign body giant cells, inflammatory cell infiltration or disturbance of bone repair around the hydroxyapatite, while these findings suggest that there are no biocompatibility problems associated with use of hydroxyapatite, but care should be taken to stabilize implanted bydroxyapatite, because implantation of hydroxyapatite in the muscles of rats results in its encapsulation by inflammatory connective tissues (Fig.1). Such fibrous encapsulation developed in response to the presence of the chemical irritants such as metals. The stronger the irritant, the thicker the encapsulation, so that the relative thickness of the fibrous capsule is an indicator of the relative biocompatibili-

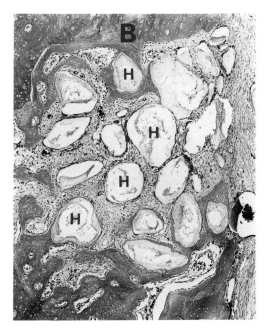

Fig.1. Hydroxyapatite and newly formed bone tissue. H: Hydroxyapatite granules, B: Bone tissue

ty of the material. However, irritation is not the only cause of encapsulation, which can occur in response to the continuous joggling force exerted on a material implanted in alveolar bone, even though the material may possess high biocompatibility. If such a material is stabilized, however, there is no encapsulation, showing that lack of stabilization will lead to fibrous encapsulation even of highly biocompatible materials. In clinical application it is not possible to achieve effective functioning of implanted materials unless they are stabilized.

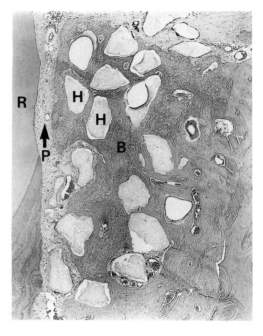

Fig.2. Hydroxyapatite and repaired alveolar bone. H: Hydroxyapatite granules, B: Bone tissue, P: Periodontium, R: Root

Repair of periodontal tissues

After hydroxyapatite granules are implanted in alveolar bone defects with chronic inflammation in dogs, the bone defects are repaired by newly-formed bone tissue around the hydroxyapatite granules (Fig.2). There is no other tissue between this bone tissue and the hydroxyapatite, and these two materials are directly bonded (Fig.3a and 3b). There are many mesenchymal cells as well as osteoid formation around the hydroxyapatite granules (Fig.4). These findings suggest that osteogeny is activated around hydroxyapatite. This suggestion is supported by following reasons. When MC3T3-E1 cells, which have the capacity to differentiate to osteoblast and mineralize in vitro[1], are cultured with hydroxyapatite granules, the alkaline phosphatase activity and mineralization of these cells are more activated than those cultured without the hydroxyapatite. Furthermore, between the alveolar bone repaired with hydroxyapatite and the dental root there are such tissues as periodontal ligaments and addition of cementum. After hydroxyapatite granules implantation into wide three wall defects in jaws of dogs, there are no hollows at the center of the repaired bone, though sites without

hydroxyapatite shows
hollows. But bone
tissue with few or no
periodontal ligaments
does not form in bone
defects, parhaps because
new periodontal ligaments
from the periodontium
are formed after repair
of alveolar bone.

Bone tissues formed
around hydroxyapatite

The bone formed around
hydroxyapatite is the
same as the natural bone,
meaning that if peri-
odontitis reccurs it will
resorbed, and the
hydroxyapatite granules
will be encapsuled with
inflammatory granulation
tissues and discharged
out of the periodontal
tissues. Thus careful
maintenance, with or
without hydroxyapatite
implantation, is recom-
mended.

Three months after
hydroxyapatite implanta-
tion into the jaws of
dogs, bone repair around
hydroxyapatite granules
is apparently completed,
but there is a distinct
border between repaired
and pre-existing bone
tissue. In addition,
bone marrow, which can
be seen in pre-existing

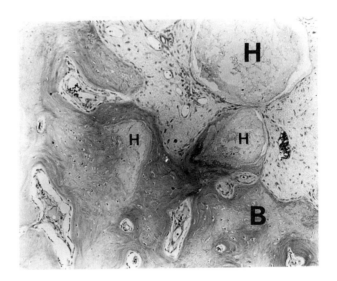

Fig.3a. Hydroxyapatite granules and newly formed bone tissue. H: Hydroxyapatite granules, B: Bone tissue

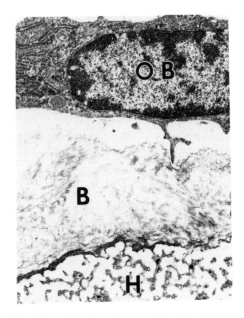

Fig.3b. Electromicrograph of Hydroxyapatite and bone tissue. H: Hydroxyapatite, B: Bone tissue, O: Osteoblast

72

bone, is not observed. But twelve months after implantation, the border becomes indistinct, and bone marrow can be seen within the repaired bone. These findings suggest that in bone tissue repaired around hydroxyapatite there is remodeling of interior[2].

Orthodontic force applied to bone repaired around hydroxyapatite brings osteoclastic bone resorption at the pressure zone and bone addition from bone at the tension zone. However, at the pressure zone hydroxyapatite cannot be resorbed because it is not biodegradable, root resorption compensates for this (Fig.5).

After root resorption, during the retension period, repaired bone spreads along the hydroxyapatite granules and

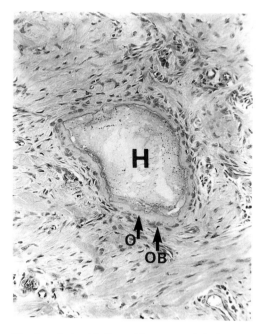

Fig.4. Osteoid formation around hydroxyapatite granule. H: Hydroxyapatite granules, O: Osteoid, OB: Osteoblasts

attaches to the adjacent root, which finally results in ankylosis, because osteogeny is activated around the hydroxyapatite. These findings imply that hydroxyapatite implantation in the pressure zone should be avoided. It is effective in the tension zone, where hydroxyapatite implantation produces more bone repair, while in controls bone defects become filled with connective tissue[3].

CLINICAL APPLICATION OF HYDROXYAPATITE

Hydroxyapatite is implanted during flap operation after debridement of inflammatory granulation tissue and root planing, as in osteoplasty and ostectomy.

Hydroxyapatite is sterilized by a dry heat sterilizer or an autoclave, mixed with saline to form a mixture with the consistency of wetsand, and implanted into bone defects with a spoon excavator or an amalgam carrier.

Biocompatibility in clinical application

The symptoms seen after hydroxyapatite granule implantation are redness and

swelling of the gingiva,
pain, increased tooth mobility, opening of wounds, and
discharge of hydroxyapatite
granules. Of these symtoms,
the first three are often
seen after usual flap operation without hydroxyapatite
implantation. Soon after
hydroxyapatite implantation,
tooth mobility sometimes
decreased and other symptoms
disappear early. These findings suggest that the biocompatibility of hydroxyapatite
in clinical application is
satisfactory.

Effectiveness and clinical
findings

  Case 1: Tooth mobility of
the two lower central incisors is Mobility-2. After
initial preparation pocket
depths were from 3 to 11mm,
and flap operation was indi-

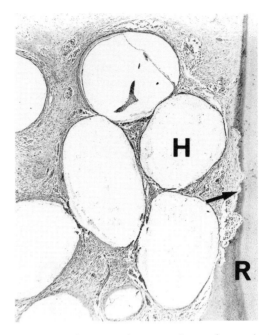

Fig.5. Hydroxyapatite granules and resorbed
dental root. Arrow indicates root resorption.
H: Hydroxyapatite granules, R: Root

cated. Hydroxyapatite granules were implanted into 2-wall bone defects. One
month after operation tooth mobility was Mobility-1, four years after operation
pocket depths are from 1 to 2mm and attachment gains are from 5 to 6mm.

  On dental X-ray films revealed findings not usually seen after standard
operations. First, a demarcation line between hydroxyapatite granules and bone
tissues appeared after 2 weeks, but it was not an important problem because it
disappeared 6 months after operation without the need for additional hydroxyapatite. This phenomenon may be caused by bleeding from the bony wall after
implantation. X-ray also revealed that a lamina dura did not appear after
implantation (Fig.6a and 6b). On X-ray films hydroxyapatite appeared as radio-
opaque granules, and the horder between hydroxyapatite and alveolar bone was
indistinct but could still be distingguished. Though bone tissue repaired
around hydroxyapatite seems to be the same as normal bone, careful maintenance
is needed, as in follow-up for conventional surgery.

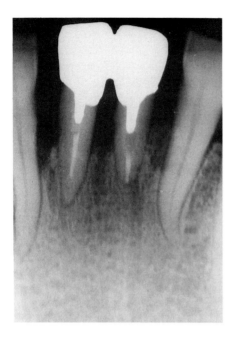 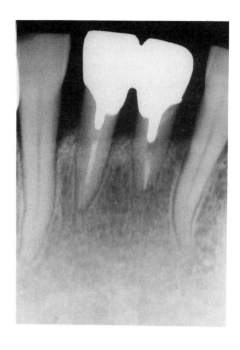

Fig.6a. Dental X-ray film before hydroxyapatite implantation.

Fig.6b. Dental X-ray film three years after hydroxyapatite implantation.

Case 2: Opening of wounds, which results in loss of some implanted hydroxy-apatite, are sometimes observed (Fig.7). However, this is not a clinical problem. because the wounds heal within 1 month after implantation. In the healing of wounds of the skin, epithelial cells from the edges of the wound invade the coagulum along fibrin. But after hydroxyapatite implantation, in which complete closure by gingival flaps cannot be achieved, the material filing the defect is not fibrin but hydroxyapatite. As a consequence, open wounds remain until the defect is completely covered with fibrin.

Case 3: This case shows discharge of hydroxyapatite granules, which rarely occur (Fig.8). While this symptom results in delayed wound healing, it is not a serious condition. We obtained similar findings in our animal experiments (Fig.9). Such discharge represents epithelial elimination of a foreign body, but its cause in these rare cases in still unclear. It is closely associated with inflammation, so complete debredement of inflammatory granulation tissue and chemical irritants like bacterial endotoxins, as well as complete plaque control are needed. Finally hydroxyapatite granules should be coverd with mucogingival flaps.

ACKNOWLEDGEMENTS

Some parts of this work are supported by the Department of Periodontics and Endodontics, the Faculty of Dentistry, Kyushu University.

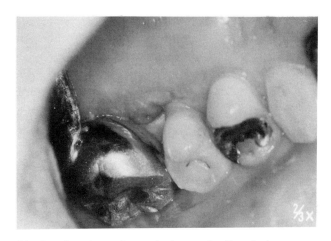

Fig.7. Opening of wound observed after hydroxyapatite implantation

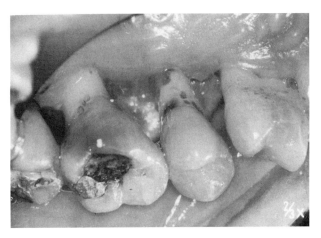

Fig.8. Discharge of hydroxyapatite granules from gingiva by epithelial elimination.

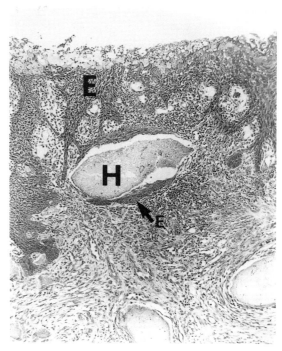

Fig.9. Epithelial elimination of hydroxyapatite observed in dogs gingiva. H: Hydroxyapatite granule, E: Epithelial cells

REFERENCES

1. Kodama H (1983) Jpn J Oral Biol 23:899-901

2. Hara Y (1988) In: Ishikawa J, Kawasaki H, Ikeda K, Hasegawa K (eds, Recent
    Advances in Clinical Periodontology, Excerpta Medica, Amsterdam, pp251-254)

3. Hara Y (1988) J Dent Res 68 (Abst): 962

© 1991 Elsevier Science Publishers B.V.
Recent advances in periodontology Vol. II,
S.I. Gold, M. Midda and S. Mutlu, eds.

CREVICULAR ANTIBIOTIC THERAPY FOR PERIODONTAL DISEASE

YOJI MURAYAMA

Department of Periodontology and Endodontology, Okayama University Dental School, Okayama 700, Japan

INTRODUCTION

A modern system of periodontal therapy is basically characterized by controlling resident mass of microbes. However, it has been shown that the various types of periodontal microorganisms are not equally susceptible to the several forms of periodontal therapy (Christersson et al., 1985, Kornman and Robertson, 1985). A mechanical control method, i.e., scaling, root planing, or curettage has the effect of reducing microbial mass and may benefit the inflamed tissues adjacent to it. The method will also be successful at controlling the specific organisms considered to be periodontal pathogens, even if it is not specifically aimed at these particular species (Theilade 1986). In some case, however, particularly juvenile periodontitis, specific pathogens still composed the resident flora and the disease progressed despite mechanical debridement and acceptable oral hygiene (Slots and Rosling, 1983; Christersson et al., 1985; Bragd et al., 1985). A number of recent studies have suggested that certain antibiotic control method may also be useful for treatment of periodontal disease, particularly since the antibiotics used may be effective in controlling specific microbiota.

The purpose of this review is to investigate the antibiotic therapy for periodontal disease. Reports from the literature have shown that crevicular administration of a minocycline ointment which is so prepared as to be slowly released in its active form may be useful pharmacokinetically, microbiologically and clinically for the treatment and management of periodontal disease (Nakashima et al., 1987; Isoshima et al., 1987; Naora et al., 1987; Kurimoto et al., 1987; Murayama et al., 1988a and 1988b).

A CONCEPT OF ANTIBIOTIC THERAPY

Loesche (1976) has referred to the relation between plaque microbes and pathologic changes of periodontal lesions as the non-specific theory in the microbial etiology of periodontal disease. It is assumed that the qualitative features of the microbiota are of minor importance and that the amount rather than the composition of the plaque is crucial to the pathogenesis of periodontal disease. However, at present it is strongly suggested that a certain degree of specificity exists between the microbiotas associated with health, gingivitis and various forms of periodontitis (Listgarten, 1988).

In a fundamental sense, the objective aim of the antimicrobial therapy for periodontal disease is to reduce the pathogenecity in the subgingival area. There are theoretically two approaches to making the subgingival area less pathogenic. The first approach is to reduce the total amount of plaque microbes. The procedure of mechanical debridement of the plaque mass and the use of antiseptic agent against non-specific microbiota will suit this purpose. The other is to reduce the level of pathogens in the plaque. In which case, antibiotics may be considered as an effective measure.

It is true that mechanical instrumentation has been the most successful method for the treatment of periodontal disease, since scaling and root planing provides not only removal of the microbial mass in subgingival pocket but also induce consistent alterations in the subgingival ecosystem and hence reduce the proportions of spirochetes and other periodontopathic microorganisms. Furthermore, the recolonization with the periodontal disease-associated microbiota may be prevented for a prolonged period of time, if adequate supragingival plaque control is performed (Siegrist and Kornman, 1982; Smulow, Turekey and Hill, 1983; Magnusson et al., 1984). Successful treatment of marginal periodontitis is based on a substantial reduction of the periodontal disease-associated microbiota concomitant with a change in the composition of the subgingival element. In this context, presumptive periodontopathic microorganisms should be suppressed substantially thereby affording the subgingival region to be recolonized with microorganisms more often encountered in conjunction with gingival health. Thus the non-specific control of the microbiota is effective in the majority of cases where access to the plaque deposits is possible. However, it is well known that patients who fail to achieve acceptable levels of plaque control during or after therapy frequently suffer recurrent periodontitis in spite of properly executed treatment (Nyman, Lindhe and Rosling, 1977; Becker, Becker and Berg, 1984; Lindhe and Liljeberg, 1984). Actually the non-specific control of the periodontal microbiota is not effective in controlling the microbial deposits located in deep pockets, furcation defects, such as grooves, created by root proximity (Listgarten, 1988).

Antibiotic therapy may be regarded successful in the management of the above-mentioned problems. Many studies have suggested that chemotherapy for periodontal disease by systemic administration of an antibiotic such as tetracycline or metronidazole can change the composition of the periodontal microflora by rapidly reducing the total subgingival microbial counts, taking into account the increase in coccoid cells and the decrease in gram-negative anaerobic cells including spirochetes and motile rods for varying periods, and in due course, promote rapidly clinical improvements of the diseased periodontal tissues (Ciancio, 1976; Listgarten, Lindhe and Hellden, 1978; Slots et al., 1979; Williams, Osterberg, and Jorgensen, 1979; Genco, 1981). However, the antibiotic measure comparative to mechanical debridement is inferior in terms of reducing the total amount of plaque microorganisms nevertheless it is directly effective toward the elimination of the specific pathogens. Consequently, the antibiotic therapy must become useful by utilizing the concept of shifting the microbial flora in healthy gingiva.

TOPICAL USE OF ANTIBIOTIC

Even though antibiotics often have proven effective against acute lesions elsewhere in the body, it has been difficult to demonstrate a similar efficacy in the treatment of periodontal diseases. For practical purposes, the effective approach to the delivery of antibiotics into deep periodontal pocket has been dependent on the systemic route so far recently. However, the clinical use of antibiotics from systemic route is associated with a number of critical problems. Most of these problems are related to the specific antibiotics used, the dosage of administration and the duration of the treatment, definitely including the development of hypersensitivity, induction of resistant strains of microorganisms and superinfection by fungal organisms. Taking these problems into consideration, topical administration seems to be for more superior to systemic administration. However, an antibiotic administered by a rinse will not reach the depth of the periodontal pocket. Even if the antibiotic is professionally administrated at the bottom of the periodontal pocket, the effectivity of the antibiotic will be limited only within the period of administration.

Various devices of placing antibiotics directly into subgingival pocket have been developed for sustained release of agents to the oral cavity. The mode of release of antibiotics from several fiber types made of antibiotic-loaded biocompatible polymers. Nevertheless, these carrier substances are still unsatisfactory for clinical use because the carrier substances which consisted of insoluble polymers must be removed from the periodontal pocket following the release of the agent and may also serve as physical stimulators in periodontal pocket. To overcome the problems posed by these non-soluble carrier substances, several investigators have devised various carrier substances to allow antibiotics to stay in periodontal pocket for a long time.

In order for topical antibiotic therapy to become an effective means in periodontal therapy, the following features of the carrier substance must meet these requirements: (1) excellent biocompatibility; (2) ability to be dissolved and absorbed in the periodontal pocket after a certain period; (3) guaranteed ability to reach the bottom of the periodontal pocket; (4) ease in clinical handling.

TRIAL OF CREVICULAR MINOCYCLINE THERAPY FOR PERIODONTAL DISEASE

We have recently conducted a series of studies to assess and establish a crevicular therapeutic system for periodontal disease by using minocycline hydrochloride (Lederle [Japan] Ltd, Tokyo, Japan) prepared as a slow releasing ointment (MINO) (Kurimoto et al., 1987). Subsequently, we conducted a follow study to evaluate clinically and microbiologically an effective crevicular minocycline therapy.

The effect of MINO containing 2% minocycline hydrochloride was compared with that of a placebo using two pairs of contralateral sites with periodontal destruction in each subject. The agent was administrated into periodontal pockets once in a week for 4 consecutive weeks. Sixteen periodontitis patients (48 teeth with periodontal pocket depth of over 4 mm) participated in this study. The subject received ultrasonic scaling immediately before the first administration of the agent and then no professional plaque control within the experimental period. The periodontal sites were examined clinically and microbiologically extending for a period of 15 weeks. The clinical examination included assessments of plaque accumulation, gingival inflammation, pocket depth and bleeding on probing. Bacterial density and the proportion of motile rods were determined on a Petroff-Hauser Counting Chamber (C.A.H. and Son, Philadelphia, PA). The organisms of black-pigmented <u>Bacteroides</u> (BPB) were identified according to a DNA-DNA hybridization assay method.

TABLE 1. Clinical findings before and after administration of MINO and placebo

Clinical parameters	Agents	Clinical findings (mean±SD)				
		0W (n=48)	4W (n=48)	7W (n=48)	11W (n=34)	15W (n=34)
Plaque index (Silness and Löe, 1964)	MINO	1.40±0.86	0.63±0.42**^{a}	0.54±0.45**^{a}	0.35±0.70**^{a}	0.38±0.60**^{a}
	Placebo	1.19±0.92	0.58±0.64*^{a}	0.56±0.50	0.47±0.54	0.47±0.62
Gingival index (Sidi and Ashley, 1984)	MINO	1.64±0.57	1.29±0.40*^{a}	1.14±0.49*^{a}	1.11±0.57*^{a}	1.05±0.67*^{a}
	Placebo	1.58±0.53	1.46±0.59 **^{b}	1.43±0.52 **^{b}	1.32±0.42 **^{b}	1.19±0.49
Probing depth of pocket (mm) (Isoshima et al, 1987)	MINO	5.01±1.20	4.19±1.01**^{a}	3.90±1.01**^{a}	3.69±0.96**^{a}	3.72±0.99**^{a}
	Placebo	4.67±1.16	4.46±1.15	4.28±1.35*^{a}	3.92±1.10**^{a}	3.91±1.08**^{a}
Presence of bleeding on probing (%)	MINO	94.7	68.4 *^{c}	94.1	75.0	81.8
	Placebo	100	95.2	100	90.0	100

statistical analysis: ^{a} Wilcoxon signed rank test, ^{b} Wilcoxon rank sum test, ^{c} Fisher exact probability test. * P<0.05, ** P<0.01.

There were significant changes in all our clinical parameters over 15 weeks after administration of MINO, and also in plaque accumulation at 4-week and in pocket depth at 7-, 11- and 15-week even after administration of placebo. Statistical differences were present between the MINO and placebo group in gingival inflammation up to 11-week, and in bleeding on probing at 4-week (Table 1). The microbial density showed a marked decrease up to 11-week in the MINO group and up to 7-week in placebo group (Table 2). However, there

TABLE 2. Bacterial density before and after administration of
MINO and placebo

Agents	Bacterial density ($\times 10^7$/ml) (mean$\pm$SD)				
	0W (n=48)	4W (n=48)	7W (n=48)	11W (n=34)	15W (n=34)
MINO	5.17$\pm$5.28	0.56$\pm$0.69**[a]	0.96$\pm$1.23**[a]	1.57$\pm$1.53**[a]	2.56$\pm$3.23
		**[b]		**[b]	
Placebo	4.56$\pm$8.51	2.16$\pm$2.48*[a]	2.78$\pm$4.57*[a]	2.67$\pm$2.83	4.20$\pm$5.59

statistical analysis: [a] Wilcoxon signed rank test, [b] Wilcoxon rank sum test.
* $p < 0.05$, ** $p < 0.01$.

was no significant decrease in the proportion of motile microorganisms at 4-week in the placebo group, whereas a decrease in significance was noted in the MINO group up to 15-week (Table 3). Furthermore, regarding microbial

TABLE 3. Percentage of motile organisms before and after administration of
MINO and placebo

Agents	Motile organisms (%) (mean$\pm$SD)				
	0W (n=48)	4W (n=48)	7W (n=48)	11W (n=34)	15w (n=34)
MINO	38.26$\pm$21.32	8.85$\pm$10.81*[a]	12.97$\pm$13.21*[a]	24.88$\pm$21.00	24.38$\pm$18.36*[a]
		*[b]		*[b]	
Placebo	34.74$\pm$18.27	28.61$\pm$19.44*[a]	27.20$\pm$22.35*[a]	32.93$\pm$22.72	29.39$\pm$23.99

statistical analysis: [a] Wilcoxon signed rank test, [b] Wilcoxon rank sum test.
* $p < 0.01$.

density and proportion of motile organisms there were statistical differences between the MINO and placebo group at 4- and 7-week. The major bacterial strains isolated at 0-week were <u>Actinobacillus</u>   <u>actinomycetemcomitans</u>, BPB (<u>B.</u>

melaninogenicus, B. intermedius, B. gingivalis), Eikenella corrodens, Fusobacterium nucleatum and Capnocytophaga spp. There was a rapid increase in the density of BPB after administration of placebo, mean while there was a gradual decrease up to 11-week after administration of MINO (Table 4).

TABLE 4. Density of black pigmented *Bacteroides*(BPB) before and after administration of MINO and placebo

Agents	Density of BPB ($\times 10^4$CFU/ml)(mean$\pm$SD)			
	0W	7W	11W	15W
MINO	11.54$\pm$21.14 (n=6)	0.06$\pm$0.11** (n=4)	1.20$\pm$2.40* (n=5)	37.21$\pm$73.86 (n=4)
Placebo	5.38$\pm$9.54 (n=6)	18.77$\pm$29.59 (n=6)	67.21$\pm$120.11 (n=6)	67.62$\pm$103.32 (n=6)

statistical analysis: Mann-Whitney test.   * P<0.05, ** P<0.01

The results of our study revealed that the microflora shifted to a typical population associated with a healthy gingiva at least for 11 weeks and that the clinical symptoms of periodontal pathology were reduced or eliminated over 15 weeks after crevicular treatment by MINO.

CONCLUSION

It is currently becoming possible to discuss successful treatment in terms of quantitative and qualitative microbial changes identified in samples of subgingival plaque. The mechanical debridement appears generally unproductive at suppressing specific organisms as resident flora in subgingival pocket, nevertheless it is most expedient for non-specific removal of plaque mass located in relatively superficial pocket. Therefore the antibiotic therapy has been advocated for the qualitative improvement of microbial plaque in advanced periodontal lesions. The results from our study indicate that the crevicular antibiotic therapy using minocycline is able to create microbiologically and clinically favorable conditions in periodontal lesions and may be proposed as a measure for the management of patients unresponsive to the conventional mechanical therapy. In this study the mechanical instrumentation was limited to rough scaling immediately before the administration of minocycline in order to reduce its beneficial effects to the minimum. However, properly speaking, the periodontal therapy should be aimed at the quantitative as well as qualitative improvement of the microbial plaque in subgingival pockets. In sum, our devised crevicular minocycline therapy may exert more favorable results microbiologically as well as clinically if it is combined with conventional mechanical debridement.

It is then assumed that the crevicular use of antibiotic offers particular value on a course of the treatment of periodontal disease. The scheme of future antibiotic clinical trials should include emphasis on shifting the microbial flora on a safety level where potential pathogens are nonexistent within the subgingival plaque with or without decreasing the total plaque mass.

REFERENCES

Becker B, B Becker and L Berg (1984) J Periodontol 55:505

Bragd L et al (1985) J Clin Periodontol 14:95

Christersson LA et al (1985) J Clin Periodontol 12:465

Ciancio SG (1976) J Periodontol 47:155

Genco RJ (1981) J Periodontol 52:545

Isoshima O et al (1987) J Japan Ass Periodont 29:472

Kornman KS and PB Robertson (1985) J Periodontol 56:443

Kurimoto K et al (1987) J Japan Ass Periodont 29:930

Lindhe J and B Liljenberg (1984) J Clin Periodontol 11:399

Listgarten MA, J Lindhe and L Hellden (1978) J Clin Periodontol 5:246

Listgarten MA (1988) J Clin Periodontol 15:485

Loesche WJ (1976) Oral Sciences Reviews 9:65

Magnusson I et al (1984) J Clin Periodontol 11:193

Murayama Y et al (1988a) J Japan Ass Periodont 30:206

Murayama Y et al (1988b) In: J Ishikawa et al (eds), Recent advances in clinical periodontology. Excerpta Medica, Amsterdam, pp215-218

Nakashima K et al (1987) J Japan Ass Periodont 29:463

Naora Y et al (1987) J Japan Ass Periodont 29:484

Nyman S, J Lindhe and B Rosling (1977) J Clin Periodontol 4:240

Siegrist BE and KS Kornman (1982) J Dent Res 61:936

Slots J et al (1979) J Periodontol 50:495

Smulow JB, SS Turesky and RG Hill (1983) J Am Dent Ass 107:737

Theilade E (1986) J Clin Periodontol 13:905

Williams BL, SK Osterberg and J Jorgensen (1979) J Clin Periodontol 6:210

© 1991 Elsevier Science Publishers B.V.
Recent advances in periodontology Vol. II,
S.I. Gold, M. Midda and S. Mutlu, eds.

CLINICAL AND MICROBIAL EVALUATION OF DENTAL IMPLANTS - A RETROSPECTIVE
ANALYSIS OF SUCCESS AND FAILURE

VINCENT IACONO,[1] LUDOVICO SBORDONE,[2] GABRIELLA SPAGNUOLO,[3] RENATO
CIAGLIA,[3] BLASCO GOMES,[1] AND PAUL BAER[1]
Department of Periodontics, School of Dental Medicine, State University of New York at Stony
Brook, Stony Brook, New York, 11794-8703;[1] and the University of Calabria[2] and Naples,[3] Italy

INTRODUCTION

Endosseous osseointegrated dental implants are increasingly being used to replace missing teeth in
both fully and partially edentulous patients (1). This is due, in part, to their rates of success reported
in case series studies (2,3). There are several implant systems available which achieve
osseointegration. One system which has become quite popular is the Core-Vent or Spectra-System.
The Core-Vent System is a comprehensive system which is marketed for use in both fully and
partially edentulous patients. Although the success rates for Core-Vent implants have been reported
to be high, there are few studies on partially edentulous patients (4). This is especially true for those
patients where the remaining teeth are periodontally compromised. One concern is the possible
colonization of the subgingival peri-implant space by periodontopathic microorganisms which could
lead to implant failure. Such a phenomenon could show similarities with the development of
periodontal disease around the dentition (5). In an attempt to address this possibility a longitudinal
study was designed (a) to determine if osseointegrated Core-Vent and other root form implants can
be maintained among periodontally compromised teeth and (b) to determine and compare the clinical
parameters and subgingival microflora of osseointegrated and failing implants with those of healthy
and periodontally compromised teeth.

MATERIALS AND METHODS
Patient selection

The study population initially consisted of 9 patients, 4 females and 5 males, with an average age
of 58.1 years (40-78 years). The patients received from 1 to 6 implants for a total of 29 implants with
14 of mandibular and 15 of maxillary location. They were used as abutments for overdentures,
implant, and implant-tooth supported fixed bridges. The patients were and are being maintained on
a 3-4 month recall schedule. As shown in Table 1, implants and teeth were examined and microbial
samples were obtained from 1 to 19 months after exposure and loading (T1) and again 11 months later
(T2).

Panoramic and periapical radiographs were obtained, and the peri-implant and periodontal sites
were scored clinically using the following measurements: probing depth (PD), attachment level (AL),
gingival index (GI)(6), and plaque index (PLI)(7), and mobility. The AL for the natural dentition was
measured from the cementoenamel junction, and for implants from the joining site between the
abutment and the fixture.

TABLE 1

Patient number (age/sex)	Implant type (number/location)	Sampling time (months)	
		T1	T2
1. 61/F	NP[1],6/mandible	19	30
2. 40/M	CV[2],4/maxilla, mandible	3	-[3]
3. 66/M	CV,4/maxilla	1	12
4. 78/M	NP,3/mandible	17	28
5. 64/F	CV,1/mandible	1	12
6. 63/M	CV,6/maxilla	5	16
7. 44/F	CV,2/mandible	1	12
8. 55/M	CV,2/maxilla	1	12
9. 52/F	CV,1/maxilla	5	16

[1]NP, Nobelpharma.
[2]CV, Core-Vent.
[3]-, patient exited from study at T1.

Microbiological techniques

Microbial samples were collected from the apical portion of periodontal and peri-implant pockets. Care was taken to obtain sampling with minimal or no contamination from micro-organisms of the supragingival plaque and/or mucosal surfaces. Bacterial samples was performed with a sterile curet. Subgingival plaque samples were immediately transferred into 2 ml of prereduced sterile anaerobic 1/4 strength Ringer's solution supplemented with 0.1% sodium metaphosphate. The samples were then dispersed by vortexing for 10 seconds, and a 0.1 ml aliquot was analyzed by phase-contrast microscopy. An additional dispersion by means of 20 seconds sonication was carried out, and an aliquot of 0.1 ml of this second dispersion was Gram-stained.

Further microbiological manipulations were then carried out by using a continuous anaerobic technique in Brewer Jars containing 85% N_2, employing full strength Ringer's solution containing 0.05% L-cysteine and 0.0001% resazurin. Aliquots of 0.1 ml of appropriate dilutions were plated onto non-selective and elective media. Plates were incubated in appropriate atmospheres at 35°C for 4-7 days and subsequently examined for the presence of colonies typical of the species sought. Where possible, at least 10 colonies were subcultured until pure, and speciated on the basis of colony morphology, aerotolerance, Gram staining and biochemical tests (8-22).

Preparations for phase-contrast microscopy were viewed by means of a Phase Star Microscope. At least 200 bacterial cells were counted in 10 randomly selected fields and assigned to the following 8 bacterial morphotypes; cocci, rods, fusiforms, filamentous forms, motile rods, and small, large and intermediate spirochetes.

RESULTS

The clinical characteristics of the sampling sites for 9 and 8 periodontally treated teeth at T1 and T2, respectively; and for 14 and 12 osseointegrated implants at T1 and T2, respectively, are shown in Table 2.

TABLE 2

Clinical characteristics of sampling sites (mean ± SD)

	Teeth		Implants	
	T1(9 sites)	T2(8 sites)	T1(14 sites)	T2(12 sites)
Gingival index	1.8±0.4[1]	1.9±0.4	1.7±0.5[2]	1.7±0.5
Plaque index	1.2±0.4	0.8±0.9	1.4±1.0	1.3±1.1
Probing depth[3]	4.4±0.5	3.8±0.7	3.5±0.6	3.6±1.2
Attachment level[3]	4.7±0.7	4.5±1.3	1.5±1.2	2.4±1.2

[1] 78% of sites displayed bleeding upon probing at T1; 87.5% at T2.
[2] 64% of sites displayed bleeding upon probing at T1; 66.7% at T2.
[3] mm.

The values for gingival index, plaque index, and probing depth were similar for both teeth and implants with no significant changes occurring between the two sampling points. With regard to attachment level, the attachment level for implants was measured from the joining site between the abutment and titanium fixture to crestal bone. The mean value for implants was 1.5mm, as compared with 4.7mm for teeth at T1, and 2.4 mm for implants and 4.5 mm for teeth at T2. All implants exhibited no clinical mobility.

After clinical indices were obtained, subgingival plaque samples were collected from the periodontal and peri-implant sulci and evaluated by phase contrast microscopy and culturing on non-selective and selective media. Implants had a microflora similar to that of the treated teeth. Cocci and non-motile rods predominated with up to 85.2% around teeth and 95.9% around implants at T1. At T2, they comprised 79% of the morphotypes around teeth and 81.9% around implants. Unlike that observed for natural teeth, spirochetes were rarely observed at implant sites.

When the composition of the cultivable microflora was compared for all teeth and implants, the similarities were striking. This can be seen in Table 3, where for example, Gram-positive facultative cocci averaged 41.7% and 40.0% of tooth associated flora at T1 and T2, respectively; and 42.4% and 52.2% of implant associated flora at T1 and T2, respectively.

TABLE 3 Composition ($\bar{X}$%±SD) of cultivable microflora in subgingival plaque samples associated with natural teeth and implants

	Teeth[1]		Implants[2]	
Bacteria	T1	T2	T1	T2
Gram-positive facultative cocci	41.7±30.0	40.0±35.1	42.4±35.6	52.2±38.0
Gram-negative facultative cocci	7.0±20.8	11.8±19.4	8.9±19.1	12.7±19.2
Gram-positive facultative rods	14.0±19.6	9.1±16.7	2.4±7.8	0.9±1.5
Gram-negative facultative rods	21.3±25.4	20.1±29.6	18.0±35.2	12.3±19.2
Gram-positive anaerobic cocci	6.1±18.3	1.8±3.6	13.3±28.3	6.8±20.8
Gram-negative anaerobic cocci	1.1±2.4	4.6±9.0	0.0	5.6±9.9
Gram-positive anaerobic rods	0.0	7.7±16.2	9.7±18.3	1.0±2.9
Gram-negative anaerobic rods	1.6±11.2	5.0±11.6	3.4±8.2	7.4±13.6

[1] Teeth; T1 = 9 sites, T2 = 8 sites.
[2] Implants; T1 = 14 sites, T2 = 12 sites.

When positive sites were compared, similar microfloras were also observed, but with some minor differences. For example, unlike teeth at T1 which exhibited no Gram-positive anaerobic rods, four of the implant sites averaged 34% Gram positive anaerobic rods.

Procedures were employed to identify 9 specific bacterial species at all sampled sites. Shown in Table 4 are their percentages of the cultivable microflora isolated at positive sites around the teeth and implants.

TABLE 4

Specific bacterial species ($\bar{X}$%±SD) at positive sites isolated from sub-gingival plaque samples

Bacterial species	Teeth[1] T1	T2	Implants[2] T1	T2
F.nucleatum	1[3] 6.70	1 0.02	5 3.39±6.04	5 0.22±0.38
A.a.[4]	0.05±0.04	3 0.56±0.58	1 0.03	3 0.16±0.11
H.aphrophilus	3 0.30±0.26	0 0.0	3 0.58±0.93	0 0.0
B.gingivalis	1 0.07	4 1.38±2.13	3 **3.09±2.97**	9 **0.76±1.32**
B.intermedius	0 0.0	1 0.03	2 0.43±0.01	2 0.34±0.37
B.melaninogenicus	0 0.0	0 0.0	2 0.03±0.04	0 0.0
Capnocytophaga	1 0.18	0 0.0	3 2.38±2.01	1 2.30
E.corrodens	2 0.58±0.35	0 0.0	1 **12.50**	2 **0.20±0.01**
E.lentum	0 0.0	0 0.0	2 **18.33±2.36**	1 **0.03**

[1]Teeth; T1 = 9 sites sampled, T2 = 8 sites.
[2]Implants; T1 = 14 sites sampled, T2 = 12 sites.
[3]Number of positive sites.
[4]A.actinomycetemcomitans.

Note that although clinically healthy at T1, 3 of the implant sites averaged 3.09% *B. gingivalis*, 1 site consisted of 12.5% *E. corrodens* and 2 sites averaged greater than 18% *E. lentum*. At T2 each of these and the other species, with the exception of *Capnocytophaga*, averaged less than 1% at the positive sites.

Of the 29 implants which were inserted in these patients, two implants in one patient had sites which exhibited a loss of attachment at T1 (i.e., 7mm and 5mm) and shortly thereafter became mobile and were extracted. The composition of the subgingival microflora at these two sites was compared to that of a natural tooth with severe attachment loss and found to consist of as many as 76.6% gram negative anaerobic rods. As shown in Table 5, when the plaque samples were cultured to identify specific bacterial species, *B. gingivalis* comprised 15%, 23.7%, and 1.9% of the cultivable microflora from samples obtained from the periodontally involved tooth and failing implants, respectively. The other species were either not detected or were present at very low levels.

TABLE 5

Specific bacterial species(%) isolated from subgingival plaque
samples associated with a diseased tooth and failing implants

Bacterial	Tooth	Implants	
species	#30DB	#8M	#9D
	(PD9,AL9)[1]	(PD9,AL7)	(PD8,AL5)
A.a.[2]	0	0.4	0
B.gingivalis	15	23.7	1.9
B.intermedius	0.35	1.1	0
B.mel.[3]	0.15	1.1	0.6
Others[4]	0	0	0

[1]PD, pocket depth; AL, attachment level.
[2]A.actinomycetemcomitans.
[3]B.melaninogenicus.
[4]F.nucleatum, H.aphrophilus, Capnocytophaga species,
E.corrodens, and E.lentum.

Those implants at T1 which had sites having a significant percentage of presumed periodontal
pathogens were evaluated for both clinical and microbial changes at T2. The findings were then
compared to those for the tooth with severe loss of attachment. As seen in Table 6, the tooth with
attachment level of 9 at T1 had 15% *B. gingivalis* which was reduced to 0.1% at T2. At T1, each
of three clinically immobile implants had as many as 20% *E. lentum*, 12.5% *E. corrodens*, and
16.7% *E. lentum*, respectively. At T2 these bacteria were not detected and the remaining species
were not detected or were present at very low levels.

TABLE 6

Specific bacterial species(%) isolated from subgingival plaque samples
associated with a treated tooth and implants

	Tooth				Implants			
Bacterial	#30DB		#4M		#20M		#21M	
species	T1(AL9)[1]	T2(AL9)	T1(AL3)	T2(AL3)	T1(AL0)	T2(AL1)	T1(AL0)	T2(AL1)
F.nucleatum	0	0	0	0	0.75	0	14.17	0.01
A.a.[2]	0	0	0	0.06	0	0	0	0
H.aphrophilus	0	0	0	0	0.08	0	1.66	0
B.gingivalis	15	0.1	0	0.01	0	0.1	0	0.76
B.intermedius	0.35	0	0	0	0	0.08	0	0
B.mel.[3]	0.15	0	0	0	0	0	0	0
Capnocytophaga	0	0	0	0	0	0	0	0
E.corrodens	0	0	0	0	12.5	0	0	0
E.lentum	0	0	20	0	0	0	16.66	0

[1]AL, attachment level.
[2]A.actinomycetemcomitans.
[3]B.melaninogenicus.

DISCUSSION

Our results indicate that with the exception of mobility, which would indicate implant failure,
attachment level should be considered the most clinically relevant parameter for implants, as the
gingival index and probing depth were often affected by the thickness and quality of the

mucoperiosteum surrounding fixtures at the time of their exposure. Indeed, as was often the case, implants with the same attachment level at the time of abutment connection had minimal to quite significant probing depths with a variable gingival index. In addition the quality of the tissue at the perimucosal region appeared to have little effect on the clinical indices. This is not unlike that reported by Apse and coworkers (23) who observed that the lack of keratinized gingiva around implants did not result in higher gingival and bleeding indices or greater probing depths.

Only two of the 29 implants examined in this study became mobile and were subsequently extracted (Table 5). This would suggest that osseointegrated implants can be maintained among periodontally compromised teeth. However, as a caveat, unlike teeth which can be maintained in a mobile state (Table 6), mobile implants are considered to be failures and are usually extracted. The pattern of destruction which occurred around the two failing "osseointegrated" implants was probably due to the combined factors of the colonization by periodontopathic bacteria and characteristic host responses. However, as reported in earlier studies (5, 24), we observed that there are several differences in the microflora between the peri-implant pocket and the periodontal pocket. The former harbors coccoid cells and few spirochetes irrespective of pocket depth, while the latter harbor as reported, significant numbers of motile rods and spirochetes. However, with this exception, implants tend to acquire the patient's characteristic indigenous microflora. The significance of the microbiology of failing implants is difficult to assess due to the small number of implant failures which results in inadequate sample size for statistical analyses. The expansion and continuation of studies of this type will help in this regard.

ACKNOWLEDGEMENTS

This work was supported in part by C.N.R. (Italian Research Council) grant #86.00143.04 to Dr. Sbordone and a Core-Vent Corporation grant to Dr. Iacono.

REFERENCES

1. Iacono, VJ (1990) In: Genco RJ, Goldman HM, Cohen DW (eds) Contemporary Periodontics. The C.V. Mosby Company, pp 653-667.

2. Adell R, Lekholm U, Rockler B, Branemark PI (1981) Int J Oral Surg 10:383

3. Branemark PI, Hansson BO, Adell R, Breine U, Lindstrom J, Hallen O, Ohman A (1977) Scand J Plast Reconstr Surg 11: Suppl 16

4. Patrick D,Zosky J, Lubar R, Buchs A (1989) J Oral Implantology 15:1

5. Iacono VJ, Sbordone L, Spagnuolo G, Baer P, Gomes B (1989) J Dent Research 68 (Sp Issue): 912

6. Loe H, Silness J (1963) Acta Odont Scand 21:533

7. Sillness J, Loe H (1964) Acta Odont Scand 22:112

8. Socransky SS, Holt SC, Leadbetter ER, Tanner ACR, Savitt ED, Hammond BF (1979) Archs Microbiol 122:29

9. Matsuda Y (1976) Bulletin of the Tokyo Medical and Dental University 23:27

10. Cowan SJ (1974) In: Cowan SJ, Steel B (eds) Cowan and Steel's Manual for the Identification of Medical Bacteria (ed 2). Cambridge University Press

11. Socransky SS, Manganiello AD, Propas D, Oram V, Van Houte J (1977) J Periodont Res 12:90

12. Walker CB, Ratcliff D, Muller D, Mandell R, Socransky SS (1979) J Clin Microbiol 10:844

13. Slee AM, Tanser GM (1978) J Clin Microbiol 8:459

14. Kilian M (1974) Acta Path Microbiol Scand (Section B) 82:835

15. Mandell RL, Tripodi LS, Savitt E, Goodson JM, Socransky SS (1986) J Periodontol 57:94

16. Slots J (1982) J Clin Microbiol 15:606

17. Mandell RL, Socransky SS (1981) J Periodontol 52:593

18. Rogosa M (1964) J Bacterol 87:162

19. Alcoforado GAP, McKay TL, Slots J (1987) Oral Microbiol Immunol 2:35

20. Zambon JJ, Reynolds HS, Slots J (1981) Interest Immun 32:198

21. Slots J, Reynolds HS (1982) J Clin Microbiol 16:1148

22. Holdemann LV, Cato EP, Moore WEC (1977) In: Anerobe Laboratory Manual (ed 4). Virginia Polytechnic Institute and State University, Blacksburg, VA

23. Apse P, Ellen RP, Overall CM, Zarb GA (1989) J Periodont Res 24:96

24. Adell R, Lekholm U, Rockler B, Branemark PI, Lndhe J, Eriksson B, Sbordone L (1986) Int J Oral Maxillofac Surg 15:39

© 1991 Elsevier Science Publishers B.V.
Recent advances in periodontology Vol. II,
S.I. Gold, M. Midda and S. Mutlu, eds.

GINGIVAL AND LATERAL PERIODONTAL CYSTS

BERNARD S. MOSKOW, D.D.S., M.Sc.D.

Clinical Professor of Dentistry, Center for Clinical Research in Dentistry,
Columbia University, School of Dental and Oral Surgery, New York, N.Y. 10032

HISTORICAL BACKGROUND

Prior to 1955 there were no reports in the world literature of gingival cysts
with distinctive clinical symptoms and the lateral periodontal cyst was considered
a rare odontogenic lesion with few reported cases. The former lesion, in fact,
was considered to be a rare academic curiosity, inadvertently encountered in the
routine examination of gingival biopsies. They were considered to be microcysts
with no clinical implications at all. Lateral periodontal cysts, on the other
hand, were usually found only during radiographic examination. In 1970, Moskow,
et al reviewed the characteristics of 62 gingival and lateral periodontal cysts
found in the literature and reported 25 new cases from the files of Columbia
University School of Dental and Oral Surgery. Since that time, virtually hundreds of similar lesions have been published in the world literature indicating
that these cysts are considerably more common than previously thought. This is
not the first instance in which lesions or diseases previously thought to be
extremely rare, begin to be seen in increasing frequency once they are brought
to the attention of the profession. Obviously, their diagnosis was missed or
they were confused with other clinical entities.

EMBRYOGENESIS AND PATHOGENESIS

Histologic studies on 10 pairs of human fetal jaws were done by Moskow and
Bloom (1983) to assess the histogenesis of gingival cysts. Cystic proliferation
of the dental lamina was noted as early as 10 weeks in utero and rapid growth
and proliferation of these lesions continued into the morphodifferentiation
stage of tooth development after fragmentation of the lamina had occured. Islands,
nests and strands of odontogenic epithelium were dispersed into extra and intraosseous locations and demonstrated histomorpholgic characteristics similar to
odontigenicallyrelated epithelium seen in adult gingiva. The authors concluded
that dental lamina epithelium appears to have a particular predisposition for
cystic degeneration and was probably the major source of cysts, hamartomas and
neoplasms encountered in the periodontal structures. Other sources of gingival
and periodontal cysts include transplanted surface epithelium ("epidermal
cysts"), cystic degeneration of down growing rete ridges from gingival epithelium,
degenerating mucous glands, cystic degeneration of pulpal granulomas in a lateral
position on the root, epithelial remnants associated with decidious teeth,

lateral dentigerous cysts and primordial cysts which occur along the side of the root. Gingival cysts in infants and newborn include: Epstein's pearls, Bohn's nodules, Eruption cysts and dental lamina cysts (Glands of Serres).

HISTOLOGIC APPEARANCE OF CYSTIC DEBRIS FOUND IN GINGIVAL TISSUES

Islands, nests and strands of epithelial cells of obvious odontogenic origin can be noted frequently in human gingival tissue. This material undergoes progressive degeneration and the following histomorphologic changes can be noted: 1) Intracellular hydropic degeneration, pyknosis of cell nuclei, nuclear fragmentation, intracellular keratinization and mucin production. Odontogenic epithelium found in the gingiva has also been associated with dystrophic calcification. Ulmansky (1965) has suggested that this is an inductive phenomenon.

CLINICAL CHARACTERISTIS

Gingival cysts are most commonly seen in the 40-60 year old age group and do not appear to have any sex or racial predilection. They usually are noted in the area of the mucogingival junction and appear as dome-shaped, bullous-like lesions with a clear grey-blue cast. Generally, they are approximately 5-10mm in diameter and their borders are well-defined. They are compressible and exude a clear fluid when pressed. The patient usually presents a history of the intermittent presence of a "bubble on the gums". Gingival cysts usually present themselves on the facial surface, but on rare occasions have been seen on the lingual gingiva. There is usually an egg-shell depression in the bone underlining the cyst, but radiographic symptoms are rarely seen in the gingival cyst. They have an uncanny predisposition for the mandibular cuspid-bicuspid region and this may be explained on an embryologic basis. Ossificiation of Meckel's cartilage, which is the precursor of the mandible, begins in the cuspid area and it is concievable that epithelial debris from the fragmentation of the dental lamina is entrapped in this part of the jaw. This could present an nidus for cystic degeneration in the future.

Lateral periodontal cysts rarely present overt clinical systems and are usually discovered on radiographic examination. They are commonly seen adjoining the periodontal ligament somewhere along the mid-point of the root, although in some instances, they can approach the apical region.

Radiographically, they appear as a typical radiolucent cystic lesion with a hyperostotic border. They can be round or tear-drop in shape and usually vary in size from 3 to 7mm in diameter. In some instances, they can be multilocular. They have been known to occur bilaterally. Lateral periodontal cysts have the same predilection for the lower-bicuspid area as the gingival cyst. Both gingival and lateral periodontal cysts are slow growing and their behavior is relatively benign. If the lesion tens to be more rapid in growth, it is in all probability

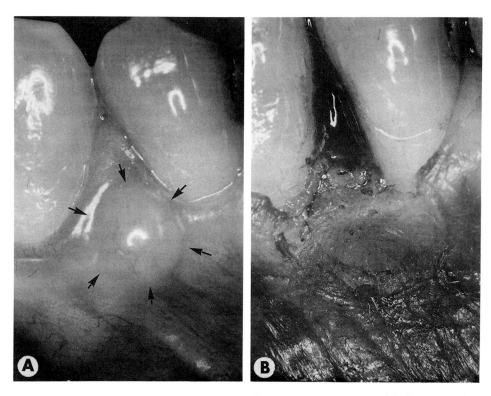

Fig. 1 (A). Typical clinical appearance of gingival cyst in mandibular cuspid-bicuspid region. The limits of the lesion are clearly defined.

(B). Note depression in underlinig cortical bone associated with the gingival cyst.

an odontogenic keratocyst. This lesion is similar in its clinical appearance to the lateral periodontal cyst, but can be rapidly destructive and tends to recurr.

CHARACTER OF LINING EPITHELIUM IN GINGIVAL AND LATERAL PERIODONTAL CYSTS

These lesions tend to be lined with a single or double layer of flat, cuboidal or short columnar squamous, epithelial cells, which are either keratinizing or parakeratinizing. Plaque-like thickenings of the cyst wall are not an uncommon microscopic finding.

TREATMENT

Gingival cysts should be exposed by a small muco-periosteal flap and the lesion cleanly curetted from the surface of the bone. Irregularities that may be present on the bone that contained the cyst need not be disturbed, as spontaneous remodeling of the cortical surface occurs. The flap should be carefully

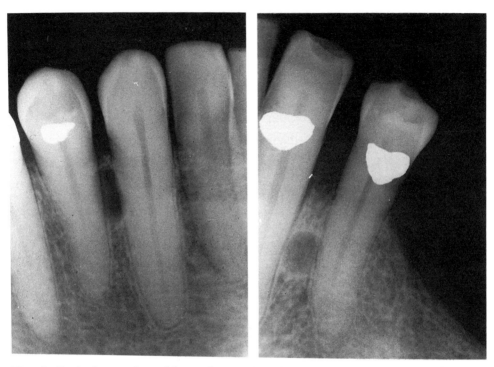

Fig. 2. Typical examples of lateral periodontal cysts in mandibular cuspid-bicuspid area. They appear as a clearly defined radiolucent areas with hyper-stotic borders.

sutured into place so as to not disturb the normal marginal contours of the gingiva.

It is important in the treatment of lateral periodontal cysts to be certain of its interproximal location in order to determine whether surgical access should be attempted from the facial or the lingual approach. This can be accomplished by sequential x-rays, taken at different horizontal angles. Following a flap exposure of the cortical alveolar bone, access to the cyst lesion can be usually accomplished by means of a small round bur or sharp instrument. Once the cystic cavity is exposed, its contents should be thoroughly removed with small curettes. It is best not to create a large opening into the cystic lesion in order to facilitate healing of the periodontal tissues after removal of the cystic tissues. Tissue removed from either type of cyst should be placed in fixative and sent for patholgic examination to be certain that the clinical diagnosis was correct.

SUMMARY

Tooth formation is a complex embryologic process which commonly results in errors in tooth development, number of teeth, etc. Retrograde changes can occur during tooth or jaw development which could result in residual entrapped odonto-genic material. Such debris of Malassez is theorized as being the main source of the large variety of odontogenic tumors, cysts, hamartomas and choristomas encountered in jaws. The boundary between developmental anomalies, cysts and tumors is not always clearly defined and many intermediate and transitional forms can be found. For example, adnexal structures such as sebaceous glands and hair follicles have been described in the gingiva.

REFERENCES

1. Bhaskar SN, Laskin, PM (1955) Gingival cysts, report of 3 cases, Oral Surgery, Oral Medicine and Oral Pathology 8, 803-807

2. Baden E., Moskow BS, Moskow R (1968) Odontogenic gingival epithelial hamar-toma. Journal of Oral Surgery 26, 702-714

3. Moskow BS (1966) The pathogenesis of the gingival cyst. Periodontics 4, 4-5

4. Moskow BS, Siegal K, Zegarelli EV, Kutsher AH, Rothenberg F (1970) Journal of Periodontology 41, 249-260

5. Moskow BS, Weinstein MM (1975) Further observations on the gingival cyst. Journal of Periodontology 46, 178-182

6. Buchner A, Hansen LA (1979) The histomorphologic spectrum of the gingival cyst in the adult. Oral Surgery, Oral Medicine and Oral Pathology 48, 531-539

7. Wysocki GP, Brannon RB, Gardner DG, Sapp P (1980) Histogenesis of the lateral periodontal cyst and the gingival cyst of the adult. Oral Surgery, Oral Medicine and Oral Pathology 50, 327-334

© 1991 Elsevier Science Publishers B.V.
Recent advances in periodontology Vol. II,
S.I. Gold, M. Midda and S. Mutlu, eds.

STUDIES IN PERIODONTAL WOUND HEALING WITH
GUIDED TISSUE REGENERATION.

JACK CATON, TIMOTHY BLIEDEN, CHARLES WAGENER, CARLOS QUINONES,
GARY GREENSTEIN AND URS ZAPPA*

Department of Periodontology, Eastman Dental Center, 625 Elmwood Avenue,
Rochester, NY 14620, USA.
*Department of Periodontology, University of Bern, Bern, Switzerland

Introduction

There is ample evidence that guided tissue regeneration (GTR) results in the formation of new bone and periodontal ligament, on and adjacent to a pathologically exposed root surface. In GTR, a physical barrier is placed between the gingival flap and root surface which prevents gingival epithelium and connective tissue from gaining access to the wound. At the same time, the barrier guides cells from the periodontal ligament and alveolar bone to populate the root surface and adjacent blood clot.

Several significant questions related to GTR have been studied in our laboratories and our preliminary results will be described in this paper. These questions include: 1) Is GTR possible in the interproximal area? 2) How long must a barrier be in place to maximize GTR? 3) How much of the exposed root surface, apical to the barrier, is at risk for regeneration? and 4) Can a biodegradable barrier facilitate guided tissue regeneration?

Experiment #1 - **Wound healing in interproximal sites using guided tissue regeneration.**

Previous studies on GTR have shown the potential for regeneration of the periodontium. However, studies in interproximal sites and at early time points were lacking. This investigation examines the potential of GTR in interproximal defects at 1 and 3 months after placement of Gore-Tex Periodontal Material®.

Methods and Results - Interproximal periodontal lesions were created in 4 Macaca fascicularis monkeys using the method of Caton and Kowalski (1976). At the time of periodontal surgery, the experimental sites were covered using Gore-Tex Periodontal Material® to facilitate GTR. Sham-operated sites did not receive barriers. The operated sites received postoperative maintenance 3 times weekly consisting of toothbrushing with a 2% chlorhexidine solution and interdental flossing. The design of the study was such that a total of 48 sites were available for histological examination, 24 sham-operated and 24 GTR sites. These groups were further subdivided into 12 experimental sites with corresponding control sites for histological examination at 1 and 3 month time points.

Specimens were processed using standard histological methods. Sections were cut in a mesio-distal plane at 6 micron thickness. Step-serial sections at 144 micron intervals were used to make histologic observations and histometric measurements of the entire bucco-lingual width of the interproximal areas.

At 1 month, the control sites demonstrated periodontal wound healing which was typical of nonregenerative surgical procedures. A long junctional epithelium extended apically along the entire length of the instrumented root surface. An angular bony defect remained with only small amounts of new bone occurring only in the most apical portions of the defects. Gingival connective tissue was interposed between the bony defect and the junctional epithelium.

In experimental sites, junctional epithelium was not seen apical to the level of barrier placement, indicative of its effectiveness at epithelial exclusion from the periodontal wound. Along the root surface, new cementum formed with attached connective tissue fibers. This was seen extending from the apical level of root planing coronally to the level of the barrier. This new connective tissue attachment was representative of an immature periodontal ligament attached to new cementum. More coronally, this new layer of cementum underwent a transition to a cell and fiber layer with no distinct cementum. Immediately subjacent to the barrier a further transition to an attached fibrillar layer was seen. In comparison to the one month control sites, there was strong histologic evidence of regeneration of new bone in these sites. A connective tissue attachment was seen between the new bone and cementum.

The one and three month control sites were similar in appearance. The apical downgrowth of junctional epithelium along the root surface with no evidence of a new connective tissue attachment was indicative of healing by repair rather than regeneration.

Experimental specimens from the three month time point exhibited definitive histologic evidence of regeneration. Apical to the level of barrier placement, new cementum lined the root surface to the apical level of root planing. The angular bony defects, which persisted in the control specimens, were almost totally filled with new bone. Within the periodontium of these specimens the new cementum had characteristics of cellular cementum. The periodontal ligament which was interposed between the new cementum and the new bone had a normal morphology. Representative sections from these tissues were stained for fiber relationships using a reticulum stain. This revealed the presence of a functionally oriented fiber attachment system in the periodontal ligament connecting the new cementum to the new bone.

Histometric analysis of these sections were performed to verify the histologic observations. To this end, the magnitude of cementum formation as well as the overall amount of regeneration that occurred was measured.

Figure 1 shows the cementum width at the middle (fig. 1A) and apical (fig. 1B) areas along the root surface. In general, the new cementum width was always greater in the experimental groups compared to control. The greatest width of cementum was measured in the 3 month experimental group. This indicates that barrier placement in experimental sites facilitated new cementum formation, and that maturation of the cementum occurred over time.

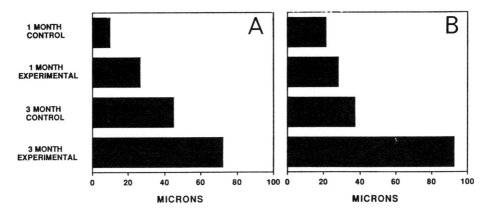

Figure 1.Cementum width at the middle (1A) and apical (1B) areas of the root surface. Values represent the mean of the 1 month and 3 month control and experimental groups.

Examination of experimental specimens with the least amount of regeneration showed that the barrier material was lying within the infrabony defect. This occurrence limited the amount of area available for regeneration. In order to compare the relative amounts of regeneration that had occurred, the percentage of the root surface covered with new cementum was calculated. In all experimental sites, coronal new attachment extended to the level of the barrier on the root surface. This is represented graphically in figure 2. Within the 1 and 3 month experimental groups, virtually 100% of the root

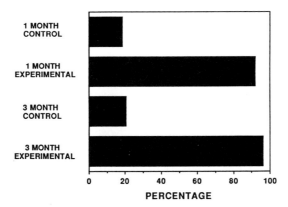

Figure 2. Mean percentage of new cementum formation in the area available for regeneration.

surface was covered with new cementum. In contrast, control sites had only 20% or less new cementum formation at both time points. These data show that while the area of regenerative potential was variable in the experimental sites, the placement of Gore-Tex Periodontal Material® ensured exclusion of epithelium and resulted in regeneration of the periodontium in interproximal sites. In addition, the amount of regeneration that occurred was only limited by the location of the Gore-Tex Periodontal Material® in the interproximal defect.

Experiment #2 - **Evaluation of a synthetic biodegradable barrier to facilitate guided tissue regeneration.**

Periodontal wound healing using GTR has been shown to result in the formation of new cementum, periodontal ligament and alveolar bone. Different materials have been used to facilitate GTR, however, these materials are nonresorbable and require a second surgical procedure for removal. Vicryl Woven Mesh® is a synthetic biodegradable polymer which has been used in the medical field as a tissue supportive material. A biodegradable barrier would be ideally suited for GTR procedures if the biodegradation of the material had no adverse effects on regenerative wound healing. It was the purpose of this study to evaluate GTR using Vicryl Woven Mesh® barriers.

Methods and Results - A fenestration wound model was used for the purpose of determining the effectiveness of Vicryl Woven Mesh® in GTR. A total of 20 teeth, 10 maxillary lateral incisors and 10 mandibular canine teeth were used in 5 adult male Macaca fascicularis monkeys. Ten teeth served as experimental sites while the remaining were used as control sites. A semilunar incision was made through the alveolar mucosa and a full thickness flap was elevated in order to expose the buccal alveolar bone. At approximately midroot level a fenestration was created through the alveolar bone, periodontal ligament, and cementum of standardized dimension: 5mm apico-coronally by 7mm mesio-distally by 2mm in depth. The experimental fenestration wounds were then covered with a Vicryl Woven Mesh® barrier which extended 2 to 3 mm beyond the wound margin and was secured with cyanoacrylate. Control fenestrations received no barriers. The flap was repositioned and sutured. After one month of healing, the animals were sacrificed and specimens from each fenestration were processed using standard histological procedures. Five micron serial sections were cut parallel to the occlusal plane. Step-serial sections taken at 150 micron intervals were stained with hematoxylin and eosin. Histologic observations and histometric measurements were performed. The histometric analysis consisted of linear measurements of the root planed surface (the area available for regeneration), periodontal ligament, new cementum, new alveolar bone, and observations of ankylosis and root resorption within the root planed area. Mean values were calculated from section measurements of individual specimens, and these values were used to calculate means for experimental and control groups. Group values were compared using a paired t test.

Histologic observations of the control specimens at one month showed minimal new cementum or bone formation. This was always seen at the edges of the wound margin. Gingival connective tissue was seen in close approximation to the root planed surface and did not form a connective tissue attachment to the tooth. In contrast, the experimental specimens displayed new cementum formation across the entire area of root planing. The new cementum was observed over old cementum as well as over the root planed dentin. Newly regenerated bone had bridged the edges of the wound formed by the fenestration. The bone had characteristics of immature woven bone. The periodontal ligament was fibrillar and highly vascular and attached the new cementum to the alveolar bone. At the one month time point, the barrier was still evident. No foreign body reaction or encapsulation was observed.

Control specimens exhibited 45.0% ± 13.1% new cementum formation while experimental specimens showed 96.7% ± 1.7% new cementum. Bone formation in control specimens was 20.9% ± 6.5% of the total area available while experimental specimens showed 86.5% ± 8.3% new bone. Both of the values from the experimental groups were significantly greater than the corresponding values from the control group. There was no observation of ankylosis or root resorption in any of the specimens.

In conclusion, GTR using Vicryl Woven Mesh® barriers facilitated the formation of new cementum, periodontal ligament and alveolar bone at one month. It was also found that while the barrier was still present at 1 month, its biodegradation did not appear to affect the wound healing process.

Experiment #3 - **Synthetic biodegradable barrier for regeneration in human periodontal defects**.

Vicryl Woven Mesh® was shown in experiment #2, to have potential in guided tissue regeneration. It was the purpose of this study to test the ability of this biodegradable material used as a barrier to promote guided tissue regeneration in humans.

Methods and Results - Forty adult human subjects, mean age 44.4 years, have thus far been included in the study. The nature of the study was explained to each subject, who then signed an informed consent approved by the Institutional Review Committee for Human Experimentation. Each subject required surgical therapy for treatment of periodontitis and had a class II facial or lingual furcation involvement in a molar tooth. In 20 experimental sites, the class II furcation was treated by flap-debridement and placement of a Vicryl Woven Mesh® barrier over the furcation defect prior to flap closure. Twenty control class II furcation defects were treated by flap-debridement alone. Post-operatively, patients took penicillin for 14 days, maintained the treated sites with 0.12% chlorhexidine rinses 3 times per day and toothbrushing, and received a weekly supragingival prophylaxis for 6-8 weeks. Measurements were taken just prior to treatment, at 1.5 months, and monthly intervals thereafter to 6 months postoperatively.

Measurements included: the presence or absence of plaque, visual signs of inflammation and bleeding after probing for pocket depth, gingival margin location, clinical attachment level and gingival width. For purposes of comparison, mean values were calculated for experimental and control groups at each time point. In addition, the horizontal furcation depth and the resolution of class II furcations for experimental and control sites were compared at baseline and 6 months.

Postoperatively, experimental and control sites healed uneventfully unless the barrier became exposed due to gingival recession. These sites were characterized by increased gingival inflammation which persisted as long as the barriers were clinically detectable. No adverse reactions or infections were observed. Barriers were detectable at one month but were not observed after 6 weeks. Pocket closure occurred at approximately 6 weeks in sites that received barriers.

The plaque, gingival and bleeding indices in both experimental and control sites were reduced to less that 20%, with experimental sites having significantly lower values than control sites at six months. Figures 3A and 3B summarize mean probing depth and clinical attachment level values respectively, for experimental and control sites. Significantly greater pocket depth reduction and gain in clinical attachment

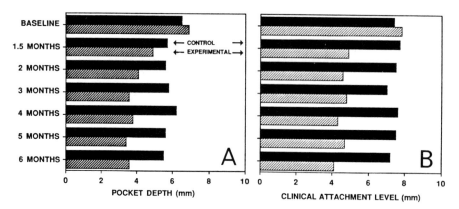

Figure 3. Summary of probing depths (3A) and attachment level (3B) for baseline through six months, for control and experimental sites. Each bar represents the mean value for each time point.

occurred in the sites receiving barriers. Table 1 summarizes mean horizontal furcation depth at baseline and six months. Mean horizontal furcation depth for experimental sites receiving barriers was reduced from 4.3mm to 1.8mm, whereas control sites were only reduced from 3.8mm to 3.3mm. Table 2 summarizes the fate of class II furcation involvements. In the experimental sites, 13 out of 20 were converted to class I or completely resolved, whereas in the control sites, only 1 of the 20 sites was converted to a class I furcation involvement.

TABLE 1

MEAN HORIZONTAL FURCATION DEPTH (mm)

Comparison between horizontal furcation depth at baseline and 6 months in experimental and control sites.

	EXPERIMENTAL	CONTROL
BASELINE	4.3	3.8
6 MONTHS	1.8	3.3

TABLE 2

FATE OF CLASS II FURCATIONS

Number of class II furcations present at baseline compared to 6 months for the experimental and control sites.

	EXPERIMENTAL	CONTROL
BASELINE	20	20
6 MONTHS	7	19

Conclusions

Clinical evaluation of Vicryl Woven Mesh®, used as a barrier to promote guided tissue regeneration, has shown it to be effective in class II furcation defects in humans. These clinical results, combined with the histological evidence of regeneration in animal studies, suggests that this biodegradable barrier may be suitable for clinical management of human periodontal defects produced by periodontitis.

In conclusion, this series of experiments answered several questions related to periodontal wound healing with guided tissue regeneration. These include:

1. Guided tissue regeneration does occur in interproximal sites with Gore-Tex Periodontal Material®.

2. Apical migration of epithelium was always limited by the position of the barrier.

3. The coronal extent of regeneration corresponded to the coronal extent of the barrier.

4. The coronal third of the regeneration was immature at 1 month, but fully mature at 3   months

5. The biodegradable barrier, Vicryl Woven Mesh®, facilitated guided tissue regeneration in experimental fenestration wounds in monkeys.and class II furcation defects in humans.

6. No adverse tissue reaction with the biodegradable barrier was observed in monkeys or man.

© 1991 Elsevier Science Publishers B.V.
Recent advances in periodontology Vol. II,
S.I. Gold, M. Midda and S. Mutlu, eds.

THE APPLICATION OF IMPLANTS IN PERIODONTAL PRACTICE

MINORU TSUHA

8-3 Shimoitouzu 4-Chome Kokurakita-ku Kitakyushu Fukuoka 803 japan

For the treatment of edentulous sites, normally, bridges or dentures are used.
However, there are problems such as the patient's comfort with the attachment,
pronunciation, and the fact that we don't want to grind off an adjacent healthy
tooth. In the event of a missing free end, there are many cases where the
toothless area has been left as it is. As a result, secondary periodontal
problems often occur as well as TMJ trouble both of which are caused by shifting
and inclination of adjacent teeth and the extrusion of antagonistic teeth, and
the deflection of the mandible, in its turn.

Also, when using a long-span bridge, there are problems with fragility and
lack of stability, often resulting in the patient and the dentist spending a lot
of energy on therapy. However, we can avoid this by increasing the number of
abutment teeth on either side of the bridge.

I'm not an implant expert, but a general dentist. I started doing implants in
1981, 9 years ago, because the operation is comparatively easy and can be
carried out in a clinic. Also, according to reports from predecessors, the
prognosis is fairly good.

With regard to the materials for implants, there are various kinds of
materials available for use such as titanium, and titanium alloy, ceramic and
hydroxy apatite, as well as various forms of blade, plate, screw, cylinder and
cone. Many methods of operation have been reported, but unfortunately, at
universities in Japan, we rarely have general lectures about implantology.
Thus, we learn new technology from seminars held over a period of days or
acquire fragmentary knowledge from manufacturers via printed materials. There
is a big demand from patients in clinics, and so, I hope to be able to make
good selections for them from the various applications available and not to be
bewildered by commercialism accompanying new products on the market.

There is a consensus of opinion that a factor which makes implants successful
is the ability to generate bone adhesion and bone ankylosis. For this, it is
agreed that titanium and apatite have the most tissue compatibility.
Particularly in recent years, Branemark's osseo-integrated implant has become
remarkably popular and has proved its satisfactory progress in the long term in
clinics.

On the other hand, blade type has been the most commonly used endosseous implant, and it has a wide scope of application to thin and low mandible bones, although all endosseous implants improved the working base.

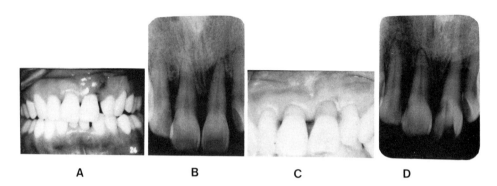

A   B   C   D

Fig. 1. A.,B. A intra-oral view and a radiograph of a 37 year-old female with periodontal disease of #21. Gingiva is inflamed and pocket depth is 10mm deep. C.,D. Ten years and 6 months after an endodontic endosseous implant insertion.

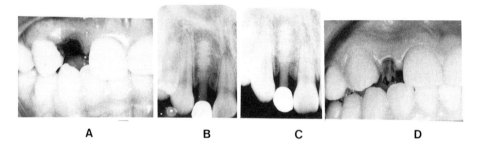

A   B   C   D

Fig. 2. A. An 8-year-old girl at the time of her initial examination. The #12 tooth was lost as the result of an accident.
B. Five years after a single-crystal sapphire implant insertion.
C. Nine years after the implant insertion. Note the excellent adaptation to the root portion of the implant.
D. The implant with the crown removed. Clinical observation shows no pathological pocket formation, that the free gingival margin is closely adapted to the implant and does not exhibit any inflammation or disease process. Plaque accumulation on the implant was less than on the natural teeth. This phenomenon probably represents the fact that the implant had a highly polished surface.

In order to establish a base line for success the following criteria for single-crystal sapphire implants were developed;

1) a bleeding index of two or less

2) a crevicular fluid volume of not greater than 10 units

3) a mobility of one or less, and

4) no radiographic evidence of bone loss.   (Mckinney in 1982)

If these clinical criteria were met, the implant was considered clinically successful. The epithelium forms hemidesmosome and it seems to attach to the basement-plate like granule with high electro-density.

Ogiso's study on apatite reports that its adhesion to the epithelium is the same as that of natural teeth and that osseo-integration occurs in relation to the bones.

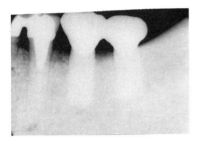 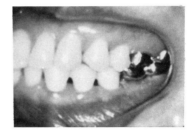

Fig. 3. Five years after hydroxy apatite implant insertion. Inflammation of the gingiva can hardly be seen.

I like to use implants fabricated from space age nickel-titanium alloy. Its design is based upon the shape memory characteristic of this alloy. On applying heat at 42°C the implant recovers its trained shape, that is, the implant blades open to 30 degrees.

The advantages of SMI are that;

It shows good biocompatibility,

bone adhesion,

and excellent fixation.

Until now, the one operation method has been used. However, because a rest after the operation is advantageous, it is being replaced by the two operation method.

It goes without saying that we should not cause a burn during drilling and consideration should be taken so as to avoid excessive occlusal pressure and to disperse that pressure.

For good initial fixation and prevention of subsidence, a shape memory implant is effective.

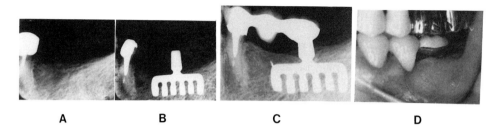

| A | B | C | D |

Fig. 4. Shape memory implant. A. Before treatment. C.,D. Five years after SMI insertion.

With implants, we can't expect to compensate for feeling in the periodontal membrane, and lack of pressure sensation makes it impossible to control occlusal pressure. Though it is controlled by the surrounding jaw muscle and the temporo-mandibular joint, there is a tendency to occlude strongly on an implant part. Shock absorbers such as inter-mobile elements have been developed, but they are still insufficient.

Therefore, in attempting to control occlusal stress, we try to reduce bucco-lingual width, to clarify spillways, and to use a material which will correct the occlusal surface spontaneously.

I agree with the opinion that the standard of success in implants should be clarified, however, I don't think that osseo-integration and fibro-integration can be judged by the same standard.

CONCLUSION

For the success of implants, selection of indications, careful operation method, upper construction and hygiene are important as well as selection of material and forms.

As I mentioned before, in periodontal practice, I believe that the scope of application of implants will become wider and wider in the future.

CASE I

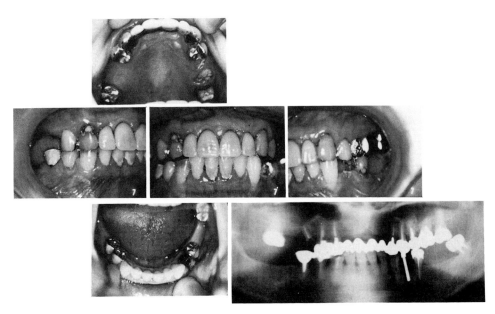

Fig. 5. A 43 year-old female. Before treatment.

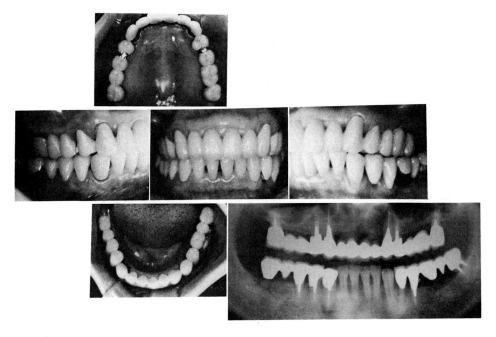

Fig. 6. Nine years and 6 months after single-crystal sapphire implant insertion.

112

CASE II

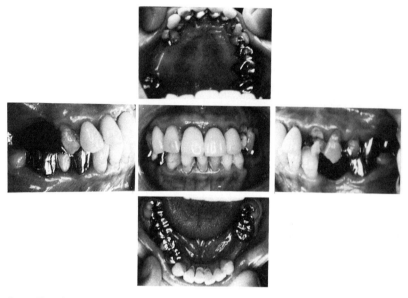

Fig. 7. A 51 year-old female. Before treatment.

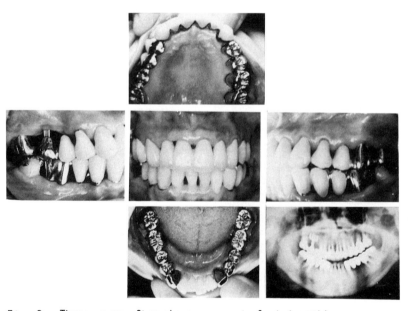

Fig. 8. Three years after shape memory implant insertion.

CASE III

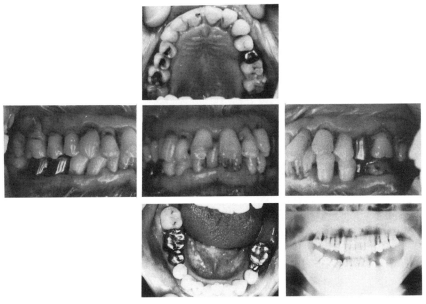

Fig. 9. A 62 year-old male. Before treatment.

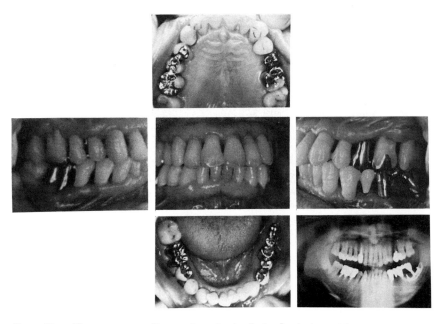

Fig. 10. Three years after subperiosteal implant insertion.

114

CASE IV

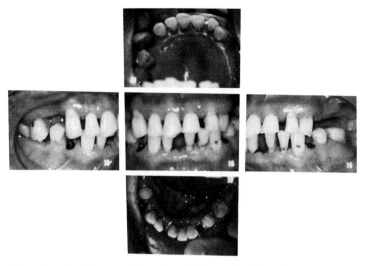

Fig. 11. A 50 year-old male. Before treatment.

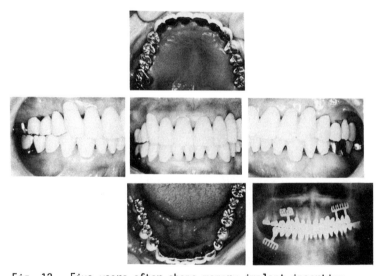

Fig. 12. Five years after shape memory implant insertion.

REFERENCES

1. Tsuru H (1989) Int J Oral Maxillofac Implants 2-6:329-335
2. Iwata T (1989) Int J Oral Maxillofac Implants 2-3:337-349
3. Yamagami A (1989) Int J Oral Maxillofac Implants 2-3:353-361
4. Ogiso M (1989) Int J Oral Maxillofac Implants 2-2:363-370

© 1991 Elsevier Science Publishers B.V.
Recent advances in periodontology Vol. II,
S.I. Gold, M. Midda and S. Mutlu, eds.

APPLICATION OF ENDODONTIC IMPLANT AND TRICALCIUM PHOSPHATE IMPLANT TO PERIODONTALLY INVOLVED TEETH IN HUMANS AND DOGS

H.YOSHIE, H.NAKAMURA, K.YAMASHITA, T.WADA, M.SHIMIZU, K.HARA, A.OKAMOTO*, and M. IWAKU*
Department of Periodontology, and *Operative Dentistry and Endodontics, Niigata University School of Dentistry, Niigata, (Japan)

I ENDODONTIC IMPLANT

EFFECTS OF ENDODONTIC IMPLANTS ON PERIODONTALLY INVOLVED TEETH IN PATIENTS

The purpose of this study was first to estimate changes of tooth mobility, probing depth and crown to root(C/R) ratio, and secondly to evaluate radiographic findings around the implant and root apex over a period of 4 years.

Material and methods

Nineteen periodontally involved mobile teeth from 12 patients were used. Three kinds of endodontic implants; single crystal Sapphire, Vitallium and Titanium alloy were inserted in root canals and alveolar bone extending approximately 10mm. Six months after implantation, some teeth were fixed and others were free standing. Digital tooth mobility, dislocation of a tooth loaded with 500g force,and probing depth were measured, and radiographs were taken 3 and 6 months and 1, 2, and 4 years after implantation.

Results(Table 1, 2)

0.7mm of tooth dislocation immediately before implantation decreased dramatically to 0.3mm after 6 months. The mobility index also decreased. C/R ratio was 2.6 before the implant, but decreased to 0.7 at 4 years after surgery. Mean probing depth did not change significantly during any periods tested. Concerning of radiolucent findings around the implant pin, there was 5 cases at 4 years after implantaion. Enlargement of periodontal ligament spaces was observed in 7 cases over the 4 year period. These seven cases consisted of 2 cases in Sapphire, 2 cases in Vitallium and 3 cases in Titanium implants.

Table 1

TOOTH MOBILITY CHANGES AFTER IMPLANTATION

	0	3 months	6 months
disloca-tion(500g) n=16	0.7 ±0.3	0.3* ±0.1	0.3* ±0.1
mobility index n=19	1.8±0.4	1.1±0.5*	0.8±0.5*

*:significant difference from 0 time at P<0.05.

Table 2

CROWN ROOT RATIO,PROBING DEPTH AFTER IMPLANTATION

	0	3months	1year	2 years	4years
C/R ratio n=19	2.6 ±0.6	0.6* ±0.1	0.8* ±0.1	0.7* ±0.1	0.7* ±0.1
probing depth n=94	1.7 ±1.0	1.7 ±0.9	1.9 ±0.9	2.3 ±0.9	2.2 ±0.9

*:significant difference from 0 time at P<0.05.

Discussion and conclusion

Cranin et al. reported 91% success rates(less than 1mm bone loss from radio-

116

graph) after 5 years of treatment using Vitallium and Titanium implants on 253 teeth. Many researchers have indicated that radiolucent findings around the root apex may depend on imperfect sealing or corrosion of the implant surface. In conclusion:

1. Reduction of both tooth mobility and C/R ratio were observed.

2. Clinical healthy conditions were maintained in 84% of the cases.

3. Pathological changes from the radiograph occurred in 28-38% of the cases.

4. There was no difference of findings among the three kinds of implant.

CASE   PRESENTATION

A 43 year old woman received a Sapphire implant at the left central incisor of the maxilla. At the first visit, prominent gingival inflammation and pathological tooth migration were observed. Ten millimeters probing depth, 4.8 C/R ratio and almost 100% of alveolar bone loss were estimated in the left central incisor(Figure 1,2). After treatment of plaque control, scaling and root planing, and gingival curettage, a Sapphire implant was inserted at the left central incisor. Prosthetic treatment was carried out 6 months after implantation, and maintenance therapy was performed at every 3 month intervals. Four years after implantation, gingival inflammation, pathological changes from the radiograph had not been noted. Excellent improvement of alveolar bone around the root apex occurred. A three millimeters probing depth, and 0.8 C/R ratio were estimated(Figure 3,4).

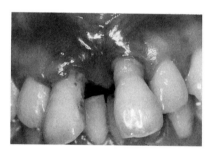

Figure 1. Severe gingival inflammation at the first visit.

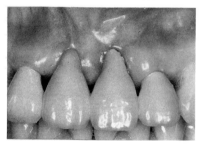

Figure 3. Four years after implantation.

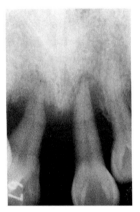

Figure 2. Severe bone loss at the first visit.

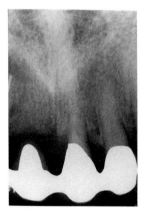

Figure 4. Excellent bone improvement 4 years after implant.

EFFECTS OF ENDODONTIC IMPLANTS ON PERIODONTALLY INVOLVED TEETH IN DOGS

There were three purposes of this study; 1) to observe the interface between implants and tissues, 2) to estimate inflammation around the root apex, and 3) to evaluate the surface corrosion of the implant materials.

Material and methods

Two mongrel dogs received periodontal surgery and half of the alveolar bone in premolar regions of the mandible was removed. One month after surgery, Sapphire, Vitallium and Titanium endodontic implant pins were inserted in 16 premolar roots extending beyond the root apex 10 mm. The dogs were sacrificed one year after implantation. Tissues for light microscopical observation were fixed with 10% neutral formalin and decalcified with Plank-Rychlo solution, and embedded with paraffin. Blocks were serially sectioned in 6 um, and stained with H-E. In order to analyze on SEM/EDX, inserted implant pins were washed and prepared with a carbon coating. Implant surface morphology and components were observed by a scanning electron microscope and energy dispersed X-ray analyzer.

Results (Figure 5-8)

Fibrous connective tissue encapsulated three kinds of implants. The fibers were oriented perpendicularly against the surface of implants like a periodontal ligament(Figure 5, 6; Sapphire implant pin). There was no inflammation in these fibrous zones. Slight to moderate inflammation with mono-nuclear cells was observed around the root apex. There were no findings of surface corrosion with the exception of one Titanium pin. The surface appeared concave by SEM. and sulfur was detected by EDX in one Titanium pin(Figure 7, 8).

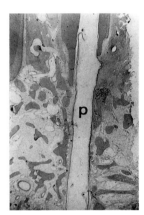

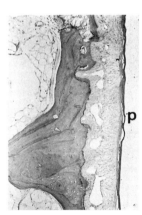

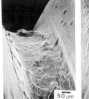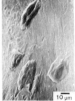

Figure 7. Surface corrosion of a Titanium pin.

Figure 5. Sapphire implant pin(P).
X 3, H-E stain.

Figure 6. Fibro-osseous integration.
P : Sapphire pin
X 25, H-E stain.

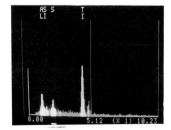

Figure 8. Sulfur detection from surface of a Titanium pin

Discussion and conclusion

Many researchers have reported that thin to thick collagen fiber capsules exist around the endodontic implant pin. In periapical tissue findings, localized slight to moderate inflammation was observed in dogs and monkeys and patients. These inflammations may have resulted from the imperfect sealing of the root apex. Regarding surface corrosion, Seltzer et al. emphasized the presence of sulfur, phosphorus, chlorine and speculated that periapical inflammation was due to the corrosion of implants.

In conclusion:

1. Fibro-osseous integration existed between implant pin and bone.
2. Slight to moderate inflammation was observed around the apex.
3. There was no surface corrosion with the exception of one Titanium pin.

FUTURE DIRECTION OF ENDODONTIC IMPLANT

1. Improvement of apex sealing

The most significant disadvantage of endodontic implants is apical inflammation due to the imperfect apical sealing. The development of root canal sealer materials may eliminate these inflammations.

2. Implant surface design

The second point is improvement of implant surface design. For example, porous type endodontic implants interact well with alveolar bone.

3. Implant surface treatment

The third point is implant surface treatment, such as, hydroxyapatite or bioglass coating. With these coatings, biointegration can be established.

II TRICALCIUM PHOSPHATE(TCP) IMPLANT

RECONSTRUCTION FOR VERTICAL BONE DEFECTS BY TCP IMPLANT IN PATIENTS

The purpose of this study was to estimate clinical attachment gain and reduction of probing depth, as well as radiographic improvement of alveolar bone over a period 5 years after implantation.

Material and methods

Twelve patients with moderate adult periodontitis participated in this study. After the initial treatment consisting of plaque control, scaling, and root planing, the remaining two or three wall vertical bone defects were selected. Beta-TCP(Synthograft) was implanted in these defects during flap surgery and the patients were followed up for 5 years at 3 month intervals. Probing depth, loss of attachment, and tooth mobility were measured. Dental radiographs were taken at 3 months and every one year until 5 years after implantation.

Results (Table 3, 4)

Mean 7.3mm probing depth and 7.8mm loss of attachment before surgery decreased significantly to 2.9mm, and 4.6mm 5 years after implant. Subsequently the tooth number of mobility index 0 increased. More than 70% of the filling in vertical bone defects was observed from radiographic findings in 78% of the cases 5 years after implantation. Disappearance of TCP particles from the radiograph was approximately one year after surgery.

Table 3

PROBING DEPTH, LOSS OF ATTACHMENT

	0	3months	1year	3years	5years
probing depth n=18	7.3 ±2.7	3.8* ±2.0	4.0* ±1.8	3.3 ±1.4	2.9* ±1.5
loss of attach- ment	7.8 ±3.2	5.1* ±2.5	5.4* ±2.5	5.1* ±3.0	4.6* ±1.6

n=18   *:significant difference from 0 time at P<0.05.

Table 4

TOOTH NUMBERS OF EACH MOBILITY INDEX

n=18 teeth

mobility index	0	3months	1year	3years	5years
0	5	7	8	10	13
1	5	6	8	8	3
2	8	5	2	0	2

Discussion and conclusion

Many researchers have indicated that 1.8 – 5.2mm pocket reduction and 1.3 – 2.7 mm attachment gain were obtained at from 4 to 18 months after implantation. None of the researchers demonstrated adverse side effects, or clinical complications and symptoms.

In conclusion:

1. Mean 3.2mm of attachment gain and mean 4.4 mm pocket reduction were observed.
2. Filling in the vertical bone defects was observed in all of cases.
3. Disappearance period of TCP particles was approximately 1 year.
4. No clinical complication was noted in any cases.

CASE   PRESENTATION

A 47 year old man received a TCP implant at the left lateral incisor of the mandible. At the first visit, 6mm of probing depth and 7mm of loss of attachment, as well as alveolar bone loss around the root apex were observed(Figure 9, 10). After the initial treatment of plaque control, scaling and root planing, TCP particles were filled in a 4 wall defect of the left lateral incisor during flap surgery. Maintenance therapy of 3 month intervals was then carried out. At 8 years after surgery, the probing depth decreased remarkably to 1mm, and 3mm of clinical attachment gain was observed. New bone formation seems to have occurred with normal findings from the dental radiograph(Figure 11,12).

TCP IMPLANTATION IN VERTICAL BONE DEFECTS IN DOGS

There were three aims of this study; 1) to evaluate osseous repair in vertical defects implanted with TCP, 2) to determine the attachment pattern between root surface and gingival tissues, and 3) to identify and characterize TCP resorbing cells in bone defects.

120

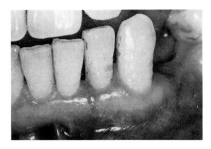

Figure 9. Gingival inflammation at the first visit.

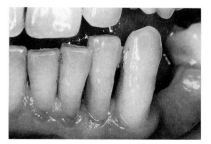

Figure 11. Eight years after implant surgery.

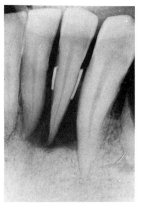

Figure 10. Severe bone loss at the first visit.

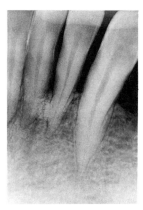

Figure 12. Bone formation 8 years after surgery.

Material and methods

Twelve dogs were used, and 23 vertical bone defects and 12 furcation defects were created. These bone defects were exposed to bacterial plaque for one month. Beta-TCP(Synthograft) was implanted in these bone defects during flap surgery. Some dogs were injected with three kinds of fluorescent dye(tetracycline;15mg/kg;1 week after surgery, calcein;2mg/kg;5 weeks after surgery, alizarin red;20mg/kg;10 weeks after surgery). Dogs were sacrificed at 5, 10, 15 weeks after surgery. For light and fluorescence microscopy, implanted tissues were removed and fixed with 10% neutral formalin. The block were decalcified and embedded with BPS or paraffin and sectioned in 7-50um thick. H-E or Azan stained sections were observed by a light microscope and undecalcified sections were observed by a fluorescence microscope. Some dogs were sacrificed and fixed with perfusion of paraformaldehyde. The blocks were decalcified with EDTA and post-fixed with osmium tetraoxide, then embedded with epon. Ultrathin sections were observed by a transmission electron microscope. Acid phosphatase activity was identified in decalcified sections with or without tartarate treatment.

Results (Figure 13-16)

Figure 13,14 show high magnification of alveolar crestal areas at 15 weeks after implantation. An alizarin red line surrounded the calcein green line throughout the areas in the implanted site(Figure 13). In the control site(Figure 14), red line was layered with limited coronal portion of alveolar crest. TCP particles remained in vertical defects and some particles united with new bone at 15 weeks after surgery. New cementum formation and fiber attachment occurred in the implanted site at 15 weeks after implantation. Multinucleated giant cells attached to the TCP particles at 5 weeks after surgery were noted by electron micrograph(Figure 15). Giant cell processes penetrated into the crystal spaces of the particles. Giant cells and mononuclear cells(macrophages) around TCP particles revealed acid phosphatase activity(Figure 16a). Tartarate treatment inhibited acid phosphatase of giant cells and macrophages(Figure 16b).

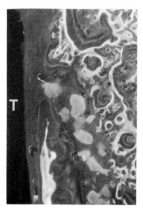

Figure 13. Diffused and broad bone formation in TCP implanted site. T : tooth. X 10.

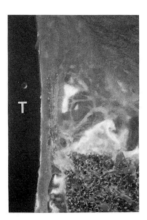

Figure 14. Layered bone formation in control site. T : tooth. X 10.

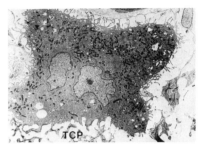

Figure 15. Multinucleated giant cells attached to the TCP. X 5300.

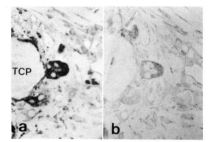

Figure 16. Inhibition of acid phosphatase of giant cells by tartarate treatment. X 100.

Discussion and conclusion

Many reports have been indicated that TCP was resorbed and replaced by normal bone in non-periodontal tissues. Levin et al., Nery et al. showed that excellent tissue tolerance and no toxic reaction to TCP, and regeneration and bone ingrowth were observed 24 weeks after implantation. Stahl and Froum were unable to demonstrate any stimulation of bone formation with TCP application. They then reported that most attachment pattern was long epithelial adhesion.

In conclusion:

1. The bone formation pattern was diffused and broad in bone defects.

2. TCP particles directly united with new bone.

3. New attachment was observed at the apical part of the bone defects.

4. TCP resorbing cells were multinucleated giant cells and macrophages. These cells had tartarate sensitive acid phosphatase activity.

FUTURE DIRECTION OF TCP IMPLANT

1. Combination therapy with TCP and osteoinductive factors.

There is no evidence that TCP have a osteoinductive activity. Osteoinductive protein, for example bone morphogenetic protein, can be useful in therapy.

2. Combination with TCP and guided tissue regeneration(GTR) method.

One of the disadvantage of TCP is development of long epithelial attachment. GTR method can prevent the migration of epithelium.

3. Combination with TCP and connective tissue substance.

Connective tissue matrix substances, e.g. collagen gel or fibrin are useful. Recent reports indicated that these therapy obtained good results.

REFERENCES

ENDODONTIC IMPLANT

1.	Nakamura, H.	et al. ;	Japan.J.Conserv.Dent.,	32,	696-712,	1989.
2.	Frank, A. L.	et al. ;	JADA,	78,	520-524,	1969.
3.	Chino,S.	et al. ;	Tsurumi Univ.Dent.J.,	1,	51-57,	1975.
4.	Lafkowitz,P.M.	et al. ;	J. Endodon.,	3,	319-321,	1977.
5.	Cranin, A.N.	et al. ;	JADA,	94,	315-320,	1977.
6.	Silverbrand,H.	et al. ;	Oral Surg.,	45,	920-929,	1978.
7.	Maeda,Y.	et al. ;	J.Osaka Univ.Dent.Sch.,	24,	131-144,	1984.
8.	Larsen, R.M.	et al. ;	J. Endodon.,	15,	496-500,	1989.
9.	Scopp, I.W.	et al. ;	J. Periodontol.,	42,	717-720,	1971.
10.	Maniatopoulos,C.	et al. ;	J.Biomed.Mater. Res.,	20,	1309-1333,	1986.
11.	Seltzer, S.	et al. ;	J. Endodon.,	2,	267-276,	1976.
12.	Kato, H.		Japan.J.Conserv.Dent.,	29,	692-751,	1986.
13.	Simon, J.H.	et al. ;	J. Endodon.,	6,	450-455,	1980.
14.	Zmener, O.	;	J. Endodon.,	9,	486-490,	1983.

TRICALCIUM PHOSPHATE IMPLANT

15.	Hara, K.	et al. ;	J.Oral Implantol.,	12,	68-79,	1985.
16.	Shimizu, M.	et al. ;	J.Oral Implantol.,	13,	196-202,	1987.
17.	Shimizu, M.	;	J.Japan.Ass.Periodont.,	28,	1028-1043,	1986.
18.	Wada, T.	et al. ;	J.Oral Implantol.,	15,	231-236,	1989.
19.	Wada, T.	et al. ;	J.Periodont.Res.,	24,	391-401,	1989.
20.	Nery, E.B.	et al. ;	J. Periodontol.,	49,	523-527,	1978.
21.	Strub, J.R.	et al. ;	J. Periodontol.,	50,	624-629,	1979.
22.	Snyder, A.J.	et al. ;	J. Periodontol.,	55,	273-277,	1984.
23.	Baldock, W.T.	et al. ;	J. Periodontol.,	56,	1-7,	1985.
24.	Blumenthal,N.M.	et al. ;	J. Periodontol.,	59,	18-22,	1988.
25.	Stahl, S.S.	et al. ;	J. Periodontol.,	57,	211-217,	1986.
26.	Froum, S.	et al. ;	J. Periodontol.,	58,	103-109,	1987.
27.	Bhaskar, S.N.	et al. ;	Oral Surg.,	32,	336-346,	1971.
28.	Levin, M.P.	et al. ;	Oral Surg.,	38,	344-351,	1974.
29.	Nery, E.B.	et al. ;	J. Periodontol.,	46,	328-347,	1975.
30.	Metsger, D.S.	et al. ;	JADA,	105,	1035-1038,	1982.
31.	Barney, V.C.	et al. ;	J. Periodontol.,	57,	764-770,	1986.
32.	Bowers, G.M.	et al. ;	J. Periodontol.,	57,	286-287,	1986.

SYMPOSIA

© 1991 Elsevier Science Publishers B.V.
Recent advances in periodontology Vol. II,
S.I. Gold, M. Midda and S. Mutlu, eds.

THE NATURE AND ROLE OF DENTAL PLAQUES IN PERIODONTAL DISEASE

LARS A. CHRISTERSSON, JOSEPH J. ZAMBON & ROBERT J. GENCO

Periodontal Disease Clinical Research Center, School of Dental Medicine,
State University of New York at Buffalo,
3435 Main Street, Buffalo, N.Y. 14214, USA.

INTRODUCTION

The first scientist to describe oral bacteria (animacules) was Anthonie van Leeuwenhoek in 1683. In a letter to the Royal Society in London, he described his oral hygiene efforts, and concluded that, despite these, he could observe more living organisms in his oral cavity than human beings in his home country, The Netherlands. He also made the observation that he had exceptionally good oral health, and that his gums did not bleed when cleaned. Despite this remarkable accomplishment it took almost 200 years until mankind realized the relationship between bacteria and disease.

PLAQUE FORMATION

The development of dental plaque on exposed tooth surfaces begins with the precipitation of a salivary derived pellicle which contains few bacteria in its early stages (1).

Microbiological studies of developing plaque have shown that bacterial adhesion takes place very rapidly, within a few minutes of cleaning the tooth surface. The first types of organisms found on a tooth surface are cocci and rods, mainly *Streptococcus sanguis*, and Gram-positive facultative pleomorphic rods like *Actinomyces viscosus* and *Actinomyces isrealii.* (2,3,4).

Studies of plaque formation in healthy oral cavities over a period of 2 to 3 weeks led to the description of microbial maturation of plaques associated with experimental gingivitis (5).

The first phase (days 0 - 2) exhibits is a proliferation of Gram-positive cocci and rods and an addition of 30% Gram-negative cocci and rods, proportions reflecting the usual distribution of these components in whole saliva. The second phase (1 to 4 days) is characterized by the appearance and increase in numbers of fusobacteria and filaments and the third phase (4 to 9 days) is characterized by the appearance of spirilla and spirochetes. Gingivitis is clinically detectable at the time of formation of these complex, mature supragingival plaques found in 4 - 9 days.

CLINICAL ASSESSMENT OF DENTAL PLAQUES

Supragingival plaques are readily detectable with the naked eye after reaching a certain thickness. When too sparse to be detected, the presence of dental plaque may be determined by the use of disclosing solution. Subgingival plaques are usually thin, contained within the periodontal pocket or gingival crevice, and hard to visualize *in situ*. There are several sampling procedures for the microbial assessment of the periodontal flora. The most commonly used is sampling of the subgingival plaques with absorbent sterile paper points (6).

Plaque indices are often used in experimental situations to demonstrate rather small changes and to obtain manageable data suited for statistical analyses (7, 8). However, in clinical practice as well as in research on periodontal therapy, dental plaque is often scored as a dichotomy, i.e. presence or absence of clinically detectable plaque.

MICROBIAL COMPOSITION

In the normal state of periodontal health the microbial flora consists of a relatively thin layer of adherent bacterial cells. These are predominantly coccoid in shape, with a majority exhibiting cell wall features of Gram-positive microorganisms. Few flagellated cells or spirochetes are observed. A variety of microorganisms including coccoid as well as filamentous forms and cells with Gram-positive and Gram-negative cell wall patterns are present adjacent to sites exhibiting gingivitis. The deeper layers of the adherent bacterial mass have undergone lysis, and mineralization of cells and zones in these plaques is common (9). Filamentous bacteria are relatively more numerous than in the normal samples, and the dense masses are occasionally covered with "corn-cob" formations comprised of long filaments covered with cocci (10). In periodontitis, subgingival plaques extend from the supragingival area into pockets bordered by the root surface and epithelium. Filamentous forms are prominent, however, the morphological cell types encountered in the gingivitis sample are also observed in the periodontitis sample.

BACTERIAL SPECIFICITY IN GINGIVITIS AND PERIODONTITIS

The factors which cause gingival inflammation may be different from those which cause loss of connective tissue attachment. Therefore, gingivitis should not indiscriminately be considered a precursor of periodontitis. Indeed gingivitis does not always lead to periodontitis.

The concept of microbial specificity in the etiology of periodontal disease has recently emerged (11). Previously, it was believed that periodontal disease resulted from the gross non specific accumulation of dental plaques. Cross-sectional and longitudinal studies of the predominant cultivable microflora reveal that of the many hundreds of bacterial species which can inhabit the human oral cavity only a small number are associated with human periodontal disease (12).

A variety of predominantly Gram-negative organisms have been implicated in the etiology of periodontal disease, including *Actinobacillus actinomycetemcomitans, Bacteroides gingivalis, Bacteroides intermedius, Fusobacterium nucleatum,* and *Wolinella recta,* as well as certain gram-positive bacteria such as *Eubacterium* species (13).

A. actinomycetemcomitans is one of the oral microorganisms which has been strongly implicated in the pathogenesis of localized juvenile periodontitis (14). This microorganism is also associated with cases of periodontitis in adults in which alveolar bone loss occurs at an unusually rapid rate (15) and periodontitis which continues to progress after meticulous scaling, root planing, plaque control, and even periodontal surgery (16, 17).

B. gingivalis is found in high frequency and in high numbers, often as a major component of the subgingival flora, in adult periodontitis lesions (18). In contrast, this organism is usually not detectable in the subgingival flora of patients with gingivitis who are not affected by periodontitis (19).

SUMMARY AND CONCLUSIONS

The concept that periodontal diseases are associated with specific microorganisms, which are not regularly found in the healthy gingival sulci and/or oral cavity, raises questions as to the nature of these species. Those organisms for which the oral cavity is a primary habitat and which do not normally cause disease, are the indigenous or resident flora. Whilst those which are not part of the resident microflora and which cause disease, are exogenous pathogens. However, *indigenous* microorganisms which are normally non-pathogenic bacteria can, under circumstances such as of reduced host resistance or overgrowth, cause disease in which case they may be considered opportunistic pathogens.

REFERENCES

1. Dawes J, Jenkins GN, Tonge GH (1963) Brit Dent J 115: 65-68

2. Krasse B (1954) Odont Rev 5: 203-211

3. Gibbons RJ, Kapsimalis B, Socransky SS (1964) Arch Oral Biol 9: 101-103

4. Carlsson J (1967) Odont Rev 18: 55-74

5. Löe H, Theilade E, Jensen SB (1965) J Periodontol 36: 177-187

6. Slots J, Reynolds HS, Genco RJ (1980) Infect Imun 29: 1013-20

7. Silness, J., Löe, H. (1964) Acta Odont Scand 22: 112-135

8. Turesky.S., Gilmore, N., Glickman, I. (1970) J. Periodontol 41: 41-43

9. Listgarten, M. A. (1976) J Periodontol 47: 1-18

10. Gibbons RJ, Gibbons NM (1970) Arch Oral Biol 15: 567-573: 1397-1400

11. Socransky SS (1977) J Periodontol 48: 497-504

12. Moore WEC, Holdeman LV, Cato EP, Smibert RM, Burmeister JA and Ranney
    RR (1983) Infect Immun 42: 510-515

13. Socransky, S. and Haffajee, A. (1990) In: Bader J.D. ed. Risk assessment in
    dentistry. Chapel Hill: Univ of North Carolina, Dental Ecology, 79-90

14. Zambon JJ (1985) J Clin Periodontol 12: 1-20

15. Tanner AC, Haffer C, Bratthall GT, Visconti RA, Socransky SS (1979) J Clin
    Periodontol 6: 278-307

16. Slots J, Bragd L, Wikstrom M, Dahlén G (1986) J Clin Periodontol 13: 570-7

17. Van Winkelhoff AJ, Rodenburg JP, Goene RJ, Abbas F, Winkel EG (1989) J
    Clin Periodontol 16: 128-31

18. Slots J. (1986) J Clin Periodontol 13: 912-17

19. Christersson LA, Zambon JJ, Dunford RG, Grossi S, Genco RJ (1989) J Dent
    Res 68: 1633-1639

© 1991 Elsevier Science Publishers B.V.
Recent advances in periodontology Vol. II,
S.I. Gold, M. Midda and S. Mutlu, eds.

ANTI-PLAQUE AGENTS FOR SUPRA-GINGIVAL PLAQUE CONTROL - RATIONALE AND OUTLOOK

FRANS J.G. VAN DER OUDERAA

Unilever Dental Research, Port Sunlight Laboratory, Bebington, Wirral,
United Kingdom

INTRODUCTION

A number of reviews of extensive population studies carried out in many
countries to evaluate periodontal health show a high prevalence of
plaque-associated marginal gingivitis as well as more advanced periodontal
disorders (1,2,3,4). The data indicate that only a small percentage of
those examined can be classified as healthy. The majority of people
assessed were found to have gingival bleeding-on-probing, calculus and
shallow pocketing, which puts them at risk of more advanced periodontal
disease. This holds true even in countries where regular oral hygiene
practices are well established. For instance, Brown etal (4) conclude that
only 15% of the US population is free of signs of periodontal disease.

A further factor which should be considered with respect to future
disease levels, is that because of the considerable reduction in the
prevalence of dental caries (5,6), a substantial reduction in edentulousness can be expected and has indeed been observed (Fig 1.) (7). This trend
and the above mentioned results of worldwide assessments suggest that Gum
Disease will become a more prominent public health problem (8).

RATIONALE

What about the potential of plaque control for prevention of disease?
There is strong evidence that good supra-gingival plaque control reduces
and may even prevent colonization of sub-gingival areas (9,10). These
findings are obviously of considerable significance in view of the fact
that advanced periodontal disease is mediated by oral anaerobes.
Furthermore clinical evidence suggests that excellent plaque control can
stop the progression of periodontal disease (for a review see ref 11).
Consequently the case for supra-gingival plaque control as a means of
preventing periodontal disease is well established. From the population
data obtained in field studies it must be concluded that the average

130

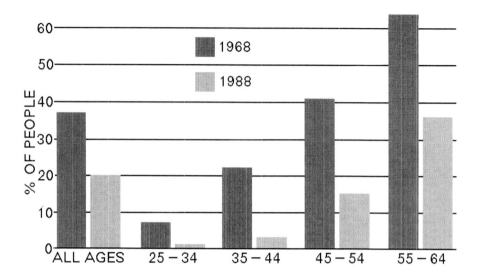

Fig. 1. Development of Edentulousness in England and Wales 1968-1988.

individual does not exercise the degree of plaque control required to maintain a healthy periodontium. It has also been observed that there is a low degree of interest and compliance with respect to prevention of oral disease (12).

Behavioural factors have been shown to influence personal oral hygiene, oral plaque levels and dental disease. In order to understand the current disease levels it is vital to analyse attitudes and behaviour. There are limited data on oral hygiene and behavioural factors such as frequency of tooth brushing, duration of toothbrushing and frequency of use of dental floss. Results of a number of studies which report brushing frequency are shown in Fig. 2. It has been found that approximately 50% of the populations interviewed brush twice a day or more.

In a study carried out in Italy (12) it was found that the average brushing time, observed at the subjects home, was 37 seconds with a quarter of the sample brushing for less than 20 seconds. Additionally the prevalence and frequent use of dental floss has been found to be fairly low (48). The pattern of these observations on oral hygiene habits are in agreement with the poor state of oral hygiene found in the above population studies.

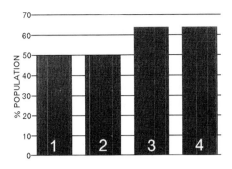

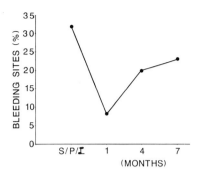

Fig. 2. Brushing frequency distribution compiled from a number of
recent studies. The bars show the
percentage of people brushing twice
a day or more; study 1 ref. 13,
study 2 ref. 14; study 3 ref. 15;
study 4 ref. 16.

Fig. 3. Gingival condition after
Dental Prophylaxis, brushing
instruction and patient motivation
(S/P/I). Bleeding-on-probing was
assessed at the start of the study,
1, 4 and 7 months in a panel of
72 volunteers (18).

Nevertheless, as shown by the study depicted in Figure 3 dental
prophylaxis followed by oral hygiene instruction and patient motivation can
very effectively reduce the level of gingival bleeding over one a one month
period (18). However, in the following six months of the same study, and
also in other similar studies, considerable deterioration occurred in all
cases of groups using a fluoride containing control toothpaste without
anti-plaque agents (19,20,21). Given these behavioural considerations and
the role of supra-gingival plaque in periodontal disease, there is
therefore, a clear rationale for the use of anti-plaque agents to augment
the effect of daily mechanical plaque control.

CRITERIA FOR APPROPRIATE AGENTS

Different patient needs require different strategies with respect to the
delivery of appropriate agents to augment plaque control (22). The main
delivery routes for agents for supra- and sub-gingival plaque control
either for self or professional application have been reviewed recently
(17,23). This paper will focus on agents and system to control
supra-gingival plaque which are suitable for self application. It could be

postulated that agents for control of supra-gingival plaque mass should
have the following properties:

i)   Sufficient intrinsic anti-microbial potency (24).
ii)   A broad spectrum of activity against plaque bacteria in view of
        the non-specific nature of the organisms involved in the etiology
        of gingivitis (25).
iii)   Toxicological safety.
iv)   Absence of adverse reactions.
v)   Substantivity at the site of action (24,23).
vi)   Their use should not lead to development of resistant organisms
        (26).
vii)   Chemical stability.

   A number of reviews of anti-plaque agents have been presented recently
(17,22,27,28). The above criteria and the information contained in these
reviews, can be used to identify agents which may be suitable for incorporation in product forms for daily prevention of dental plaque. However, the
final formulation must not only be optimised for bioavailability and
release of the agents in the mouth but also should have acceptable in use
properties to the patient to achieve maximum patient compliance.

AGENTS FOR SUPRAGINGIVAL PLAQUE CONTROL
i)   Positively Charged Antiseptics
        Most of these agents, such as chlorhexidine, hexetidine and cetyl-
        pyridinium chloride, have good intrinsic anti-microbial activity.
        Chlorhexidine, in particular, which has a favourable combination
        of high efficacy against oral organisms and oral substantivity, is
        widely used (29). Agents of this type are generally formulated in
        mouthrinses, but they are not compatible with the constituents of
        other product forms such as dentifrices (23). Their widespread
        use is also hampered by adverse effects such as toothstaining and
        alteration in taste sensation.
ii)   Metal Salts
        The intrinsic efficacy of these broad spectrum agents is lower
        than that of the positively charged organic molecules. The anti-
        plaque efficacy in vivo of stannous salts (30) and zinc salts
        (31,32) has been described. Their oral substantivity and, in
        particular, their uptake into dental plaque following application,

is also well documented (33,34). These agents are compatible with rinse and dentifrice formulations, however, some metal salts, are prone to precipitation into biologically inactive forms (35). Toothstaining has been observed after use of stannous fluoride (36).

iii)   Non-charged Phenolic Agents

In order to avoid the compatibility problems associated with the positively charged organic molecules, non-charged phenolic anti-microbial agents have been investigated. The rinse Listerine contains such agents. Recently triclosan has been shown to have efficacy in vivo (37,38,39,40); it has a low Minimal Inhibitory Concentration (MIC) against oral bacteria (41) and is retained in plaque after brushing for eight hours (42). No adverse reactions have been observed for triclosan (38).

iv)   Combination Systems

Recently it has been shown that the combination of two complement-tary, moderately active agents, i.e., a zinc salt and triclosan can be incorporated in a toothpaste. Studies of up to twelve months duration have shown highly significant reduction of the recurrence of gingivitis (19,20,18,21,40). No adverse reactions or changes in the ecology of mouth were found during use of the combination of these two agents (38,18).

OTHER AGENTS

Various other classes of agents, such as enzymes (43,44,45) sugar substitutes (28), peroxides (46) and surface modifying agents (47) may have promising properties for incorporation into anti-plaque systems, however, at present the evidence from in vivo studies is either non-existent or ambiguous. Also data on the stability of some of these agents, such as enzymes and peroxides, which may be prone to inactivation on storage, are not available.

CONCLUSIONS

Some agents for daily use to control plaque and gingivitis have been successfully formulated in product systems such as dentifrice and mouth-rinses. A few rinse and gel systems containing positively charged agents are available. These agents are however incompatible with the most commonly used oral hygiene system i.e., a toothpaste. Metal salts and non-charged agents, such as triclosan, are bioavailable from this vehicle. Particularly

134

good results have also been obtained in long term unsupervised brushing studies using a combination of two agents i.e., triclosan and zinc citrate (18,19,20,21,40).

ACKNOWLEDGEMENTS

The author wishes to thank Dr D Cummins and Dr D Purdell-Lewis for critically reviewing the manuscript.

REFERENCES

1. Pilot T, Barmes DE, Leclercq MH, McCombie BJ, Sardo Infirri J (1986) Comm Dent Oral Epidemiol 14: 310-312

2. Cutress TW (1986) Int Dent J 36: 146-151

3. Pilot T, Barmes DE, Leclercq MH, McCombie BJ, Sardo Infirri J (1987) Comm Dent Oral Epidemiol 15: 366-388

4. Brown LJ, Oliver RC, Loe H (1989) J Periodontol 60: 363-370

5. Brunelle JA, Carol JP (1990) J Dent Res (Spec Iss) 69: 723-727

6. Kalsbeek H, Verrips GHW (1990) J Dent Res (Spec Iss) 69: 728-732

7. Government (UK) Statistical Service (1990) OPCS Monitor 14 March SS 90/1: 1-5

8. Williams RC (1990) N Eng J Med 6: 322-382

9. Waerhaug J (1978) J Periodontol 49: 1-8

10. Waerhaug J (1981) J Periodontol 52: 30-34

11. Attstrom R (1988) Does Supragingival Plaque Removal Prevent Further Breakdown? In: Guggenheim B (ed) Periodontology Today, Basel, Karger 251-259

12. Wilson TG (1987) J Periodontol 58: 706-714

13. Berenie J, Ripa LW, Leske G (1973) J Publ Health Dent 33: 160-171

14. Burchell CK, Stephen KW, Russell JI, Creanor SL, Knoop DTM (1990) Caries Res (accepted for publication)

15. Macgregor IDM, Balding JW (1987) Br Dent J 162: 141

16. Todd JE, Walker AM (1987) Adult Dental Health Volume 1 England and Wales 1968-1979 London HMSO 47

17. Van der Ouderaa FJG (1991) J Clin Periodontol (in press)

18. Stephen KW, Saxton CA, Jones CL, Ritchie JA, Morrison T (1990) J Periodontol (in press)

19. Svatun B, Saxton CA, van der Ouderaa FJG, Rolla G (1987) J Clin Periodontol 14: 457-461

20. Svatun B, Saxton CA, Rolla G, van der Ouderaa FJG (1989) J Clin Periodontol 16: 75-80

21. Svatun B, Saxton CA, Rolla G (1990) Scan J Dent Res 98: 301-304

22. Kornman KS (1986) J Periodontal Res (Suppl) 21: 5-22

23. van der Ouderaa FJG, Cummins D (1989) J Dent Res (Spec Iss) 68: 1617-1624

24. Goodson JM (1989) J Dent Res 68: Spec Iss 1625-1632

25. Ranney RR (1986) J Clin Periodontol 13: 356-357

26. Ranney RR (1984) J Dent Res (Spec Iss) 68: 1655-1660

27. Mandel ID (1988) J Clin Periodontol 15: 488-498

28. Scheie AAa (1989) J Dent Res 68: (Spec Iss) 1609-1616

29. Gjermo P (1989) J Dent Res (Spec Iss) 68: 1602-1608

30. Svatun B (1981) In: Rolla G, Embery G and Sonju T (Eds) Tooth Surface Interactions and Preventive Dentistry London, IRL Press, 33-37.

31. Saxton CA, Harrap GJ, Lloyd APR (1986) J Clin Periodontol 3: 301-306

32. Jones CL, Stephen CW, Ritchie JA, Huntingdon G, Saxton CA, van der Ouderaa FJG (1988) Caries Res 22: 84-90

33. Afseth J, Helgeland K, Bonesvoll P (1983) Scand J Dent Res

34. Gilbert RJ, Ingram GS (1988) J Pharm Pharmacol 40: 399-402

35. Cummins D, Watson GK (1989) J Dent Res 68: (Spec Iss) 1702-1705

36. Pader M (1988) Oral Hygiene Products and Practice 1st Ed New York Dekker Inc, p469

37. Saxton CA, Svatun B, Lloyd AM (1987) Scand J Dent Res 96: 212-7

38. Gjermo P, Saxton CA (1991) J Clin Periodontol (in press)

39. Polomo F, Wantland L, Sanchez A, Alvaro S, DeVizio W, Carter W, Baines E (1989) Am J Dent 2: 231-237

40. Svatun B, Saxton CA, Rolla G, van der Ouderaa FJG (1989) Scand J Dent Res 97: 242-6

41. Marsh PD (1991) J Clin Periodontol (in press)

42. Cummins D (1991) J Clin Periodontol (in press)

43. Rotgans J, Hoogendoorn H (1979) Caries Res 13: 144-148

44. Guggenheim B, Regalati B, Schmit, Muhlemann HR (1980) Caries Res 14: 128-137

45. Groeneveld A, Kalsbeek H, Hoogendoorn H, Piessens JP (1984) Ned Tydschr Tandheelk 91: 530-533

46. Afflitto J, Gaffar A, Moreno EC (1988) In Vivo J Dent Res 67: 401

47. Glantz PO, Attstrom R (1986) In: Loe H and Kleinman DV (Eds) Dental Plaque Control Measures and Oral Hygiene Practices. Oxford, IRL Press, 185-194

48. Chen MS, Robinson L (1982) JADA 104: 43-46

© 1991 Elsevier Science Publishers B.V.
Recent advances in periodontology Vol. II,
S.I. Gold, M. Midda and S. Mutlu, eds.

THE EFFECT OF ZINC CITRATE AND TRICLOSAN ON THE CONTROL OF PLAQUE AND OF
GINGIVITIS: SHORT TERM CLINICAL AND MODE OF ACTION STUDIES

DIANE CUMMINS

Unilever Dental Research, Port Sunlight Laboratory, Bebington, Wirral,
United Kingdom

INTRODUCTION

The rationale for the use of antimicrobial/anti-plaque agents to control
supragingival plaque formation and to prevent the onset of early periodontal
disease is clear (1,2,3). In principle, toothpastes provide an excellent
vehicle for the delivery of such agents. However, very few have been
successfully formulated to give clinically active products (3,4).

We have developed a dentifrice formulation based upon the additive anti-
plaque effects of low levels of zinc citrate and triclosan, which is carefully optimised with respect to delivery and clinical activity. This paper
focusses on short term clinical microbiological mode of action and oral
delivery studies.

SHORT TERM CLINICAL STUDIES

The clinical benefits of combining zinc citrate and triclosan have been
demonstrated in a hierachy of plaque and gingivitis protocols. In both
16-hour (5,6) and 4-day (7) non-brushing studies, zinc citrate/triclosan
inhibited plaque accumulation significantly more than either zinc citrate or
triclosan alone. Numerous short-term plaque studies have subsequently
confirmed these findings: 16 hour plaque growth inhibition data show an
average reduction of over 35% for the optimised 0.5% zinc citrate 0.2%
triclosan formulation compared to a control toothpaste and less than 25% for
either zinc citrate or triclosan alone.

The effect of reduced plaque growth on the development of gingivitis has
been demonstrated in a 21-day non-brushing experimental gingivitis study;
0.5% zinc citrate alone reduced the development of gingival bleeding sites
by 20% compared to a control toothpaste. The addition of 0.2% triclosan
significantly enhanced the efficacy of the paste giving a reduction of
nearly 70% in new bleeding sites (Figure 1).

138

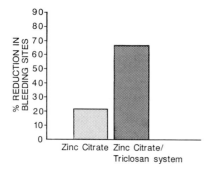

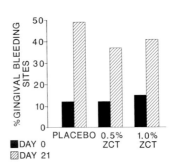

Fig. 1. Reduction in development of
gingival bleeding in the 21-day
experimental gingivitis model of a
toothpaste containing both zinc
citrate (0.5%) and triclosan (0.2%)
or zinc citrate alone compared to
a control toothpaste (23).

Fig. 2. Development of gingival
bleeding in the 21-day experimental
gingivitis model at baseline and at
21 days for zinc citrate (0.5% and
1.0% and control pastes (10).

Additional 21-day studies have confirmed the benefits of the optimised
zinc citrate/triclosan formulation (8,9) and suggest that a gingival health
benefit might be expected from a six month study using a normal oral hygiene
regime.

The same enhancement of anti-plaque and anti-gingivitis activity cannot be
achieved by using higher levels of either zinc citrate or triclosan. A
recent 21-day experimental gingivitis study of the dose-response relationship
of dentifrices containing 0.5% and 1% zinc citrate has confirmed the anti-
plaque efficacy of zinc citrate, demonstrated that zinc citrate delays the
onset of gingivitis and shown that the activity is not improved by increasing
the zinc ion concentration (10). The data for gingival bleeding are given
in Figure 2.

MODE OF ACTION OF ZINC CITRATE AND TRICLOSAN
The modes of action of zinc citrate and triclosan on plaque micro-organisms
are thought to be complementary.

Metals almost certainly act multifunctionally. In the first instance,
they may affect bacterial aggregation by modifying the surface properties of

individual plaque organisms either by altering cell proteins (11), by inhibiting protease induced adhesion (12) or by modifying electrostatic interactions (13). The major effect of metals is, however, thought to be the inhibition of glucose metabolism. The inhibitory effects of zinc have been shown to result from a combination of reduced glycolysis and glucose uptake (14-16) the former through the inhibition of the sulphydryl enzymes aldolase and glyceraldehyde dehydrogenase (17).

Zinc inhibition of glucose metabolism by Streptococcus mutans NCTC 10449 has been studied using a novel chemically defined pH-stat assay system (18) a direct relationship between inhibitory activity and zinc adsorption in the cells has been observed (Figure 3).

Importantly, it has also been shown that the chemical composition of the zinc species is the key factor in determining the biological activity of zinc as a metabolic inhibitor (19,20). Glucose metabolism by Streptococcus sanguis and Actinomyces naeslundii have also been shown to be inhibited by zinc (Watson and Cummins, unpublished data).

In contrast, triclosan is thought to act at the bacterial cell wall by increasing its permeability, ultimately leading to cell death. Mode of action studies on non-oral organisms suggest that triclosan adsorption is rapid and closely associated with the lipid fraction of the cell wall (21). At low, bacteriostatic concentrations, triclosan acts at the cytoplasmic membrane reducing intake of essential amino and nucleic acids. At higher, bactericidal levels, triclosan induces membrane lesions which lead to cell death (22).

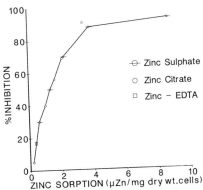

Fig. 3. Correlation between inhibition of acid production *in vitro* and zinc sorption to streptococcus mutans for systems containing zinc sulphate, citrate, or EDTA (19,20).

We have shown that triclosan inhibits the glucose metabolism of Streptococcus mutans NCTC 10449, Streptococcus sanguis and Actinomyces naeslundii.
In contrast to zinc which is bacteriostatic, triclosan is bactericidal at
90% inhibition of metabolism (Watson and Cummins, unpublished data).

In addition to the complementary effects of zinc and triclosan on
microbial metabolism and growth, their effects on the potential virulence of
peridontopathic organisms has been demonstrated (23). Zinc and triclosan
both inhibited the trypsin-like activity of Bacteroides gingivalis W50 and
Capnocytophaga gingivalis W43. Additive effects were observed for the
combination of zinc and triclosan (23).

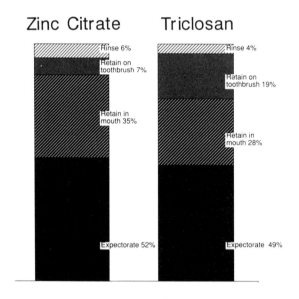

Fig. 4. Fate of zinc citrate and triclosan after use (27)

ORAL SUBSTANTIVITY OF ZINC AND TRICLOSAN

The anti-plaque and anti-gingivitis activity of the zinc citrate/triclosan
system is likely to result from the retention of the two anti-microbial
agents in micro-reservoirs in the mouth.

Oral substantivity is an important pre-requisite of any agent for
anti-plaque activity in vivo (24,25). Pharmacokinetic data demonstrate that

approximately 30% of both the zinc and triclosan dosed from the optimised
ZCT/triclosan system is retained immediately after brushing (26-29)
(Figure 4).

Saliva decay curves indicate that triclosan is cleared more quickly from
the mouth than zinc, which is consistent with the physicochemical properties
of the two agents (27). The anti-plaque agents are present in plaque for at
least 8 hours and on the oral mucosa for at least 3 hours after
toothbrushing (28) (Figure 5).

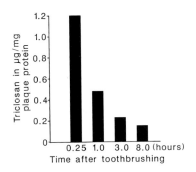

Fig. 5. Levels of triclosan in plaque
after brushing with the zinc citrate/
triclosan dentifrice (28).

In a recent study, it was found that oral retention of zinc and triclosan
is maintained when they are used for an extended period. This observation
gives additional confidence that the combined use of zinc and triclosan will
result in consistent anti-plaque activity during extended use and, hence,
will give rise to long term gingival health benefit.

REFERENCES

1.   Kornman KS (1986) J Periodontal Res 21: Suppl 16, 5-22

2.   Ciancio SG (1989) Am J Dent 2: (Sp Iss) 299-302

3.   van der Ouderaa FJG (1991) J Clin Peridontol (in press)

4.   van der Ouderaa FJG, Cummins D (1989) J Dent Res 68: (Sp Iss) 1617-24

5. Saxton CA, Lane RM, van der Ouderaa FJG (1987) J Clin Periodontol 14: 144-8

6. Saxton CA, Svatun B, Lloyd AM (1988) Scand J Dent Res 96: 212-7

7. Saxton CA (1986) J Periodontol 57: 555-561

8. Saxton CA, van der Ouderaa FJG (1989) J Periodontal Res 24: 75-80

9. Saxton CA (1989) J Dent Res 68: (Sp Iss) 1724-6

10. Saxton CA, Cummins D (1989) J Dent Res 68: (Sp Iss) 971

11. Jones CL, Purdell-Lewis DJ, van der Ouderaa FJG (1988) J Dent Res 67: (Sp Iss) 327

12. Li J, Ellen RP (1990) J Dent Res 69: (Sp Iss) 141

13. Hanke TM (1940) J Am Dent Assoc 27: 1379-93

14. Opperman RV, Rolla G, Johansen JR (1980) Scand J Dent Res 88: 389-396

15. Scheie AAa, Assev S, Rolla G (1986) in: Leech SA (Ed) Factors relating to demineralisation and remineralisation of teeth, Oxford, IRL Press, 1986: 99-104

16. Hamilton I, Bowden GW (1988) in: "Fluoride in Dentifrices" pp77-102

17. Scheie AAa, Assev S, Rolla G (1988) APMIS 96: 761-7

18. Marsh PD, Keevil CW, McDermid AS, Williamson MI, Ellwood DC (1963) Archs Oral Biol 28: 233-40

19. Watson GK, Cummins D (1988) J Dent Res 76: (Sp Iss) 402

20. Cummins D, Watson GK (1989) J Dent Res 68: (Sp Iss) 1702-1705

21. Meincke BE, Kraz RG, Lynch DL (1980) Microbios 28: 133-47

22. Regos J, Hitz HR (1974) Zbl Bakt Hyg I Abt Orig A226: 390-401

23. Cummins D (1990) J Clin Periodontol (in press)

24. Goodson JM (1989) J Dent Res 68: (Sp Iss) 1625-32

25. Gjermo P (1989) J Dent Res 68: (Sp Iss) 1602-8

26. Gilbert RJ, Fraser SB, van der Ouderaa FJG (1987) Caries Res 21: 29-36

27. Gilbert RJ (1987) J Pharm Pharmacol 39: 480-3

28. Gilbert RJ, Williams PEO (1987) Br J Clin Pharm 23: 579-83

29. Gilbert RJ, Tan-Walker RLB, van der Ouderaa FJG (1989) J Dent Res 68: (Sp Iss) 1706-7

© 1991 Elsevier Science Publishers B.V.
Recent advances in periodontology Vol. II,
S.I. Gold, M. Midda and S. Mutlu, eds.

MICROBIOLOGICAL STUDIES OF THE PREVENTION AND CONTROL OF PLAQUE
AND GINGIVITIS BY A ZINC AND TRICLOSAN-CONTAINING DENTIFRICE

P D MARSH

Pathology Division, PHLS Centre for Applied Microbiology and
Research, Salisbury SP4 OJG (England)

INTRODUCTION

The customary oral hygiene method of toothbrushing is usually
insufficient by itself for many individuals over long periods
to provide a level of plaque control compatible with oral
health. Consequently, the incorporation of antimicrobial
agents into dental products as a means of controlling dental
plaque and gingivitis has been advocated for a number of years.
A wide range of agents have been tested for antiplaque and
antimicrobial activity (1), but few have been successfully
incorporated into modern toothpaste formulations. Some
promising compounds are incompatible with ingredients of
dentifrices, while others have undesirable side-effects (2).
Recently, a toothpaste containing both zinc citrate and
Triclosan has been formulated successfully; the combination of
two agents has the advantage that additive or synergistic
interactions can occur resulting in increased clinical activity
and benefit from relatively low concentrations of each agent
(3).

DENTAL PLAQUE AND HEALTH

Dental plaque forms naturally on the tooth surface and has
properties that are beneficial to the host in that it can act
as a barrier to colonisation by exogenous, and often
pathogenic, micro-organisms. At healthy sites, the majority of
plaque bacteria are Gram-positive cocci or rods, such as
streptococci and actinomyces. Obligately anaerobic bacteria
are present only in low numbers. The function of antimicrobial
agents should be, therefore, to *control* plaque accumulation and
composition, but not to *eliminate* it.

DENTAL PLAQUE AND GINGIVITIS

Numerous studies of experimental and natural gingivitis in children and adults have shown that there is an increase in both plaque accumulation and in the diversity of the composition of the microflora (4,5). No single species is regarded as the aetiological agent in chronic gingivitis, but there is a shift in the balance of the resident microflora towards higher levels of *Actinomyces* species, particularly *A. naeslundii* and *A. viscosus*, and an increase in the isolation and proportions of capnophilic and obligately anaerobic bacteria (4,5). These include increased numbers of *Capnocytophaga* spp., *Prevotella* (formerly *Bacteroides*) *intermedia*, and *Fusobacterium nucleatum*.

ANTIMICROBIAL PROPERTIES OF ZINC SALTS AND TRICLOSAN - LABORATORY STUDIES

The conventional first stage in determining whether an agent has antimicrobial activity is to determine its minimum growth inhibitory concentration (MIC) against a wide range of relevant micro-organisms. Triclosan has activity against yeasts and a broad spectrum of oral Gram-positive and Gram-negative bacteria (Table I), including capnophilic and obligately anaerobic organisms implicated in gingivitis (6). Among the species that are most sensitive are those that have been proposed as being associated with active periodontal breakdown (*Actinobacillus actinomycetemcomitans*, *Prevotella* (formerly *Bacteroides*) *intermedia*) (7). There are few equivalent data on the activity of zinc salts against fastidious oral species due to the binding of the cation to conventional bacteriological media components. However, recently a more refined procedure using a chemically-defined medium has demonstrated the inhibition of the growth of *Streptococcus* and *Actinomyces* species at concentrations of between 0.010 and 0.015% (8). Both zinc (9) and Triclosan (10) are adsorbed to mucosal and bacterial cells, and are retained in the mouth at concentrations similar to the MIC of oral bacteria.

TABLE I

ORAL BACTERIAL INHIBITED BY TRICLOSAN*

GRAM-POSITIVE SPECIES	GRAM-NEGATIVE SPECIES
Streptococcus mutans	*Actinobacillus*
Streptococcus sanguis	*actinomycetemcomitans*
Actinomyces naeslundii	*Bacteroides oralis*
Actinomyces viscosus	*Bacteroides distasonis*
Actinomyces odontolyticus	
Actinomyces israelii	*Eubacterium lentum*
Peptococcus asaccharolyticus	*Fusobacterium nucleatum*
Peptococcus saccharolyticus	
Peptococcus magnus	*Leptotrichia buccalis*
Peptostreptococcus anaerobius	*Porphyromonas* (formerly
	Bacteroides) *gingivalis*
	Porphyromonas (formerly
	Bacteroides) *endodontalis*
	Prevotella (formerly
	Bacteroides) *melaninogenica*
	Prevotella (formerly
	Bacteroides) *intermedia*
	Veillonella parvula

*The minimum inhibitory concentration (MIC) ranged from 0.0005-
0.005% (6).

However, most successful anti-plaque and antibacterial agents used in dentistry are retained in the mouth for prolonged periods and function at sub-MIC levels. Studies on volunteers have shown that both zinc salts and Triclosan can still be detected in saliva and plaque for several hours after brushing with a dentifrice containing both agents. At equivalent concentrations in laboratory studies, it has been shown that zinc and Triclosan can interfere with metabolic traits of oral bacteria that are associated with their pathogenicity. For example, zinc can inhibit acid production by the cariogenic species *Streptococcus mutans* and *Streptococcus sanguis* (11), as well as by *Actinomyces viscosus*, which is implicated in gingivitis. Similarly, zinc salts can severely reduce (>90%) protease activity by *Capnocytophaga gingivalis* and by the periodontopathogen *Porphyromonas* (formerly *Bacteroides*) *gingivalis* (12). Zinc has also been shown to affect the ultrastructure of *S. sobrinus* (13). Triclosan has limited inhibitory effects on glycolysis and protease activity but additive effects on these properties have been found when low (sub-MIC) concentrations of zinc and Triclosan are combined (14,15).

The above studies have been performed on pure cultures of oral bacteria. In order to simulate the diversity of the plaque microflora, the effect of sub-MIC levels of zinc citrate and Triclosan, alone and in combination, on the stability of complex mixed cultures of oral bacteria has been studied *in vitro*. Ten oral bacterial species, representative of the plaque microflora in health and disease, were grown stably at pH 7.0 using continuous culture techniques (Table II) (16).

TABLE II

EFFECT OF DOSES OF TRICLOSAN (10mg/L) OR OF TRICLOSAN + ZINC CITRATE (25mg/L) ON A MIXED CULTURE OF ORAL BACTERIA

BACTERIA INHIBITED* BY:	
TRICLOSAN	ZINC CITRATE + TRICLOSAN
Actinomyces viscosus	*Streptococcus gordonii*
Veillonella dispar	*Streptococcus mutans*
Fusobacterium nucleatum	*Neisseria subflava*
Prevotella (formerly	*Porphyromonas* (formerly
Bacteroides) *intermedia*	*Bacteroides*) *gingivalis*
	*Veillonella dispar***
	*Fusobacterium nucleatum***
	Prevotella (formerly
	Bacteroides) *intermedia***

* Bacteria were statistically significantly inhibited compared
  with pre-dosing levels.
** Greater inhibition than with Triclosan alone.

After a continuous dose of Triclosan (final concentration = 10mg/L), the viable counts *Actinomyces viscosus, Veillonella dispar, Fusobacterium nucleatum, Prevotella* (formerly *Bacteroides*) *intermedia* were reduced. However, additive inhibitory effects were obtained when zinc citrate (final concentration = 25mg/L) and Triclosan were combined. There was a wider spectrum of bacteria inhibited, while those species that had been inhibited by Triclosan alone were affected to an even greater extent by the combination of agents (Table II). In contrast, organisms associated with dental health were relatively unaffected (eg *S. oralis*) and the microbial community after dosing was dominated by benign species (*S. oralis*, *S. gordonii* (formerly *S. sanguis*) and *V. dispar*). These studies showed that zinc citrate and Triclosan remain active at sub-MIC levels and have an additive but selective effect, by inhibiting primarily the bacteria associated with dental disease.

ANTIMICROBIAL PROPERTIES OF ZINC CITRATE AND TRICLOSAN - CLINICAL STUDIES

Studies with human volunteers have confirmed the promise of the laboratory data outlined above. Zinc and Triclosan appear to have complementary and additive inhibitory actions, with zinc citrate being most effective on existing dental plaque whereas Triclosan prevents plaque formation on clean surfaces (3). Similarly, in a partial mouth experimental gingivitis model, the local application of a dentifrice containing 0.2% (w/v) Triclosan and 0.5% (w/v) zinc citrate reduced the amount of dental plaque formed during the 21 day period of general oral hygiene abstention, and inhibited the development of gingivitis when compared to a placebo paste lacking both agents (17). Plaque from the test group had a statistically significantly reduced ratio of anaerobic/aerobic bacteria (Table III), and there was a trend for a reduction in the proportions of *Actinomyces* spp. compared to plaque from those using the placebo dentifrice (17). Importantly, the prolonged use of the zinc/Triclosan toothpaste by volunteers did not cause adverse shifts in the balance of the resident plaque microflora, nor did it lead to the enrichment of yeasts or enteric bacteria; likewise, there was no evidence for the selection of resistant organisms (18). Interestingly, toothbrushes from volunteers using the zinc/Triclosan toothpaste retained antibacterial activity and also had a statistically significantly lower level of contamination with environmental micro-organisms than did those from subjects using a placebo dentifrice.

TABLE III

EFFECT OF A PLACEBO DENTIFRICE OR A DENTIFRICE CONTAINING 0.2%
TRICLOSAN AND 0.5% ZINC CITRATE ON THE RATIO OF ANAEROBIC AND
AEROBIC BACTERIA IN PLAQUE AFTER A 21 DAY EXPERIMENTAL HUMAN
GINGIVITIS STUDY (17)

Dentifrice	Day	Mean viable count		Ratio Anaerobic/ Aerobic
		Anaerobic Microflora	Aerobic Microflora	
Placebo	0	2.45×10^4	1.95×10^4	1.26
	21	5.62×10^6	9.33×10^5	6.02
Zinc citrate/ Triclosan	0	3.39×10^4	1.35×10^4	2.51
	21	2.95×10^6	8.13×10^5	3.63

CONCLUSION

The collective laboratory and clinical data suggest that zinc
and Triclosan, in combination, have additive antibacterial and
antiplaque properties that will be of therapeutic value in both
preventing and controlling gingivitis. These agents are also
active at sub-MIC levels and appear to have a valuable
selective effect by inhibiting primarily those bacteria
associated with gingivitis, while leaving relatively unaffected
those that are predominant in plaque in health.

REFERENCES

1. Scheie AA (1989) J Dent Res 68: 1609-1616

2. van der Ouderaa FJ, Cummins D (1989) J Dent Res 68: 1617-
    1624

3. Saxton CA, Svatun B, Lloyd AM (1988) Scand J Dent Res 96:
    212-217

4. Moore LVH, Moore WEC, Cato EP, Smibert RM, Burmeister JA,
    Best AM, Ranney RR (1987) J Dent Res 66: 989-995

5. Savitt ED, Socransky SS (1984) J Periodont Res 19: 111-123

6. Ritchie JA, Jones CL (1988) In: Hardie JM, Borriello SP
    (eds) Anaerobes Today. Wiley, Chichester, pp240-241

7. Slots J, Bradg L, Wikstrom M, Dahlen G (1986) J Clin
    Periodontol 13: 570-577

8. Ritchie JA, Jones CL (1990) Letts Appl Microbiol 11: 152-154

9. Gilbert RJ, Ingram GS (1988) J Pharm Pharmacol 40: 399-402

10. Gilbert RJ, Fraser SB, van der Ouderaa FJG (1987) Caries Res 21: 29-36

11. Scheie AA, Assev A, Rölla G (1988) APMIS 96: 761-767

12. Sundqvist G, Carlsson J, Hanstrom L (1987) J Periodont Res 22: 300-306

13. Scheie AA, Fejerskov O, Assev S, Rölla G (1989) Caries Res 23: 320-327

14. Marsh PD (1991) J Dent Res 70: in press

15. Cummins D (1991) J Clin Periodontol: in press

16. Bradshaw DJ, McKee AS, Marsh PD (1990) J Dent Res 69: 436-441

17. Jones CL, Saxton CA, Ritchie JA (1990) J Clin Periodontol 17: 570-574

18. Jones CL, Ritchie JA, Marsh PD, van der Ouderaa F (1988) J Dent Res 67: 46-50

© 1991 Elsevier Science Publishers B.V.
Recent advances in periodontology Vol. II,
S.I. Gold, M. Midda and S. Mutlu, eds.

REVIEW OF THE CLINICAL EFFECTS OF DENTIFRICES CONTAINING TRICLOSAN

PER E GJERMO[1] and CHARLES A SAXTON[2]

1) Department of Periodontology, Dental Faculty, University of Oslo, Norway
2) Unilever Dental Research, Port Sunlight Laboratory, Bebington, Wirral, United Kingdom

INTRODUCTION

Good oral hygiene and freedom from gingivitis are important both for individual personal comfort[1] and a healthy dentition. Moreover, socially acceptable oral hygiene does not necessarily require the removal of all plaque, but rather a degree of cleanliness which most people could achieve by diligent use of currently available oral hygiene aids.

Most individuals seem to have difficulty in achieving perfect control by mechanical means and research has been directed towards the development of safe and effective chemical anti-plaque agents. In spite of changing concepts of the etiology and natural history of periodontal diseases over the last few decades, plaque control is still regarded as essential in the prevention and treatment of periodontitis[2].

The purpose of the present paper is to review clinical data on the effects of zinc ions and the anti-microbial compound triclosan separately and in combination on plaque, gingivitis and calculus. Particular emphasis has been placed on dentifrice formulations, including those containing chlorhexidine.

CHLORHEXIDINE DENTIFRICES

The remarkable effect of chlorhexidine on plaque and gingivitis was first documented in simple rinses; which in addition highlighted the unsightly toothstaining caused by this cationic material.

The advantage of including chlorhexidine in a dentifrice base which contains abrasives could be that the abrasive would control the toothstaining.

Long term studies which have included the assessment of plaque and gingivitis have been unimpressive, with neither plaque levels nor gingival health being improved by the chlorhexidine dentifrice[3,4]. Furthermore, the dentifrice abrasive was largely ineffective in preventing toothstaining[5].

The overall view appears to be that such dentifrices have met with limited success[6].

ZINC

Zinc, most often as the citrate salt, has been incorporated in many commercially available dentifrices[7-10]. An overall impression from the literature is that zinc ions exert a moderate effect upon plaque formation. Studies on the effect of zinc on gingivitis have not yet been reported.

The combination of zinc salts and anti-microbial agents and/or surfactants has been suggested to have additive or synergistic effects[11-13] indicating that their modes of action are different and/or support each other.

TRICLOSAN

Several studies indicate that triclosan alone, in spite of its anti-bacterial spectrum, has only a moderate effect on plaque formation[8,14,15]. Plaque inhibition is not directly correlated with *in vitro* anti-microbial activity and it would appear that triclosan like some other anti-microbial agents with good MIC values has limited bio-activity in *in vivo*.

Animal studies[16] have indicated that the effects of triclosan were enhanced when it was delivered in a lipophilic gel formulation. Recently, this principle has been pursued by incorporating triclosan, which is lipid soluble, in a co-polymer of methoxyethylene and maleic acid.

Human studies on the effect of the combination of 0.3% triclosan and 2% of the co-polymer indicate a moderate effect upon plaque in studies of up to six weeks duration[17,18]. Palomo *et al*[19] confirmed the anti-plaque effects in a fourteen week study and in addition reported a 50% difference in mean gingivitis values between test and control groups. A seven month gingivitis study has been recently published[20] showing promising data in support of the triclosan/co-polymer product.

ZINC AND TRICLOSAN COMBINED

An alternative approach to utilising the potential of triclosan and, in addition, increasing the activity of a dentifrice against plaque and gingivitis is to incorporate a combination of zinc and triclosan in the formulation. This combination is attractive because of low toxicity and few reported side-effects of the agents when applied in therapeutic doses[21].

Initial clinical studies were performed to investigate the potential efficacy of various concentrations and doses of these agents.

Saxton *et al*[10] found that a combination of 1% zinc citrate and 0.5% triclosan in a dentifrice in four week cross-over studies resulted in statistically significant reductions of both plaque and gingival indices so confirming that the anti-plaque effect was sufficient to benefit gingival health. A one year unsupervised clinical study comparing the effect of a fluoride dentifrice containing 1% zinc citrate and 0.2% triclosan with a control dentifrice was then undertaken on one hundred subjects with good baseline standards of oral health[24,25]. Plaque and gingivitis scores approached zero following prophylaxis and brushing instructions. After six months, only 7% of the control group had less than 5% bleeding sites in contrast to 60% of the test group. The authors concluded that the use of the test dentifrices maintained a higher level of gingival health and could compensate for absence of mechanical interdental cleaning.

Recently, studies using the twenty-one day experimental gingivitis model have shown that the level of zinc citrate could be further reduced to 0.5% without loss of anti-gingivitis activity. Moreover, the same model has been used in two further studies to demonstrate that this combination of zinc citrate and triclosan was much better at delaying the onset of gingivitis than either zinc alone or triclosan with co-polymer (Fig. 1).

However, other published reports from short term human plaque studies have concluded that there is little benefit from a triclosan over a placebo toothpaste when used alone or in combination with zinc citrate[14,15]. In the experimental gingivitis model, 0.5% zinc citrate in combination with 0.2% triclosan has, however, shown promising results[25,27,30].

In a six month unsupervised toothbrushing clinical trial, the gingival health of the test group was significantly better than the control group. In this study, the authors used the same protocol and similar populations to those of their previous investigations using 1% zinc citrate[24]. The similarity of the results support the twenty-one day data that no loss of clinical effect occurred as a result of reducing the level of zinc from 1.0 to 0.5% (Fig. 2).

The relatively good results of the Norwegian study achieved with a young age group, with good oral hygiene, prompted a further study in which the dentifrice was used by a wider age range of adults with poorer oral hygiene. A similar result was observed, thus indicating that the dentifrice was equally effective in older people with higher initial levels of disease. The data for both studies showed that, at the start,

154

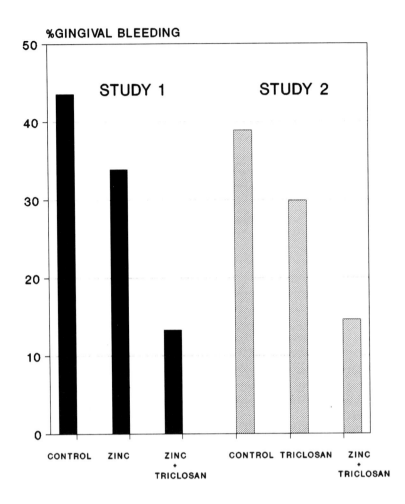

Fig. 1. Comparison of dentifrices containing; zinc citrate alone,
triclosan and co-polymer and a combination of zinc citrate and triclosan.

both study groups exhibited relatively poor gingival health on molar
teeth and lingual surfaces; sites known to be difficult to clean. On
completion, these sites again exhibited high levels of inflammation in
the placebo group. In contrast, these sites were significantly healthier
in the test group (Fig. 3) suggesting that the active agents are
delivered to sites which are normally inadequately brushed and have a
stabilising influence on gingival health.

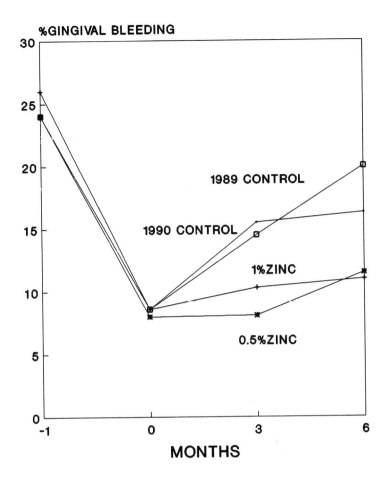

%GINGIVAL BLEEDING

1989 CONTROL

1990 CONTROL

1%ZINC

0.5%ZINC

MONTHS

Fig. 2. Comparison of two Norwegian Studies testing dual active
dentifrices. 1% zinc was used in 1989 and 0.5% in 1990.

Clinical Significance

The authors have also examined the data from these studies in an
attempt to judge the clinical significance of the results. Clinical
relevance might be expressed as the proportion of people who, on
completion of the six month study, had derived a certain level of
improved gingival health as a result of participation. If gingival
health could be expressed as less than 10% gingival bleeding sites[3] more
than 50% of users of the test dentifrice could be so classified compared
to only approximately 20% of the fluoride containing placebo group
(Fig. 4).

156

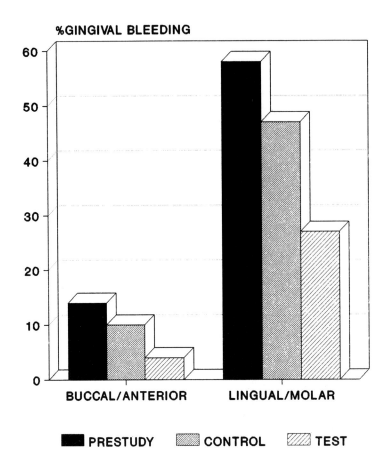

Fig. 3. The distribution of gingivitis according to tooth surface
before and after use of placebo or test paste.

ADVERSE EFFECTS

It is equally important that the effectiveness of preventive and
therapeutic measures when used at the population level are not
compromised by the emergence of adverse side effects. Participants in
long term clinical trials using dentifrices, with the combination of zinc
salts and triclosan, have been free of any subjective or clinically
detectable side effects[26,24,30], nor have substantial shifts in the oral
flora, or any development of bacterial resistance against triclosan been
observed[29,31].

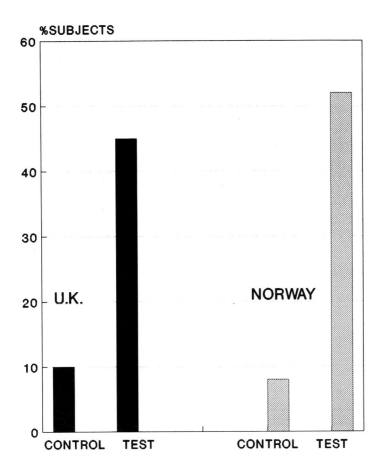

Fig. 4. The proportion of participants with < 10% gingival bleeding sites after using dentifrices for six months.

CONCLUSION

At present, there are two commercially available dentifrices claiming to have clinical effects on plaque and gingivitis, with triclosan as one of the active ingredient. Both formulations contain additives aimed at maximising the effect of triclosan. One uses a co-polymer in order to provide an extended release phase of the active agent and the other a metal salt to enhance the attack on the plaque flora. The former formulation has been tested up to seven months and the latter has been demonstrated to be efficacious in promoting gingival health in twelve month studies. The studies reviewed in this paper represent promising approaches to improving oral health.

158

REFERENCES

1) Gjermo P (1984) In: Frandsen A (ed) Public Health Aspects of
    Periodontal Disease, Quintessence, Berlin, pp 121-134

2) Glavind L, Nyvad B (1987) In: Gjermo P (ed) Promotion of Self Care
    in Oral Health Dental Faculty, Oslo, pp 77-92

3) Dolles OK, Gjermo P (1980) Scand J Dent Res 88: 22-27

4) Johansen JR, Gjermo P, Erikson HM (1975) Scand J Dent Res 83:
    288-292

5) Dolles OK, Eriksen HM, Gjermo P (1979) Scand J Dent Res 87: 268-274

6) Kornman KS (1986) J Periodontal Res 21 (special suppl) 5-22

7) Addy M, Willis L, Moran J (1983) J Clin Periodontal 10: 89-99

8) Saxton CA (1986) J Periodontol 57: 555-561

9) Saxton CA, Harrap GJ, Lloyd AM (1986) J Clin Periodontol 13: 301-306

10) Saxton CA, Lane RM, van der Ouderaa FJG (1987) J Clin Periodontol
    14: 144-148

11) Saxer UP, Muhlemann HR (1983) A review. Schweiz Monatsschr
    Zahnheilkd 93: 689-704

12) Giertsen E, Scheie AAa, Rolla G (1989a) Caries Res 23: 278-283

13) Giertsen E, Scheie AAa, Rolla G (1989b) Scand J Dent Res 96: 541-550

14) Jenkins S, Addy M, Newcombe R (1989a) Am J Dent 2: 211-214

15) Jenkins S, Addy M, Newcombe R (1989b) J Clin Periodontol 16: 287-385

16) Muhlemann HR (1973) Helv Odontol Acta 17: 99-103

17) Clerehugh V, Worthington H, Clarkson J, Davies TGH (1989) Am J Dent
    2: 221-224

18) Singh SM, Rustogi KN, Volpe AR, Petrone M, Kirkup R, Collins M
    (1989) Am J Dent Res 2: 225-230

19) Palomo F, Wantland L, Sanchez A, de Vizio W, Carter W, Baines E
    (1989) Am J Dent 2: 231-237

20) Garcia-Godoy F, Garcia-Godoy F, de Vizio W, Volpe AR, Ferlauto RJ,
    Miller JM (1990) Am J Dent 3 special issue 515-526

21) Scheie AAa (1989) J Dent Res 68: 1609-1617

22) Saxton CA, Svatun B, Lloyd AM (1988) Scand J Dent Res 96: 212-217

23) Svatun B, Saxton CA, van der Ouderaa FJG, Rolla G (1987) J Clin
    Periodontol 14: 457-461

24) Svatun B, Saxton CA, Rolla G, van der Ouderaa FJG (1989) J Clin Periodontol 16: 75-80

25) Saxton CA, van der Ouderaa FJG (1989) J Periodontol Res 24: 75-80

26) Saxton CA (1989a) J Dent Res (Sp Iss) 68: 743

27) Jones CL, Saxton CA, Ritchie JA (1990) J Clin Periodontol (in press)

28) Svatun B, Saxton CA, Rolla G (1990) Scand J Dent Res (in press)

29) Stephen KW, Saxton CA, Jones CL, Ritchie JA, Morrison T (1990) J Periodontol 61: 674-679

30) Saxton CA (1989b) J Dent Res 68: 1724-1726

31) Jones CL, Ritchie JA, Marsh PD, van der Ouderaa FJG (1988) J Dent Res 67:46-50

FREE PAPERS

© 1991 Elsevier Science Publishers B.V.
Recent advances in periodontology Vol. II,
S.I. Gold, M. Midda and S. Mutlu, eds.

THE TREATMENT OF DEEP INFRABONY DEFECTS BY THE USE OF AUTOGENOUS CANCELLOUS BONE AND MARROW COMBINED WITH FREEZE-DRIED BONE

OFER MOSES,[1] YUVAL ZUBERY,[1] HAIM TAL,[1] SANDU PITARU[2]

[1]Department of Periodontology and [2]Department of Oral Biology,
The Maurice and Gabriela Goldschleger School of Dental Medicine,
Tel Aviv University, Israel

The treatment of advanced periodontal cases with multiple vertical bony defects enables a more effective treatment providing we take advantage of the special topography of the bony defects, the potential of osteo-inductive materials and the changes in the root surface that may enhance regeneration. The ultimate goal of periodontal regenerative therapy is the re-establishment of a new attachment apparatus including new cementum, alveolar bone and functionally oriented periodontal ligament just apical to the cemento-enamel junction.

One of the most potent osteo-inductive materials to induce reconstitution of connective tissue attachment is autogenous cancellous bone and marrow. However, post-operative problems associated with grafting of fresh autogenous material, such as root resorption, exfoliation sequentration, rapid recurrence of defect, and infection have been discussed by Schallhorn and others. Viable bone marrow elements present at or coronally to the crest of the bone may be related to the resorption phenomena. This phenomena has not been reported in clinical cases treated with frozen autogenous bone and marrow.

Since freeze-dried bone and autogenous bone marrow are potent osteo-inductive material, it is logical to assume that mixing them together will form a grafting material which will result in improved healing without significant side effects. Root conditioning may improve healing. The further use of saturated solutions of tetracycline, an acidic preparation capable of surface demineralization, was claimed to facilitate binding of fibronectin and cells participating in the creation of new attachment apparatus.

The following presentation will demonstrate the treatment of advanced periodontitis with multiple vertical defects using the following materials and principles:

a. Frozen autogenous cancellous bone and marrow harvested from the anterior iliac spine, with a combination of freeze-dried bone

b. Root conditioning with tetracycline

c. Adjusting our treatment to the special topography of the multiple vertical bony defects

Case Presentation

A 47-year-old woman suffering from advanced adult type perio-dontitis, was referred to the Periodontal Department at Tel Aviv University Dental School. Clinical examination revealed a probing depth of 6-9 mm in all four molar regions. Radiographic examination showed deep vertical infrabony pockets. During the past 15 years, the patient had three full mouth surgical periodontal procedures. Initial preparation produced only minor reduction of probing depth and the next surgical procedure was considered for this case. Based on the fact that the patient was highly motivated with excellent plaque control, it was decided to harvest bone and bone marrow from her anterior iliac crest region.

Under local anaesthesia, a skin incision in the right anterior iliac spine region was performed reflecting the bone. Through this incision, a punch biopsy was inserted, and cores of cancellous bone was harvested, followed by aspiration of 20 cc of bone marrow, which clotted in a short time. The material was put in 15% glycerol in minimum essential medium as a cryoprotective agent under sterile condition, and was divided into several vials. These samples were first frozen to -4°C and later to -79°C for storage. Healing of the biopsy area was without any complaint or discomfort.

In all four quadrants, inverse bevel full thickness mucoperiosteal flaps were reflected. An effort was made to retain the marginal gingivae to ensure maximum soft tissue coverage of the graft material. Site preparation included debridement of defects and root planing. This was followed by rubbing tetracycline solution pH-1 for 1 minute with a cotton pellet. Meanwhile, vials containing plug of cancellous bone and bone marrow were let to thaw to room temperature. Mixing bone marrow with 1 g freeze-dried bone made the consistency of the mixture comfortable to handle and place it into the bony defects. The grafting procedure included placement and crushing of cancellous bone plug, vertically to the base of the bony defect followed by placement of the marrow and freeze-

dried bone mixture to the level of the bone crest. Complete closure of the soft tissue was followed. Radiographic examination,
immediately after each procedure, revealed radiolucency in the bony
defect area. Radiographic examination performed 3, 6, 9, and 12
months after the procedure, revealed a gradual growing radiopacity
in the bony defects, except in the area of MB root of tooth 16
(maxillary left molar) and MB root of tooth 26 (maxillary right
molar) (Figs. 1 and 2). Clinical evaluation showed reduction of
probing depth from 9 mm to 2-3 mm, marked bone fill of infrabony
defects, and some increase in crestal bone levels between teeth
15-16 (left maxillary molar and premolar) and teeth 25-26 (right
maxillary molar and premolar).

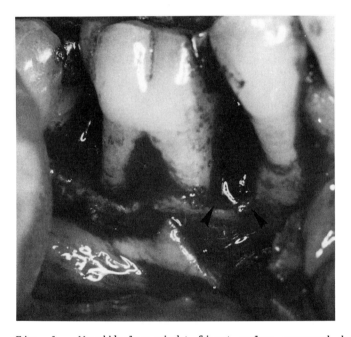

Fig. 1.   Mandibular right first molar exposed during surgery.
          Defects filled with bone marrow and FDB (arrow)

Cases with multiple vertical infrabony defects, were treated successfully with the use of autogenous cancellous bone and marrow,
combined with freeze-dried bone. This technique is advantageous in
cases of multiple deep infrabony defects, by using the topography
of the defects to support the graft material.

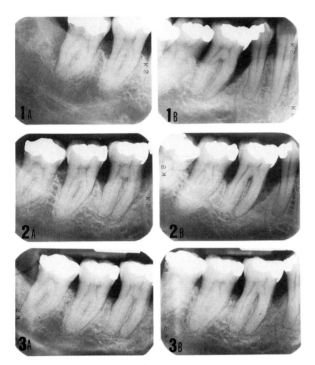

Fig. 2.   Radiographic followup
   a. Defect at the distal aspect of the 3rd molar
   b. Defect at the mesial aspect of the 1st molar
   1. At time of grafting procedure
   2. 3 months later
   3. 6 months later

Using a fresh autogenous material obliges the surgeon to harvest the bone from the iliac crest and to do the surgical periodontal procedure in a single session. A fresh autogenous material is known to cause root resorption; freezing this material to -79°C provides us with: osteogenic material without unwanted results, such as root resorption, and a long-term storage of the material and an option to use more material in re-entry grafting procedures, if needed.   Mixing freeze-dried bone and bone marrow gives us a high potent osteogenic material, as was demonstrated in this case.

REFERENCES
1.   Schallhorn RG (1968) J Periodontol 39:145
2.   Dragoo MR, Sullivan NC (1973) J Periodontol 44:599
3.   Burwell GR (1964) J Bone Joint Surg 46B:110
4.   Schallhorn RG (1972) J Periodontol 43:3

© 1991 Elsevier Science Publishers B.V.
Recent advances in periodontology Vol. II,
S.I. Gold, M. Midda and S. Mutlu, eds.

CLINICAL USE OF GUIDED TISSUE REGENERATION. CASES PRESENTATION

ANDREAS PARASHIS AND FOTIS MITSIS

Dept. of Periodontology, School of Dentistry, Athens University, 2 Thivon str.,
GR-115 27 Athens, Greece

INTRODUCTION

The goal of periodontal therapy is to maintain the natural dentition in an optimal state of health, function, comfort and esthetics for the life of the patient. It is recognized, and well substantiated, that a number of currently available therapeutic procedures are able to retain a reduced periodontium in health. However, periodontal regeneration holds the prospect of regaining support, root coverage and a return to a prediseased state.

Regeneration of periodontal tissues has always been the ideal objective of periodontal therapy. Different techniques such as subgingival curettage, flap operations, bone and synthetic grafts have been used in clinical practice to achieve this goal (1). Although, bone repair could occur in periodontal osseous lesions following grafting, the formation of new attachement is usually minimal following these procedures (2,3). The use of barrier techniques, such as membranes or filters, for selected cell repopulation have indicated that the combination of epithelial exclusion and the isolation of the root surface from the gingival connective tissue can result in significant amounts of new attachement (4-6). Recently, membranes made from teflon (Gore-tex periodontal material) are available for clinical use.

The purpose of this presentation is to discuss the use of guided tissue regeneration in clinical practice as well as to present cases where the technique has been used.

INDICATIONS

The technique is indicated for formation of connective tissue attachement in intrabony defects and in class II furcation involvements and also in class III furcation involvements and two wall defects. The clinician must always have in mind that the outcome of the procedure is also influenced by the shape and the size of the defect. Consideration must be given to the distance that the PDL cells will have to cover. Thus, in cases of shallow one wall lesions the amount of periodontal ligament cells is minimal and the distance is long. On the contrary, in deep angular bony defects with two or three walls and in furcations migration of the PDL cells is hapenning not only from the deepest point of the lesion but also from the lateral sides. Therefore the amount of cells is bigger and the distance smaller.

TECHNIQUE

There are important factors that influence success of the procedure. The need for plaque control and removal of bacterial products is universally recognized as an essential component in the sequence of periodontal therapy. The elimination of all potentially compromising agents through the efforts of both the therapist and patient is the key to success. Without elimination of the etiological agents, efforts at regeneration of the periodontium will ultimately fail. Elimination of trauma from occlusion if any is also important. The initial incision must be done in such a way to preserve as much tissue as possible for coverage of the material. After flap reflection degranulation of the area and root preparation is of paramount importance for successful regeneration. The membrane is adjusted in such a way to cover completely the bone defect. Tight adaptation of the colar with the root is necessary to preserve the epithelium from moving apically. Complete coverage of the membrane for better plaque control is also advantageous. The membrane must stay in place for 4-6 weeks. A small flap is necessary for its removal. In this stage, great attention must be given to the new granulation tissue that is forming since it is the pool for the cells that will form the new attachement. This tissue must be covered with the flap for proper protection. Problems associated with the method are technique sensitivity and the need for a second procedure. Since the formation of new attachement can not be verified in clinical practice, pocket reduction, improvement of clinical attachement level ≥ 2 mm and absence of bleeding in probing, are the criteria of clinical success. Although the formation of new attachement is predictable, significant coronal growth of alveolar bone usually doesn't occur. Thus, radiographic changes usually are not evident.

FURCATIONS

It is well known that furcations respond differently to periodontal treatment than flat surfaces. Root planning, flap surgery and osseous resective surgery have shown to be inadequate in totally controlling disease progression in this region. Regenerative therapy represents a valuable alternative of treatment for furcation areas.

Today, cases especially with class II furcation involvement can be treated successfully with the principle of GTR. Thus, more complex and constly procedures such as root amputation procedures can be avoided especially in patients with full dentitions that they will not need prosthetic reconstruction.

Even if new bone is not going to be formed the advantage of "closing" the difficult for cleaning and debridement area of the furcation gives a tremendous advantage for long term maintenance of the area.

Reports indicate complete closing of class II furcation most of the times after

using GTR procedures (7). Results for class III furcations have been less promising. Complete closing was observed in 25% of the furcations treated and partial closing in 55% (8).

Our evaluation in ten class II furcations from 6 months for up to 2 years (mean
time 13.6 months) showed the following results. The mean probing depth at the
furcation sites at the initial examination was 5.8 mm. Following treatment there
was a marked reduction in the mean probing depth to 2.7 mm. Treatment resulted
also in a marked reduction in the mean vertical clinical attachement level from
7.3 mm to 4.6 mm   (Fig. 1).

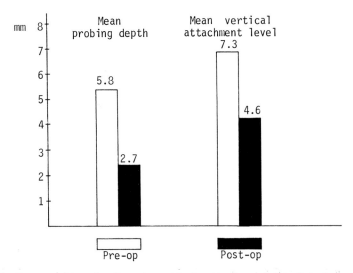

Fig. 1. Mean probing depth and vertical attachement level before and up to 2
years after using G.T.R.

Results for horizontal attachement level showed complete "closure" of the furcation in six cases. That means that in these six cases the furcation space was
occupied by tissue which prevented probe penetration. Furthermore, one defect
had a residual horizontal attachement level of no more than 1 mm. Two defects
has a residual level of 2 mm and one had 3 mm (Fig. 2).

CONCLUSION

There is evidence today that new attachement can be formed in roots previously
exposed to the disease after use of the GTR. Its clinical application in every
day practice especially for three wall bony defects and class II furcations is
a reality. Furthermore, new exiting applications of the technique for ridge augmentation and for coverage of implants put in extraction sites are in the verge

170

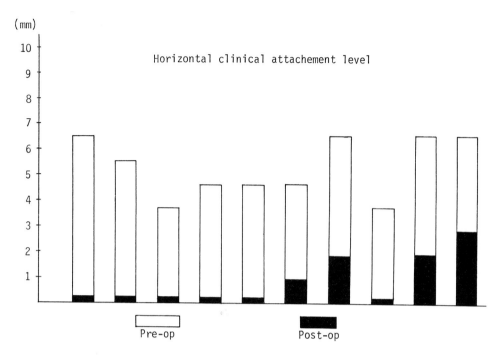

Fig. 2. Results for horizontal clinical attachement level indicate complete "closure" in six cases.

of reaching the clinical practice. The use of absorbable membranes will solve the problem of the second procedure but requires additional evaluation. We believe that is not optimistic anymore to say that a new era in regeneration therapy has evolved.

REFERENCES
1. Card S, Caffesse R, Smith B (1987) J West Soc Periodontol 35:93
2. Stal S, Froum S, Kushner L (1982) J Periodontol 53:15
3. Nyman S, Lindhe J, Karring T (1981) J Clin Periodontol 8:249
4. Nyman S, Lindhe J, Karring T, Wenstrom J (1987) J Periodont   Res 22:252
5. Auckhil I, Simpson D, Suggs C, Petterson E (1986) J Clin Periodontol 13:862
6. Gottlow J, Nyman S, Lindhe J, Karring T, Wennstrom J (1986) J Clin Periodontol 13:604
7. Pontoriero R, Lindhe J, Nyman S, Karring J, Rosemberg E, Sanavi F (1988) J Clin Periodontol 15:247
8. Pontoriero E, Nyman S, Lindhe J, Rosemberg E, Sanavi F (1987) J Clin Periodontol 14:618

© 1991 Elsevier Science Publishers B.V.
Recent advances in periodontology Vol. II,
S.I. Gold, M. Midda and S. Mutlu, eds.

CROWN LENGTHENING AND RESTORATIVE TREATMENT IN MUTILATED POSTERIOR TEETH

ANDREAS PARASHIS and ARIS TRIPODAKIS

INTRODUCTION

Crown lengthening has extensively been advocated as a treatment modality in order to restore teeth that involve reduced clinical crown due to different kinds of mutilations. This surgical approach would provide the necessary zone of healthy tooth structure coronaly to the alveolar crest for a new gingival attachment complex and the crown margins in order not to violate the biologic width of the periodontium and to preserve periodontal health in the long run (1,2). Clinically, the application of this procedure has been well established and extensively discussed in the dental literature specially for single rooted teeth (3-5).

Multirooted teeth however, present specific anatomical features that complicate surgical and prosthetic treatment. Such features are the furcation area and the corresponding interadicular bone, the retromolar pad and the external oblique line that limit the possibility for bone reduction and minimise the effectiveness of this approach. Nevertheless, multirooted teeth with reduced clinical crown may be critical distal abutments for a bridge or unique posterior teeth present in the quadrant. Consequently, their loss will require the unpleasant, for the patient, construction of a removable partial denture or the more demanding and costly placement of osseointegrated fictures. Therefore, the possibility of saving these teeth through a modified approach of crown lengthening and proper perio-prosthetic management should carefully be examined.

The purpose of this article is to underline the importance and to discuss the indications and techniques of crown lengthening procedures in multirooted teeth.

SURGICAL PROCEDURES AND SPECIAL CHARACTERISTICS

The aim of surgical crown lengthening is the exposure of at least 3-4 mm of healthy tooth structure coronaly to the alveolar crest (6). This can be achieved with surgical reduction of the attachment complex if the distance of the defect to the bone is adequate or may also involve modification of the hard tissues if the defect is in close proximity to the bone. The most widespread technique for the achievement of this goal is the apically positioned flap in combination with a distal wedge, if the distal surface of the molar must be lengthened. It is the procedure of choice since direct observation of bone is achieved, permitting the correct evaluation of the position of the defect and alveolar reduction if necessary. If ostectomy is required, care must be taken not to expose the furcation area. Furcation exposure during surgery will lead to an iatrogenic class II furcation defect and induce possibly further periodontal destruction of the area.

Ideally, ostectomy should aim to a straight horizontal line configuration with scalloping interdentally in order to promote positive architecture during healing (7). However, modification of this line by curving away from the furcation can be done without significant implications to the end result. Obviously this approach requires that the tooth structure above the furcation is intact.

When the surgery is performed in lower molars, the existence of the external oblique ridge makes the apical repositioning of the buccal flap difficult since the tissue has a tendency to move coronaly after the reflection.
In order to overcome this problem, vertical sling suturing engaging the periosteum is necessary for the tissue to be stabilised apically allowing the lengthening of the crown.

In cases that a distal wedge is necessary, care must be taken at the anatomy of the retromolar area. If the tissue in this area is fat covered by alveolar mucosa, the apical repositioning is difficult if not impossible and crown lengthening often fails.

CROWN LENGTHENING AND ROOT RESECTION

Although multirooted teeth present many difficulties during surgical crown lengthening as mentioned above, they also present the possibility of root resection that offers another valuable alternative of treatment.

Thus, in cases of deep fractures or subgingival caries present on one or two roots, the involved part of the tooth can be removed. This is preferable if it is evident that crown lengthening will require extensive ostectomy that will expose the furcation or jeopardise the support of adjacent teeth. Furthermore, root resection or separation is a must and the only solution when caries extend in the furcation area.

If root resection is necessary the following factors must be taken into consideration (8):
- bone support in the remaining roots
- root canal anatomy and access for decent endodontic therapy
- prosthetic importance of the remaining roots.
Many times the molars that require crown lengthening are also involved with periodontal disease. In such cases, the lengthening is performed in conjuction with periodontal therapy. Correct evaluation of bone support in relation with the part of the tooth involved, is necessary before surgery in order to decide which root has to be removed. This decision however, often has to be taken during surgery. In these instances, root canal therapy is also postponed but it should be performed as soon as possible after surgery.

Root resection must always be performed after raising a flap. This allows evaluation of the extent of the subgingival defect and of the bone support of the roots. After removal of the affected root, it is often necessary to reduce the height of the interadicular bone to get adequate exposure of sound tooth structure.

The above approach is also applicable in cases of root separation. The placement of an additional suture between the two roots during suturing, will help to the adaptation of the soft tissue in this area and allow healing with favorable contours and facilitate access to adequate plaque control. Thus, the final prosthetic restoration can be placed beyond the furcation area without violating the soft tissue and periodontal health can be assured.

CONCLUSION

The periodontal space in which the restorative treatment is practiced without problems is the gingival crevice (9). It is very important for the maintenance of periodontal health the restoration not to exert any violence on the epithelial attachment. If the clinical situation presents a potential of violation of this principle, surgical crown lengthening must be performed. This is particularly true for molars since their strategic value makes them very important teeth for the mouth or for the reconstruction. Although molars present specific anatomical difficulties during surgical crown lengthening, the possibility of root resection is an alternative in cases where conventional surgery is not possible.

With or without a combined approach, multirooted teeth with subgingival defects or inadequate axial height of intact clinical crown can be treated successfully, harmonizing the restorative procedures and materials with the supporting biologic environment and ensuring the longevity of the dentition.

REFERENCES

1. Gargiulo AW, Wentz FM, Orban B (1961) J Periodontol 32:261
2. Nevins M, Skurow HM (1984) Int J Periodont Rest Dent 4:30
3. Kaldahl WB, Becker CM, Wertz FM (1984) J Prosthet Dent 51:36
4. Kohavi D, Stern N (1983) Compend Cont Educ Dent 4:413
5. Sivers J, Johnson GK (1985) Quintessence Int 16:833
6. Block PC (1987) J Prosthet Dent 57:683
7. Ochsenbein C, Ross SE (1969) Dent Clin North Am 13:87
8. Newell D (1981) J Periodontol 52:550
9. Wilson RD, Maynard JG (1981) Int J Periodont Rest Dent 1:34

© 1991 Elsevier Science Publishers B.V.
Recent advances in periodontology Vol. II,
S.I. Gold, M. Midda and S. Mutlu, eds.

A TEAM APPROACH TO MALOCCLUSION WITH ADVANCED PERIODONTITIS - A CASE REPORT-

KOJI INAGAKI[1], TOSHIHIDE NOGUCHI[1], MASARU SAKAI[2], and KUNIAKI MIYAJIMA[2]

Depts. of Periodont.[1] and Orthodont.[2] ,School of Dent.,Aichi-Gakuin Univ.,2-11
Suemori-Dori,Chikusa-Ku,Nagoya,464 Japan

INTRODUCTION

Following the development of medical care and nutrition, the average age of
death has become intensely higher in Japan. These changes are involving a dramatic effect on our health as well as physical health and may change oral breakdown process to periodontal disease. In such circumstances, frequency of malocclusion associated with tooth size discrepancy is gradually increasing. Therefore, periodontal considerations following orthodontic treatment are very important and inevitable. Iatrogenic effects by orthodontic treatment are gingival
inflammation, alveolar bone and / or root resorption, loss of connective-tissue
attachment and marginal tissue recession. Surgical approach to marginal tissue
recession must be considered. In general, teeth usually have physiological mobility and continuous migration. Missing of teeth or loss of periodontal tissues,
however, create pathological tooth migration and break its physiological process.
Especially in cases of advanced periodontal diseases, destruction of supporting
structures has chance to breakdown to a level of extraction. In such cases, loss
of periodontal tissues can result in the development of diastema and / or spacing of the teeth particularly in the anterior area, and the reduction of the
bite. Malocclusion aggravated by occlusal trauma and oral habits, then, may become worse. All above symptoms in addition to the typically periodontal signs is
common in individuals with advanced periodontal disease. Therefore, combined
periodontal and orthodontic team approach should be performed for the malocclusion with advanced periodontitis.

The present case report describes the treatment of malocclusion with an extremely advanced periodontal destruction. A 23-year-old female with non contrib-
utory medical histories were reffered to an orthodontic office. After a complete
examination, the combined periodontal and orthodontic therapy was planned. Following the overall treatment, physiological occlusion, good periodontal condition as well as esthetics were achieved and are maintained for about 7 years
from her initial visit.

CASE : S.I. (23-year-old, female)

Initial visit	: Sep.29, 1983.,	Race	: Japanese
Occupation	: Nutritionist,	Marital	: Single

C.C.   : Maxillary Protrusion

P.H.   : Her medical histories were unremarkable, with only a history of uterus insufficiency.

H.P.I. : Her periodontal symptoms such as gingival bleeding appeared in her early teens, but periodontal treatment was not given so far. Therefore, she visited an orthodontic office for her malocclusion and was referred to this hospital for the evaluation of periodontal disease.

P.S. :

 General condition : General condition appeared normal. Serum chemistry and all blood counts were within normal limits.

 Local condition   : Periodontal examination disclosed the presence of an advanced destruction of the supporting tissues around most part of the dentition and the presence of angular bony defects (Fig. 1,2). Deep pockets more than 5 mm with acute gingival inflammation were measured in most teeth. The teeth of 15, 14,34 and 42 exhibited increased tooth mobility. Impacted teeth, 13 and 48 were observed on the X ray film. Upper incisors protrusion and a retrognathic mandible were displayed.

Periodontal diagnosis : Post-juvenile periodontitis was suspected.

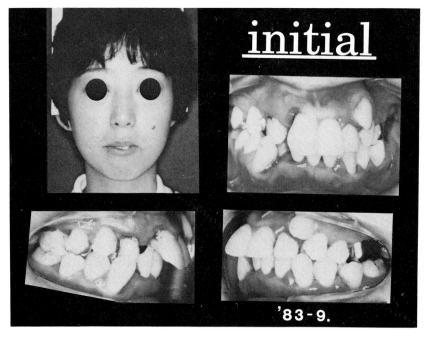

Fig. 1. Clinical views at an initial visit.

177

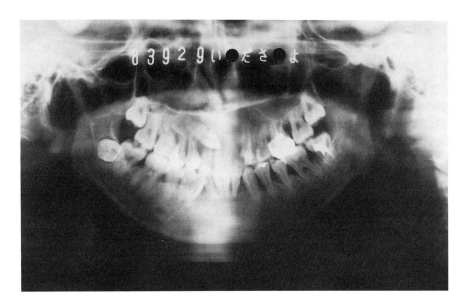

Fig. 2. Radiographs at an initial visit.

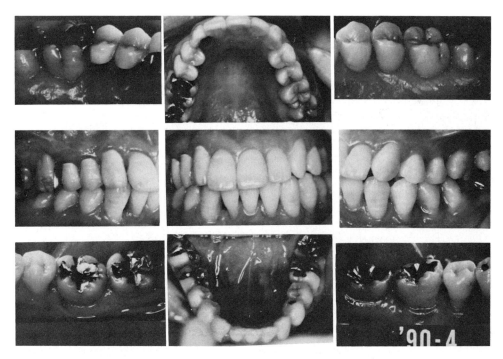

Fig. 3. Clinical views of 7 years later.

178

Orthodontic diagnosis : Angle's class II divition I with deep bite and severe crowding. Facial pattern was dolico type.

Treatment procedures : Initial therapy consisted of several sessions of scaling and root planing, oral hygiene and instruction of nutritional pattern. Following completion of initial phase, periodontal surgery for a pocket improvement was carried out on the teeth of 16-12, 24-27, 31-35 and 41-45. Vestibular extension based on Edlan's technique was performed on the tooth, 16. The teeth of 13, 26, 42 and 48 were extracted during periodontal surgeries. After the healing of periodontal tissues, orthodontic treatment based on Edgewise technique including bite raising, improvement of crowding and space closure, was applied to eatablish esthetic and physiological occlusion. After 2.5 years of orthodontic treatment, orthodontic retainer to upper teeth was placed and lower anterior teeth were splinted. The teeth of 12, 14 and 15 were fixed with full crowns.

Conclusion : Following reevaluation of the periodontal condition and craniomandibular function, the patient was recalled for maintenance care for about 7 years from her initial visit. Periodontal destruction has been ceased and physiological occlusion as well as good periodontal condition is maintained (Fig.3,4).

In the cases of a malocclusion with advanced periodontitis, combined periodontal and orthodontic team approach should be performed.

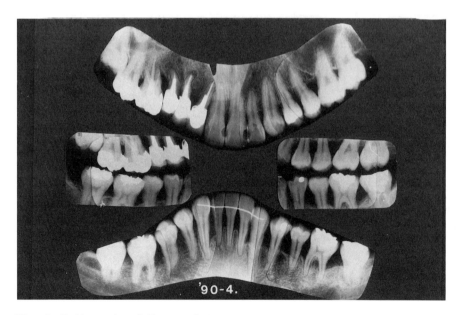

Fig. 4. Radiographs of 7 years later.

© *1991 Elsevier Science Publishers B.V.*
Recent advances in periodontology Vol. II,
S.I. Gold, M. Midda and S. Mutlu, eds.

THE EFFECT OF CYCLOSPORIN-A (CyA) ON THE ULTRASTRUCTURE OF GINGIVAL MAST CELLS (GMC) IN BEHÇET'S DISEASE (BD).

OKTAY ARDA, ÜLKÜ NOYAN*, SELÇUK YILMAZ*
İ.U. Cerrahpaşa Medical   Faculty   Histology   and   Embryology
Department.   İstanbul (Turkey).
*M.U. Dental Faculty, Periodontology Department. İstanbul (Turkey).

INTRODUCTION

Turkish dermatologist Hulusi Behçet described the triple symptom syndrome as recurrent painful oral and genital ulcers and recurrent inflammation of the uvea in 1937 (1).   It is a multisystem disease with minor effects of skin, joints, nervous, cardiovascular, renal and gastrointestinal disorders.   Evidence of cell mediated immunity to antigens extracted from oral mucosa (2), enhanced cell mediated cytotoxicity for cultural oral epithelial cells (3) and B-cell activation (patients are   hypergammaglobulinemic)   (4)   strongly points out the immunologic pathogenesis in the unknown etiology of BD recently. Yet it is not clear whether these changes are primary to the pathogenesis of disease and/or secondary to another agent or mechanism. CyA included in BD's immunosuppressive treatment newly. It suppresses cellular immune system particularly inhibiting T4 cells and some of T suppressor, T cytotoxic and interleukin-2 producing T cells. It also inhibits production or release of lymphokines or both, including interleukin-2 and interleukin-1 (5).

A side effects caused by CyA is gingival hyperplasia (GH) (6). We interested in the ultrastructure of immunocompetent target cells that affected by CyA in BD's patients' gingiva who did or didn't display GH.

MATERIAL AND METHOD

Three groups arranged in each having 5 BD patients. First group (control) didn't have CyA treatment. Patients who had CyA, but didn't show GH assembled the second group. The ones displaying GH formed the 3rd. group. The specimens prefixed in 4% glutaraldehyde mixed in Milloning phosphate buffer at pH 7.3 and 0-4oC overnight and post fixed in 1% osmium tetroxide mixed in the same buffer, pH and temperature for 1h. They embedded in Araldit following ethanol dehydration. Sections stained with uranyl acetate and lead citrate.

RESULTS

Group 1 (BD patients)

Unusually there were intraepithelial mast cells (MC) interposed among the epithelial cells close to basal lamina. Interstitial spaces of epithelium widened with moderate desmosomal destruction. Fig. 1, 2. There were many MC in lamina propria which is a typical character for BD (7). The MC granules severally altered their normal morphology Fig. 3, 4.

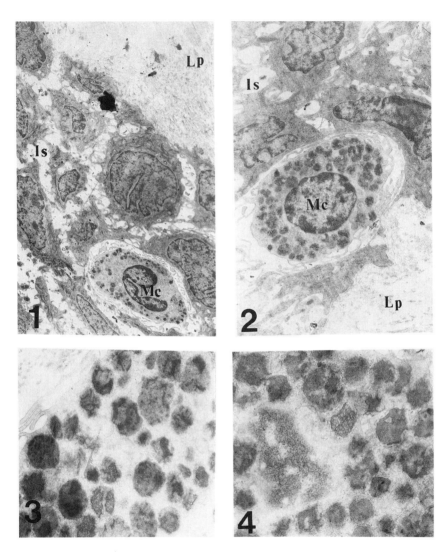

Fig. 1, 2. (Group 1). Epithelial lining of BD patients gingiva.
Lamina propria (Lp), Interracial spaces (Is), Mast Cell (MC)
Fig. 3, 4. (Group 1). Unusual MC granules of BD patients.

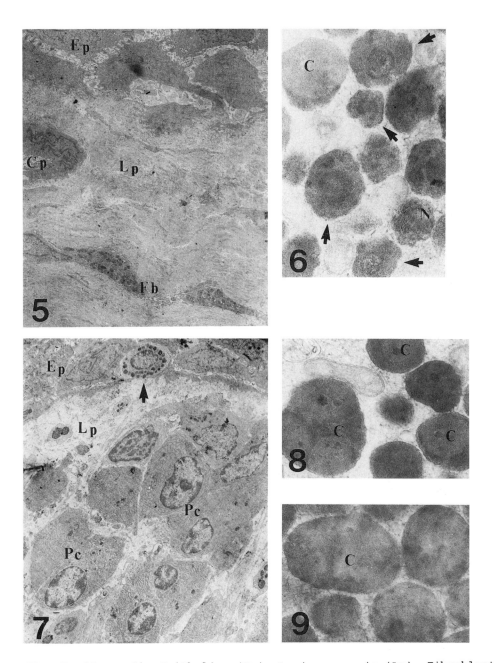

Fig. 5. (Group 2). Epithelium (Ep), Lamina propria (Lp), Fibroblast (Fb), Capillary (Cp),
Fig. 6. (Group 2). MCG with; electron dense cores (->), in crystalline form (C) and morphologically normal one (N).
Fig. 7. (Group 3). Epithelium (Ep), Lamina propria (Lp), Mast cell (->), Plasma cell (Pc),
Fig. 8, 9. (Group 3). MCG in crystalline form (C), Mitochondrion (Mt)

Group 2 (BD patients, +CyA, -GH)

The epithelium returned to its normal morphology and there were nearly no intraepithelial MC among epithelial cells. Fig. 5. MC granules changed their morphology. Some had electron dense cores, a few had crystalline form and some of them were morphologically normal. Fig. 6. These structural changes conferred initiation of supplementary cellular activity and possible maturation of new function changes. We think that the release mechanism of the granules inhibited by the action of CyA (8) and/or cellular immunosuppressive action of CyA resulted this alteration (5).

Fibroblasts and fibroblastic activity enhanced in this group Fig. 5. MC were in close neighborhood to these cells. CyA mainly inhibits cellular immune system. This reversible action suppresses T-Cell system including the lymphokines (9) that are cytotoxic for fibroblasts (10)

Group 3 (BD patients, +SyA, +GH)

There were again many intraepithelial MC present among epithelial cells neighboring basal lamina. Fig. 7. Interstitial spaces widened showing edema. Increased number of MC, plasma cells and fibroblasts located in edematous connective tissue in proximity Fig. 7. MC granules were similar to the ones described in group 2, but most of them were in crystalline form. Fig. 8, 9. We think that CyA's inhibition of granular release caused these changes.

Fibroblasts and Plasma cells were extensively active. Fig. 7 Inhibition of cellular immune system and T cell cytotoxicity to fibroblast helps gingival irritants to gain potential in provoking of GH. Absence of GH in edentulous mouth (11) or reversal of this pathological process following extraction of teeth (12), can point out the triggering role of antigens in the suppressed immune system with the action of CyA.

We believe in different populations of MC present in distinct parts of the body, as well as in different individuals, forming the different clinical effects.

REFERENCES

1. Behçet H (1937) Dermatol Monatsschir 105:1152-1157
2. Lehner T (1969) J Pathol 97:481-494
3. Rogers RS, Sams WM, Shorter RG (1974) Arch Dermatol 109:361-363
4. Takano M, Mizajuna T, Kiuchi M (1976) Tissue Antigens 8:95-99
5. American Hospital Formulary Service -Drug Information. Bethesda, MD, American Society of Hospital Pharmacists (1985) pp 826-828, pp 1731-1737, pp 612-613.
6. Friskopp J, Klintmalm G (1986) Swed Dent J 10:85-92
7. Lehner T (1969) J Path 97:481-487
8. Pedersen C et-al (1985) Allergy 40:103-107
9. Daley TD, Wysocki GP (1984) J Periodontal 55:708-712)
10. Wahl SM, Gately CL (1983) J Immunol 130:1226-1231
11. Wysocki GP, et-al (1983) Oral Surg 55:274-278
12. Rateitschak-Plüss EM, et-al (1983) 10:273-246

© 1991 Elsevier Science Publishers B.V.
Recent advances in periodontology Vol. II,
S.I. Gold, M. Midda and S. Mutlu, eds.

A STUDY OF PERIODONTAL ALTERATIONS IN REMOVABLE OVERDENTURE PROSTHESES RETAINED
BY MOLLOPLAST-B

K.SERHAN AKŞİT, VİLDAN GÖKSOY, METİN TURFANER
Istanbul University Faculty of Dentistry Department of Prosthodontics and Department of Periodontology, Çapa-Istanbul-34390 (Turkey)

INTRODUCTION

In this research of ours, attempts have been made to employ such kinds of
prostheses in the treatment of partial anodontic cases. Partial anodontics is a
frequently encountered anomaly in which the number and morphologic development of
teeth in either single or both jaws are not completed. In such cases, it is generally observed that occlusal relations are impaired vertical dimension in dynamic
occlusion is decreased, and that free-way space between the jaws is increased.
The aim in the prosthetic treatment of these cases is to preserve the existing
teeth and their periodontium in the oral cavity, thus rearranging the vertical
dimension and occlusal relations in compliance with physiologic conditions and
improving the esthetics, phonetics and function.

For about one-hundred years, various methods and materials have been suggested
and developed by authors to maintain the retainment of removable overdenture
prostheses applied in these cases: Springs, Suckers, magnets (8), various implants (6,8), telescope crown, Dolder bar, various anchors and clasps, etc.(3,12).

We have attempted for 8 years to maintain the retainment of removable overdenture prostheses by molloplast-B, which we have applied in partial anodontia cases
referring to our clinic. The procedure we employed in these cases (15), aims to
cover the abutment teeth for prostheses with Molloplast-B thick enough to attach
to prosthetic base material, and to allow the retainment of the prosthesis by
taking advantage of the elasticity of this material as in telescope system.

We present as an alternative to the prosthetic treatment of partial anodontics
our procedure which we have seen with our clinical observations (1,7), to have
functionally and physiologically positive results. We deem it useful to report
here the results obtained from those prostheses whose effects on periodontal
tissues we have found an opportunity to examine for 2 years out of those removable overdenture prostheses which we applied by this method.

MATERIAL AND METHODS

Our investigation has been realized on 5 cases of partial anodontics with 18-
20 years of age, who utilized removable overdenture prostheses retained by Molloplast-B.

Case 1: B.A, Female (protocol no.537); Case 2: I.K.,Male (protocol no.82);

Case 3: S.K., Female (protocol no.328); Case 4: A.B., Female (protocol no.298); Case 5: R.T., Male (protocol no.92).

In our cases, it was seen that no previous prosthetic or orthodontic procedure was carried out, and that no endodontic and marked periodontal problems existed except already known functional and occlusal anomaly.

In our investigation, these cases were examined by the following indices and measurements prior to the application of prostheses and at 15 days, 1 month, 3 months, 1 year, and 2 years after the prostheses were applied:

a) Quigley-Hein bacterial plaque index (by erythrocyine solutions.)

b) Gingival inflamation (SBI) index (as per Muhlemann and Son (1971)).

c) The measurement of the width of the attached gingiva (visually and by using periodontal probe and Schiller iodine solvent.)

d) The measurement of pocket depth.

e) Measurement of tooth mobility (manually)

FINDINGS

Values and averages we obtained by periodontal indice and measurements which we applied prior to and 15 days, 1 month, 3 months, 1 year, and 2 years after the application of prostheses in every 5 cases are listed in the tables below:

TABLE I

QUIGLEY-HEIN BACTERIAL PLAQUE INDEX VALUES

Number of case	Before wearing prostheses	15th Day	1st Month	3rd Month	1st Year	2nd Year
1	3.31	2.00	2.35	1.25	1.94	1.11
2	2.44	1.60	2.15	1.98	1.84	1.68
3	1.28	1.07	2.50	1.28	1.32	1.04
4	2.01	1.40	1.58	1.22	1.31	1.06
5	1.46	1.18	1.37	1.29	1.22	0.98
Average	2.10	1.45	1.99	1.40	1.52	1.17

TABLE II

FINDINGS OF GINGIVAL INFLAMATION (SBI) INDEX

Number of case	Before wearing prostheses	15th Day	1st Month	3rd Month	1st Year	2nd Year
1	1.62	1.39	1.50	0.68	1.35	1.29
2	0.23	1.95	1.99	2.38	2.97	2.66
3	1.28	3.45	2.28	2.04	0.92	0.18
4	1.45	1.28	1.40	0.77	1.19	1.12
5	1.08	1.37	1.46	1.23	1.34	1.12
Average	1.13	1.88	1.72	1.42	1.55	1.27

TABLE III
WIDTH OF THE ATTACHED GINGIVA (mm)

Number of case	Methods of Measurements	Before wearing prostheses	15th Day	1st Month	3rd Month	1st Year	2nd Year
1	Observation	7.37	7.37	6.37	6.50	5.88	6.66
	Schiller	6.62	6.50	6.00	5.87	5.66	6.44
2	Observation	4.47	4.26	4.76	4.68	4.56	4.18
	Schiller	4.31	4.15	4.71	4.32	4.06	3.80
3	Observation	6.71	5.71	5.35	4.57	3.50	3.63
	Schiller	5.00	4.71	4.71	4.07	3.59	3.83
4	Observation	6.42	6.31	5.91	6.02	5.78	5.89
	Schiller	6.28	6.16	5.73	5.84	5.63	5.82
5	Observation	5.35	5.24	5.48	5.29	5.18	4.89
	Schiller	5.04	4.81	5.01	4.69	4.38	4.22
Average	Observation	6.06	5.77	5.57	5.41	4.98	5.05
	Schiller	5.45	5.26	5.23	4.95	4.66	4.82

TABLE IV
FINDINGS OF POCKET DEPTH (mm)

Number of case	Before wearing prostheses	15th Day	1st Month	3rd Month	1st Year	2nd Year
1	2.56	2.40	2.09	1.85	2.51	2.20
2	1.07	1.75	2.39	2.42	2.74	2.25
3	1.96	2.07	2.14	1.90	1.13	0.70
4	2.63	2.48	2.33	2.16	2.35	2.19
5	1.11	1.42	1.52	1.59	1.39	1.15
Average	1.86	2.02	2.09	1.98	2.02	1.69

DISCUSSION AND RESULTS

There are opponents to those authors who report in the literature that over-denture prostheses applied by other procedures resulted in caries and periodon-tal problems (2,5,9,10,11,13).

In our investigation, although bacterial plaque index values have increased in 5 cases in the 1st month, this increase seems to have ceased at the end of 3rd months, and at the end of 1 and 2 years index values have decreased positively compared to those prior to the application of prostheses.

Regarding with SBI index whereas Ettinger, Taylor and Scandrett (4) reported that SBI values increased as a result of using overdenture prostheses produced by other method, it is understood in our cases that the changes in these values in our cases were related with hygenic factors rather than prosthetic factors. As a matter of fact, it was detected that in periods and cases when oral hygiene recei ved great care and attention, SBI values decreased positively compared to the values prior to prosthesis, but increased in otherwise cases.

In our investigation, a decrease has been determined which has been accepted to be within normal limits at the termination of two years of usage of prostheses in the measurements of attached gingiva width realized visually and by Schiller iodine solvent.

It was seen that the values of gingival pocket depth were changed depending on the hygenic factors. When we examined the changes in the tooth mobility manually, no negative difference was found in two years.

In conclusion, it was detected that overdenture prostheses retained by Molloplast-B had no negative effect on periodontal tissues, and that in the presence of a good oral hygiene, it provided positive improvements. This positive effect may be interpreted by stating that such elastic materials reported in the literature (11) allowed improvement in a short-time by stimulating blood circulation by vibro-massage on the impaired supporting tissues and that prostheses transmitted their vertical and horizontal compressions to the teeth and periodontium by reducing effects.

REFERENCES

1. Akşit KS, Göksoy V, Turfaner M (1988) Clinical investigations for removable overdenture prostheses retention achieved by Molloplast-B (This paper was read in the 5th International week for Dentistry in Istanbul, Turkey).

2. Bergman B, Hugoson A, Olsson C (1982) Caries, periodontal and prosthetic findings in patients with removable partial dentures: A ten year longitudinal study, J.Prosthet. Dent 48: 506.

3. Dolder EJ (1961) The bar joint mandibular denture, J.Prosthet.Dent 11:689

4. Ettinger RL, Taylor TD, Scandrett FR (1984) Treatment needs of overdenture patients in longitudinal study: Five-year results, J.Prosthet.Dent 52 (4):532-537.

5. Fenton AH, Hahn N (1978) Tissue response to overdenture therapy, J.Prosthet. Dent 40 (5):492-498.

6. Freedman H (1953) Magnets to stabilize dentures, J Am Dent Assoc 47:288

7. Göksoy V, Akşit KS, Turfaner M (1989) Periodontal investigations for removable overdenture prostheses in which retention was achieved by Molloplast-B in Partial Anodontia (Hypodontia) (This paper was read in the 7th scientific Congress of P.I.S in Antalya, Turkey).

8. Maghadam BK, Scandrett FR (1979) Magnetic retention for overdentures, J.Prosthet. Dent 41 (1): 26-29.

9. Reitz PV, Weiner MG, Levin B (1980) An overdenture survey: Second report, J. Prosthet. Dent.43 (4): 457-462.

10. Rissin L, House JE, Conway C, Loftus ER, Chauncey HH (1979) Effect of age and removable partial dentures on gingivitis and periodontal disease, J.Prosthet. Dent 42:217.

11. Rissin L, Feldman RS, Kapur KK, Chauncey HH (1985) Six-year report of the periodontal health of fixed and removable partial denture abutment teeth, J. Prosthet.Dent., 54 (4):461-467.

12. Thayer HH, Caputo AA (1977) Effects of overdentures upon remaining oral structures, J.Prosthet.Dent 37 (4):374-381.

13. Toolson LB, Taylor TD (1989) A 10-year report of a longitudinal recall of overdenture patients, J.Prosthet.Dent., 62 (2):179-181.

14. Turfaner M (1980) Problems of complete prosthesis and resorption, Istanbul, Turkey.

15. Turfaner M, Akşit KS (1988) The use of Molloplast-B for retention of removable overdenture prostheses in partial anodontia (Explanation of the method) (This paper was read in the 5th International week for Dentistry in Istanbul,Turkey)

© 1991 Elsevier Science Publishers B.V.
Recent advances in periodontology Vol. II,
S.I. Gold, M. Midda and S. Mutlu, eds.

Sustained Release Device Containing SrCl2 as treatment of dentinal hypersensitivity

Z. Mazor, DMD*
M. Friedman, Ph.D.**
D. Steinberg, Ph.D**
L. Brayer, D.M.D.*

* Dept. of Periodontics, Hebrew University, Hadassah Faculty of Dental Medicine, Jerusalem, Israel.

** Dept. of Pharmacy, Hebrew University, School of Pharmacy, Jerusalem, Israel.

INTRODUCTION

Dentinal hypersensitivity of cervical exposed dentin has long been a problem for both the patient and the dentist. Graf and Galasse have reported that no less than one out of seven patients suffers from hypersensitivity.

Clinical investigations for reducing cervical root hypersensitivity have shown that treatment with strontium chloride is effective. The exact mechanism whereby strontium and other desensitizing agent cause sensitivity reduction is unknown. It is assumed that its pharmacological action is by biochemical blocking of the neural transmission of stimuli through the nerve fibers, or by remineralization process. The cause for dentinal hypersensitivity can be incorrect tooth brushing, recession of the gingiva, periodontal surgery and habits. The present investigation was undertaken to reduce hypersensitivity of cervical dentin by application of strontium via sustained release device.

Slow release deevices have been used in pharmacy as a novel way of drug delivery. The use of S.R.D. is also been lately undergone research in the dental field. Sustained release devices have been used for plaque prevention and also as a an application to suppress the unmber of cariogenic bacteria in the oral cavity.

Slow release devices in the pharmaceutical form as a degradable film as non degradable film or as fibers have been used as a way of treating periodontal diseases. In this investigation a slow release device embedding strontium was applied on the surface of the teeth as a medicament for reducing dentinal hypersensitivity.

MATERIALS AND METHODS

110 teeth in twenty patients who had been reffered to the periodontal clinic due to dentinal hypersensitivity were selected. All patients have undergone oral hygiene instructions and scaling previously. Informed consent was signed by each patient. Teeth with hypersensitivity were selected and arbitrarily divided into three groups that received the following treatment modalities: strontium incorporated in a slow release device (SRD), placebo and - no treatment.

Each tooth was examined and scored according to the methods described by Gedalia et al and Minkov et al. The examination had been carried on after each sensitive tooth was isolated with a cotton wool roll and dried with an airstream. To assess the effect of thermal stimulation, cotton pellets soaked in crushed ice water were placed on the surface of the teeth. A cold temperature was chosen becuase teeth are generally more sensitive to low than to high temperatures. To assess the response to mechanical stimulation the cervical area of the tooth was carefully scratched by a standard dental explorer (S.S White no. 23).

The range of severity of the pain response for individual teeth could be classified as none, slight, or moderate according to the patient reaction. Severe pain was accompanied by closing of the eyelids, facial expression, and head movement. The pain categories were given numerical values of 1 (no pain), 2 (discomfort only), 3 (pain), 4 (severe pain) and 5 (umbearable pain).

Patients were examined and scored once a week in a double blind method by a trained periodontist who did not know to which gruop of treatment the teeth were assigned.

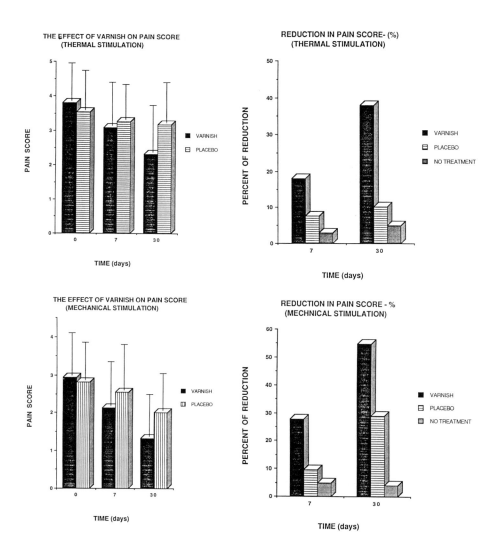

THE EFFECT OF VARNISH ON PAIN SCORE
(THERMAL STIMULATION)

REDUCTION IN PAIN SCORE- (%)
(THERMAL STIMULATION)

THE EFFECT OF VARNISH ON PAIN SCORE
(MECHANICAL STIMULATION)

REDUCTION IN PAIN SCORE - %
(MECHNICAL STIMULATION)

The application was carried out by the patients once a day for thirty days, according to the instructions given to them. Each patient was provided with codified vials for the local self applications with small nylon brush. Patients were instructed not to change their usual habits of oral hygiene during the experimental period and to record each daily application.

RESULTS

The results in our study after application of a sustained release device containing strontium indicated a reduction in dentine hypersensitivity.

The reduction was observed over the 30 days of the experiment both to the mechanical stimuli and to the thermal stimuli.

Both the sustained release varnish application containing strontium and the placebo application showed a significant decrease in hypersensitivity. Pain score reduction to thermal stimuli after 30 days was greater than after a week in the treated group (18%-38% respectively). The same trend was found with the mechanical stimuli, showing a 28% hypersensitivity reduction in pain score after a week and 54% after 30 days. The reducation in the pain score of the placebo application was also significant, however the level of pain reduction was lower compared to the treated group. It seems that the matrix of the device forms a coating over the surface of the teeth thus blocking the opening of the dentinal tubules and the presence of strontium in the matrix causes an additional improvement due to the specific pharmacological activity of the drug.

Our clinical findings indicate that a Sustained Release Device containing strontium may contribute to the treatment of dentine hypersensitivity.

© 1991 Elsevier Science Publishers B.V.
Recent advances in periodontology Vol. II,
S.I. Gold, M. Midda and S. Mutlu, eds.

THE HISTOLOGICAL INVESTIGATION OF GINGIVA FROM PATIENTS WITH CHRONIC
RENAL FAILURE AND RENAL TRANSPLANT RECEPIENTS

[1]N.YAMALIK   [2]L.DELİLBAŞI   [3]H.GÜLAY   [4]F.ÇAĞLAYAN   [5]M.HABERAL
[6]G.ÇAĞLAYAN

(1,4,6):DEPARTMENT OF PERİODONTOLOGY-FACULTY OF DENTISTRY,
        UNIVERSITY OF HACETTEPE-ANKARA-TURKEY.
(2):DEPARTMENT OF HISTOLOGY-EMBRYOLOGY,FACULTY OF MEDICINE,
        UNIVERSITY OF HACETTEPE-ANKARA-TURKEY.
(3,5):TURKISH ORGAN TRANSPLANTATION AND BURN THERAPY FOUNDATION,
        ANKARA-TURKEY.

INTRODUCTION

Many studies have investigated the effect of immunosuppressive therapy on
the various parameters of periodontal disease (1-7).It is not surprising
that drugs that alter the immune system are of considerable interest to the
periodontist.Schuller et al (1) were the first to demonstrate that immunosuppressive drugs given to renal transplant patients,reduced the inflammatory response
to bacterial plaque.There are also studies that have failed to show any significant difference in plaque accumulation,gingival inflammation or periodontal destruction when normal individuals were compared with dialysis patients and renal
transplant patients on immunosuppessive drugs (4).

Immunosuppressive agents provide an opportunity for investigating pathological
sequela of immune reactions in the gingiva. This study concerns the histological
investigation of gingiva from patients with chronic renal failure (CRF) and
renal transplant recipients (RTR) treated with immunosuppressive drugs following
renal transplantation.

MATERIAL AND METHODS

Patient selection: This study was conducted on 8 female and 12 male patients
who had undergone renal transplant procuders in the Turkish Organ Transplantation
and Burn Therapy Therapy Foundation Hospital,and 2 female and 10 male patients
with CRF who were treated in the same center with hemodialysis.Five female and 7
male patients who were in need of periodontal therapy were chosen among otherwise
healthy subjects. The mean age was $31,5 \pm 4,7$ for the RTR group, $31,6 \pm 2,12$ for
the CRF group and $31,9 \pm 1,59$ for the periodontitis group.

Clinical Studies: Plaque and Gingival Index (PI),(GI) scores of Löe (8) were
recorded in each patient. Also pocket depths were measured.Patients who had received periodontal therapy in the previous 6 months were not included in this study.

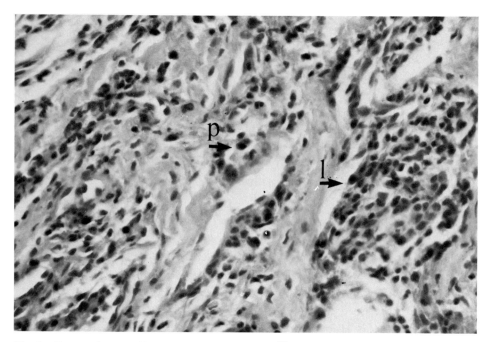

Fig.1. Mononuclear cell infiltration in the CRF group. P:Plasma cell, L:Lympocyte.

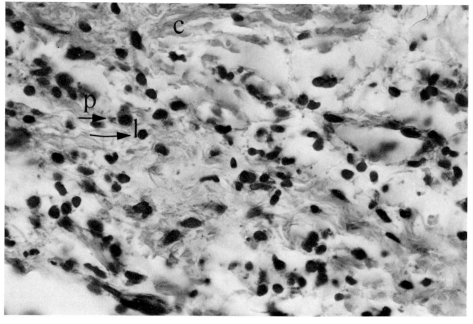

Fig.2. In the RTR group mononuclear cell infiltration and the presence of collagen. c:Collagen, P:Plasma cell, L:Lymphocyte.

Gingival biopsies were obtained from the patients following the clinical examinations.

Histological Studies: Gingival biopsies were prepared for light microscopic investigation and sections were stained with Hematoxylin-Eosin for routine observations. Additionally some of the sections were stained with Masson's Trichrome and
Verhoff-Van Gieson (9).Some sections were prepared for electron microscopic investigation and contrasted with Sato's lead nitrate,lead citrate and lead acetate
mixture (10).

Statistical Studies: Differences regarding the clinical parameters were determined by analysis of variance (11).

RESULTS

Clinical Findings: Data concerning the clinical parameters are given in the table.
The GI mean score was significantly lower in RTR group when compared to the other
2 groups ($p < 0,05$) although the PI mean scores did not differ significantly
($p > 0,05$). Pocket depths were significantly higher in the periodontitis group
($p < 0,05$).

TABLE   Data Concerning the Age,Sex and Clinical Parameters of the Patient Groups

Patient Groups	Pocket Depth $\bar{X} \pm S.E$	Gingival Index $\bar{X} \pm S.E$	Plaque Index $\bar{X} \pm S.E$
Renal Transplant Patients	$2,58 \pm 0,13$	$0,74 \pm 0,05$	$1,85 \pm 0,06$
Patients with Chronic Renal Failure	$2,58 \pm 0,19$	$1,82 \pm 0,11$	$1,98 \pm 0,08$
Patients with Periodontitis	$3,53 \pm 0,10$	$2,02 \pm 0,08$	$1,91 \pm 0,09$

$\bar{X}$:arithmetical mean

S.E:standad error.

Histological Findings: Achantosis,retepeg formation,increased vascularisation
and presence of a mononuclear cell infiltration were the common findings in all
of the specimens from the 3 groups (figure 1,2). In CRF group, prominent epithelial changes were noticed.In CRF group, in electron microscopic investigation
epithelial cells presented swollen cisternae of granular endoplasmic reticulum
(GER) (Figure 3).In RTR group, plasma cells and fibroblasts with well-developed
GER were noticed in the connective tissue. Although there is evidence that both
the uremic state and immunosuppession inhibit various immune responses, the patients were still able to mount a response to the existing bacterial plaque.

194

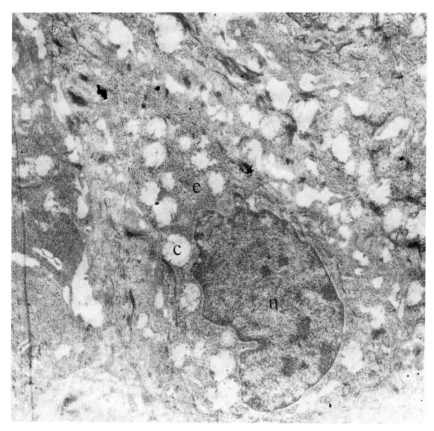

Fig.3. In the CRF group, epithelial cell which has swollen cisternae of endoplasmic reticulum resembling of vacuoles. e:epithelial cell,c:cisternae,n:nucleus.

REFERENCES

1. Schuller PD, Freedman HL, Lewis DW (1973) J.Periodontol 44:167-170.

2. Tollefsen T,Saltvedt E,Koppang HS (1975) J.Periodontal Res. 13:240-250.

3. Kardachi BJR,Newcombe GM (1978) J.Periodontol 49:307-309.

4. Oshrain HI, Mender SM, Mandel ID (1979) J.Periodontol 50:185-188.

5. Been V, Engel D (1982) J.Periodontol 53:245-248.

6. Tollefsen T, Koppang HS, Messelt E (1982) J.Periodontol Res.17:329-344.

7. Sutton RBO, Smales FC (1983) J.Clin.Periodont. 10:317-326.

8. Löe H (1967) J.Periodontol 39:610-616.

9. Mc Manus JFA,Mowry RW (1964) In:Staining Methods Histologic and Histochemical. New York,Evanston-London, pp.74.

10. Sato TA (1967) J.Electronmicroscopy 16:133-140.

11. Cohen L, Holliday,M (1982) In:Statistics for Social Scientists. London, pp.206.

© 1991 Elsevier Science Publishers B.V.
Recent advances in periodontology Vol. II,
S.I. Gold, M. Midda and S. Mutlu, eds.

FLOW VISUALIZATION OF MOUTH BREATHING IN ORAL CAVITY USING HYDROGEN BUBBLE TECHNIQUE

JUN ISHIKAWA, HITOSHI DOHKAI and HIROSHI KATO
Department of Periodontology, School of Dentistry, Hokkaido University, North 7, West 13, Sapporo, 060, JAPAN

INTRODUCTION

Nasal breathing is physiological, but mouth breathing is not. Mouth breathing is good only for auxilially purposes, for instance, hard musclular labor, heavy sports, psychial excitment, conversation and so on. Frequency of habitual mouth breathig is very high epidemiologically, and it is a big accerelating factor for periodontal disease — especially gingival inflammation. Because, it increases dental plaque accumulation and reduces tissue resistance due to gingival dehydration.[1] - [5]

Clinically, in habitual mouth breathers, the following findings are quite common; (1) lip seal insufficiency, (2) lip drying, (3) wrinkles in chin area associated with lip sealing, (4) multiple tooth decay in upper front teeth, (5) on labial side, mouth breathing line with prominent hyperplastic gingivitis, and (6) on palatal side, tension ridge, a belt-like hyperplastic swelling along with palatal gum margin, extending from front teeth to molar area.

The pupose of this study is to know three dimensional air flow pattern in oral cavity, and to make clear the relationship between tension ridge formation and air stream.

APPARATUS AND METHOD

A big water tank made of glass was prepared for this study. Its length was 120 cm, width was 20 cm and deapth was 40 cm, and a transparent three dimensional mouth model was fixed in the middle of this tank (Fig. 1 and 2).

To visualize water flow pattern, hydrogen bubble technique was used. Namely, as a cathode rays, a framed thin platinum wire (diameter 0.1 mm) was placed in front of upper incisal edge. When direct electric current passes through this intermittently, linear multiple minute bubbles are produced simultaneously from its surface, and it is called time line. To make those regular time lines repeatedly, a puls maker (made by Sugawara Co., Model 305) was used. Interval of each puls was 200 msec and its duration was 10 msec. Flow pattern of those lines were photographed and observed.

To inhale water into the transparent mouth model, the jaws were opened 2 mm in rest position, and its width was 5 cm. Accordingly, cross section of mouth opening was 1 square cm.

In water stream study, both of steady and unsteady flow pattern were examined. To reproduce inspiration phase of mouth breathing, the valve of water was controlled 12 times per minute just like human physiological respiration. Average speed of water flow was ascended and descended between 0-500 cm/sec, and its Reynold's Number was 0-667 respectively. Besides this, steady flow experiment was also made under three different speed. Namely, from high to low, 100 cm, 40 cm and 10 cm per second. To obtain equivalent Reynold's number of water stream to air flow, suction volume of water was controlled between 0-43 ml/sec. respectively.

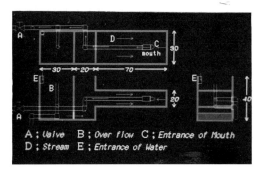

Fig. 1. Schematic drawing of experimental apparatus.   Fig. 2. Photograph of experimental apparatus.

RESULT

As the results of this experiment, we found the followings:

(1) Either in steady or unsteady flow experiments, there were no remarkable differences in their flow pattern.

(2) In steady flow experiment, water speed was changed in three stages, and basic flow pattern were almost same. However, in high speed, the pattern of time line showed one pyramidal peak, and in low speed, two peaks were observed (Fig. 3a and 3b).

(3) Three dimensional construction of flow patern was examined macroscopically and photographically, and two types of different stream were observed. Namely, one was main central flow and the other were lateral streams. From a view of sagittal direction, the main inhalation flow came into the oral cavity along the upper incisal edges, then, clashed against the palatal gum margin and ran into throat alongside the hard palate.

From a view of horizontal direction, the main stream entering through the central incisor area was same to the former pattern.

However, side streams entering through canine areas, progressed just like to join into the main stream, but these parts were separated from the main stream to right and left near the first molar teeth, then made a circle with descending motion. After making such spiral motion, side streams joined into the following central stream and progressed into the throat (Fig. 4).

(4) In order to corroborate this findings, another small experiment was made in the same apparatus using Uranin luminescent dye solution. To visualize dye solution linearly, three fine and long injection needles were fixed in front of the incisal edges. In high speed experiment, circular pattern similar in hydrogen bubble technique were observed following lateral stream, but in low speed study, there was not.

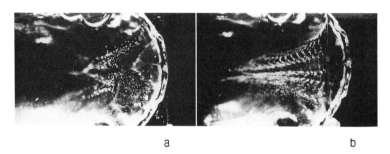

a   b

Fig. 3. Hydrogen bubble flow visualization on three dimensional mouth model viewed from horizontal direction.
a: in high speed (single projection), b: in low speed (double projections)

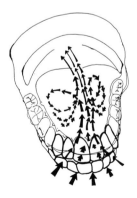

Fig. 4. Schematic drawing of inhalation stream in three dimensional mouth model.

DISCUSSION

Either in steady or unsteady stream, no remarkable difference was observed in their oral flow pattern. In steady flow observation, however, shape of time line was different according to speed.

A single pyramidal projection was observed in high speed, but two peaks were in low speed. As a reason of it, concentration power of high speed may be stronger than lower one. Concentrated main stream progressed toward the throat, but sides of it were separated in the soft palate area and turned back along the palatal surface of the molar teeth. This phenomena may mean that tension ridge extendes from the incisal to the molar region frequently.

Conclusion

To know the three dimensional pattern of inhalation stream associated with mouth breathig, a series of visualizing rheological study were made using hydrogen bubble technique in a transparent mouth model setting in a huge water tank.

The results of this study were as follows:

(1) Flow pattern in steady and unsteady stream, there were no remarkable difference.

(2) Shape of time line in steady flow experiment showed a single projection in high speed, but double peaks in low speed.

(3) The main stream after entering through incisal opening, it was concentrated and progressed to the throat, but sides of it were separated in the soft palate area and turned back along the palatal surface of the molar teeth.

(4) This turned back flow may indicate that tension ridge is not only limited in front teeth area but also extendes to the first molar region in many habitual mouth breathers.

REFERENCES
(1) Hsaio Feug HSU et al.: J.Japan.Ass.Periodont.27:554, 1985.
(2) Ichiro Kobayashi et al.: J.Flow Visualization Society of Japan, 4 Suppl:67, 1984.
(3) Toshiaki Mizuno:J.Japan.Ass.Periodont.27:739, 1985.
(4) Hitoshi Dohkai et al.: J.Japan.Ass.Periodont.29:853,1987.
(5) Jun Ishikawa: Hokkaido J.Dent.Sc.7:47,1986.

© 1991 Elsevier Science Publishers B.V.
Recent advances in periodontology Vol. II,
S.I. Gold, M. Midda and S. Mutlu, eds.

THE STUDY OF THE ORAL EFFECTS OF LEAD ON THE WORKERS WORKING IN PRESS WORKS

NURHAN AKSOY

Dicle Universty, Faculty of Dentistry, Dept. of Periodontology, Diyarbakır.

INTRODUCTION

Lead is a rare found but extensively spread metal in nature. The event that it has found a wide area of use in contemporary technology, is spoiling the natural distribution balance of the lead. In result of the activity of men, the lead is even being met at the regions of poles which are the most uninhabited places of the world.

The fact that it is necessary to spread the use of the benzine without lead, it threatens the human health directly through exhaust gases, and the fruits and the vegetables indirectly, the news about that lead existing in blood in the ratio of 50 μg/100 ml in urine 80 μg/100 ml causes death are in the agenda of our press[1,2].

In general men breath the lead from the air through respiration, foods through digestion and from the water they drink. The other sources of being exposed take their origins from the technological usage of lead. The formation of metal vapor on the employees working in lead mines and at the places where lead is processed in general the existence of the dusts of oxide of lead, cause the lead intoxication in different levels.

On the employees working in accumulator industry, lead pipe industry,press houses which are not modern, the lead exposition is pretty much. Since there isn't a hygienic work in Turkey and in the childhood begins the work the problem is important.

The lead compounds entering in the body through respiration, digestion and skin, by spreading into various organs and tissues with the blood flow accumulate especially in the bone tissue. It causes acute and chronic intoxication by making toxic effect on certain systems being clear on hematopoietic and nervous system in the body.

Besides the exposition sources such as air, water and food, it may happen to take in lead by cigarette too[2,3] The arsenic lead proportions found in tobacco show that the source of lead acetate which is used as insecticide. The quantity of lead per cigarette is between 10.4-15 μg. The quantity passing to the smoke is around 2%. So when 20 cigarettes are smoked the proportion of lead taken through inhalation is between 1-5 μg.

The clinical findings of the lead intoxication may be studied in three groups. The curable symptoms seen in early stage of intoxication, the more serious and long termed intoxication symptoms and sequela stage.

200

Some of the beginning symptoms are physical weakness, tiredness, sleeping
disorders, headache, pain in bones and ioints, constipation, pain in abdomen and
anorexia. More objective findings seen in this stage are paleness, Burton line
in dark gray blue colour about 1mm. in distance from the teeth on gingiva, me-
talic taste in the mouth, salivation and ulceration[4567] It is being arqued
that this streaking in the mouth on the ones whose mouth hygiens are insufficient
is a finding formed in result of precipitation of the lead sulphur at the submucosa after the lead unites with the hydrogen sulphide which occurs from the
waste food particles in the mouth[8] .It has been shown that the lead accumulates
on the dentin layer on the teeth by electron microscope. A weak relation has
been found between the quantities of the lead on the teeth and the bones and
hair, but a better relation with blood lead quantity
Under the light of these information we too have tried to determine the mouth
findings determined by being effected by lead among the press works employees
in Diyarbakır who are continuously in contact in their professions and the
effects of the criteria like oral hygiene, age, beginning age to work, duration
of work, professional branch, cigarette habit[9,10]

MATERIAL AND METHODS

Our study has been done on 80 men who are continuously in contact with lead
either directly or indirectly working at 23 different press houses in the province of Diyarbakır.

The names-surnames, addresses, professional branches, ages, the age of beginning work, the duration of working, habit of smoking cigarettes have been recorded on the forms beforehand by asking one by one. Intra oral examination has
been done and the plaque index (Silness-Löe) measures have been recorded from
$\frac{6 \mid 14}{41 \mid 6}$ numbered teeth. In order the date obtained in the study to be sound
and standard all these procedures have been followed by one doctor.

RESULTS

The press house workers are in touch with lead at different levels but continuously because their ages, begining ages to work, duration of work and different branches of profession.

The professional branches in the press houses are book binders, arrangers and
the other branches of work. The arrangers are the persons who deal with the
arrangement and the casting of the lead. The book binders is the group who deals
with the binding works. Their contacts with lead happen less often.

The ones who have less contact with lead and who we call the others, are the
employers, the administrators, the little children, the ones who do all the other
jobs other than arrangements, casting and binding.

All the men who have been taken in the study have been borned in Diyarbakır or around, almost the same in their socio-ecnomical conditions, not taking preventive measures and don't have means for their periodical controls to be done.

In Table. The ages, ages for beginning to work, the duration of work and the distributions according to the professional branchas are seen belonging to 80 men events.

TABLE I.

The distribution of the events according to the age, age for beginning to work, the duration of work and professional branch.

	Age Distr.		Age For Begin Work		Duration of Work(Year)		Professional Branch		
	18 and↓	18↑	15 and↓	15↑	5and ↓	5↑	Arr.,Binders,oths.		
Pers.	26	54	62	18	21	59	55	16	9

In Table II. The percentages of meeting the oral findings determined on the events are given. Burton line has been fixed in the highest proportion.

TABLE II.

The percentages of the oral findings to be met in the events.

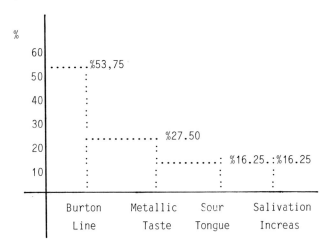

All the symptoms have been determined in higher percentages on adults, on the ones who have their durations of work over 5 years and on arrangers comparing the other groups.

We determined that the Burton line has been met in the highest proportion

(% 53.75). When we examine in accordance to the oral hygiene aspect while the plaque index avarages of the patients who have Burton lines is 1.80, the plaque index avarages of the patients having no Burton lines is 1.45. This difference is meaningful (p $<$ 0.05) (Table III). Besides when we search its relation with smoking cigarretes, we have determined that 79% of the patients showing Burton line symptom smoke cigarrettes (Table IV) (p $<$ 0,001).

TABLE III.
The comparison of the plaque scores of the two groups.

	Having Burton Lines (n = 43)		Not Having Burton Lines(n=37)	
	X	CD	X	CD
Plaque score	1.830	0.598	1.456	0.597
		t=2.59		p $<$ 0.05

TABLE IV.
The percentages of the smoking and not smoking.

Cigarrette Habits	Having Burton Line		Having No Burton Line	
Smoking	34	79%	7	18.9%
Not smoking	9	20.9%	30	81.1%

Metallic taste in the mouth, lead streaks on the gingiva, (Burton line), salivation increase are among the early stages of the lead intoxication.

In our events the Burton lines are seen in the rate of 53.75%, metallic taste in the mouth 27.50%, the salivation increase 16.25%, sour tongue 16.25%.

The appearance of the Burton line more in the persons who have insufficient mouth hygiene, supports the argument that this streaking has been formed by the hydrogen sulphide occuring from the food particles in the mouth and lead combination after lead sulphide procipitates in the submucosa. This too reveals the importance of the oral hygiene concerning individuals. This pigmentation is rather a cosmetic problem than being a medical one.

In our study all the symptoms on the cigarette smoking persons have been found high compared to the ones who don't smoke cigarette. The reason of this is bringing lead in the mouth by the hands through holding the cigarette at the moment of contact with it. Besides the cigarette gets contaminated with lead because of the usage of lead insecticides during tobacco cultivation.

Under the results of our study and the enlighment of the information in literature, on the asymptomatic persons who are are in contact with lead, the existence of the subjective and physical symptoms have to remind chronical intoxication and for the final diagnosis absorption and intoxication test have to be done. The blood lead level reflects the dynamic balance position between the lead quentities passing into the blood and accumulate on the tissues and discharged. Therefore the determination of lead in the blood, is a measurement of lead absorption in the blood. So the relation of the oral symptoms and the blood lead level has to be searchad.

At the places of work in which lead exposition exists the below indicated methods of protection have to be applied for sure.

1. In industry and in the places of work, the necessity of the arrangeement which will absorb the lead dusts and vapor immediately where they appear and throw out,

2. The cleaning of the places of work with wet means,

3. The shortening of the daily working hours of the workers working in the lead dusts and vapor and their being equipped with protective mask, (colloidal filter, fresh air current mask) protective clothing and hats,

4. The seperation of the places where the danger of meeting with lead exist from others completely,

5. The prohibition of eating, drinking and smoking at the places of work,are among these protective measures.

REFERENCES

1. "Güneş" newspaper (1990) 13 th of August.

2. Vural N, Güvendik G (1983) A survey of air and blood lead levels of population in Ankara Doğa Bilim Dergisi. 7:191-198

3. Vural N, Güvendik G (1984). Lead absorption in chuldren living in Ankara, related to environmental contamination A.Ü. Eczacılık Fakültesi Mec.Ankara. 109-115

4. Atlıhan F, Bilgin UV, Taş MA, Barış E, Gürer F (1989) A survey of toksic effects of lead on printers D.Ü.Tıp Fak. Derg. 16:2,pp 190-198

5. Environmental Health Criteria (1977) 3. Lead World Health Organization.Geneva.

6. Gazi MI (1986) Unusual pigmentation of the gingiva Oral Surg. Oral Med.Oral Pathol. 62:646-649.

7. Tal H, Landsberg J, Kozlovsky A (1987) Cryosurgical depigmentation of the gingiva. J. Clin. Periodontol 14:614-617.

8. Baloh R (1974) Laboratory diagnosis of increase lead absorption. Arch Environ Health 28:198.

9. Gilman AG, Goodman LS, Rall TW, Murad F (1985) Goodman and Gilman's the Pharmacological Basis of Therapeutics Seventh edition. Macmillan Publishery Company, New York

10.Wintrobe MM, et al.(1981) Clinical Hematology. Seventh edition, Philadelphia, Lead and Febiger, pp 662-664

© 1991 Elsevier Science Publishers B.V.
Recent advances in periodontology Vol. II,
S.I. Gold, M. Midda and S. Mutlu, eds.

PERIODONTAL HEALTH IN SJOGREN'S SYNDROME

SERDAR MUTLU, STEPHEN PORTER, ANDREA RICHARDS, KAREN PORTER, PETER MADDISON*,
CRISPIAN SCULLY

Centre for the Study of Oral Disease, University Department of Oral Medicine,
Surgery and Pathology, Bristol Dental School and Hospital, Lower Maudlin
Street, Bristol BS1 21Y (UK)
*Royal National Hospital for Rheumatic Diseases, Bath (UK)

INTRODUCTION

There is surprisingly little data on the nature and frequency of
periodontal disease in patients with Sjogren's syndrome. The only reported
study of periodontal disease in Sjogren's syndrome did not find any
increased liability to periodontal destruction, but only 14 patients were
examined and the study was not controlled (1).

Xerostomia in Sjogren's syndrome gives rise to a variety of oral
problems (2) including increased liability to sialadenitis, caries and
candidal infection, probably reflecting inadequate lubrication of mucosal
surfaces and/or quantitative and qualitative changes in salivary proteins
(3). An increased liability to periodontal disease has been noted with
xerostomia from other causes (eg post-radiotherapy and HIV-infection) (4,5).

The aim of the present investigation therefore, was to compare the
periodontal status of patients with Sjogren's syndrome with that of
individuals without dry mouth. A disease control group comprising individuals
with connective tissue disorders other than Sjogren's syndrome and without
xerostomia was included, as well as a group of healthy controls. The former
control was used to exclude any effects of anti-inflammatory or immunosuppressive therapy.

MATERIALS AND METHODS

Patient groups

The Sjogren's syndrome (SS) group comprised 28 patients (primary SS:
6, secondary SS: 22) (26 female; median age 49 years, range 26-70) with
clinical (clinically demonstrated keratoconjunctivitis sicca and xerostomia),
labial salivary gland histopathological and serological features of primary
or secondary Sjogren's syndrome (2). The disease control group comprised 37
patients (31 female; median age 48 years, range 18-76 years) with a variety
of connective tissue diseases (CTD) (similar to those in secondary SS) other
than SS, but without xerostomia and sicca syndrome. Patients in the SS and
CTD groups were receiving similar anti-inflammatory or immunosuppressive
therapies. The healthy control group comprised 25 individuals (23 females;

median age 44 years, range 24-65 years) without clinical evidence of
connective tissue disease or xerostomia, and not receiving anti-inflammatory
or immunosuppressive therapy. Xerostomia in all individuals was assessed by
whole unstimulated sialometry (2).

Assessment of gingival and periodontal health

Plaque indices were determined by the method of Silness and Loe (1964)
(6), gingival indices by the method of Loe and Silness (1963) (7) and periodontal pocket depths with a calibrated periodontal probe. Student's t-test
was employed for all statistical analyses.

RESULTS

Comparison of the plaque indices, gingival indices, and periodontal
pocket depths between each patient group are shown in Table 1. Although
there were no significant differences in plaque or gingival indices between
patient groups, those with Sjogren's syndrome and those with other connective
tissue disorders had significantly reduced periodontal pocket depths compared
with healthy control individuals. Patients with Sjogren's syndrome had
significantly greater periodontal pocket depths compared with those with
other connective tissue disorders. There were no correlations between
duration of Sjogren's syndrome or connective tissue disease, or systemic
therapy and the degree of periodontal destruction (data not shown).

TABLE 1

COMPARISON OF MEAN PLAQUE INDICES (PI), GINGIVAL INDICES (GI) AND PERIODONTAL
POCKET DEPTHS (PD) BETWEEN PATIENTS WITH SJOGREN'S SYNDROME (SS), OTHER
CONNECTIVE TISSUE DISEASES(CTD) AND HEALTHY CONTROLS

Comparisons	GI	PI	PD
SS/healthy controls	$p>0.05$	$p>0.05$	$p<0.05$[1]
CTD/healthy controls	$p>0.05$	$p>0.05$	$p<0.01$[1]
SS/CTD	$p>0.05$	$p>0.05$	$p<0.05$[2]

[1]Significantly decreased in disease groups compared with healthy controls
[2]Significantly increased in Sjogren's syndrome compared with CTD

DISCUSSION

The results of the present investigation indicate that patients with
connective tissue diseases, other than Sjogren's syndrome, have similar

plaque and gingival indices but reduced periodontal destruction compared
with healthy controls. Patients with Sjogren's syndrome have a similarly
decreased liability to periodontal destruction but have greater periodontal
pocket depths than patients with the other connective tissue diseases. The
precise pathogenic mechanism of the relatively greater periodontal disease
in Sjogren's syndrome is unclear: it may perhaps reflect alterations in
salivary constituents or a more periodontopathic oral microflora.

The reduced periodontal destruction compared with healthy controls in
all the connective tissue disorders, including Sjogren's syndrome, accords
with recent observations in rheumatoid arthritis (8), though one report
showed increased periodontal destruction in rheumatoid arthritis patients
(9). The present group of patients, unlike those previously reported with
reduced periodontal disease (8), did not have significantly better oral
hygiene than healthy control patients. This decreased liability to periodontal destruction in connective tissue diseases might be due to the effects
of long term administration of non-steroidal anti-inflammatory or immunosuppressive drugs (9). The mild immunodeficiency seen in CTD may also reduce
susceptibility to periodontal destruction (10). It is also possible that
the periodontal microflora in connective tissue disease is of lower
pathogenicity (9) but there is no evidence to support this notion at present.

In conclusion, while patients with connective tissue disorders may
have an overall reduced liability to periodontal destruction, the xerostomia
in Sjogren's syndrome appears to modulate this. Nevertheless, the level of
periodontal disease is still below that of otherwise healthy individuals.
The pathological mechanisms accounting for this observations are not, as
yet, known.

ACKNOWLEDGEMENTS

S Mutlu was supported by a Turkish Government Scholarship and the
authors wish to thank Miss Connie Blake for the careful typing of this
manuscript.

REFERENCES

1. Tseng CC, Wolff LF, Rhadus N, Aeppli DM (1990) The periodontal status
    of patients with Sjogren's syndrome. J Clin Periodontol 17: 329-330.

2. Scully C (1986) Sjogren's syndrome: clinical and laboratory features,
    immunopathogenesis and management. Oral Surg Oral Med and Oral Pathol
    62: 510-523.

3. Greaves D, Whicher JT, Bhoola KD et al (1989) Anionic salivary proteins
    associated with connective tissue disorders: sialated tissue kallikreins.
    Ann Rheum Dis 48: 753-759.

208

4. Wight WE (1985) An oral disease prevention programme for patients receiving radiation and chemotherapy. JADA 110: 43-47.

5. Porter SR, Scully C, Greenspan D (1990) In: Jones JH, Mason DK (eds) Oral manifestations of systemic disease. Balliere Tindally, London (in press).

6. Silness P, Loe H (1964) Periodontal disease in pregnancy. Acta Odont Scand 22: 121-135.

7. Loe H, Silness P (1963) Periodontal disease in pregnancy. Acta Odont Scand 21: 533-551.

8. Sjostrom L, Laurell L, Hugason A, Hakansson P (1989) Periodontal conditions in adults with rheumatoid arthritis. Com Dent Oral Epidemiol 17: 234-236.

9. Tolo K, Jorkjend L (1990) Serum antibodies and loss of periodontal bone in patients with rheumatoid arthritis. J Clin Periodontol 17: 288-291.

10. Porter SR, Scully C (1990) In: Jones JH, Mason DK (eds) Oral manifestations of systemic disease. Balliere Tindally, London (in press).

© 1991 Elsevier Science Publishers B.V.
Recent advances in periodontology Vol. II,
S.I. Gold, M. Midda and S. Mutlu, eds.

A SCANNING ELECTRON MICROSCOPIC STUDY OF THE EFFECT OF DOXYCYCLINE ON BACTERIAL INVASION IN CEMENTUM AND RADICULAR DENTIN

KÖKSAL BALOŞ-LEVENT KORALP-KAYA EREN-COŞKUN BARAN-BELGİN BAL
Periodontology Department of Dental Faculty of Gazi University
8.cad.Emek,Ankara(The Turkey)

INTRODUCTION

It has been demonstrated that the bacteria which lead to destructive periodontal disease invade the soft tissues(4-6).

Especially regarding the root surfaces,some researchers have indicated that bacterial products contaminate periodontally involved root surfaces and cause pathological changes in the cementum(3-5).

Also,there some limited reports pointing out that bacteria themselves invade the hard tissues,even in the dentinal tubules(1-2).

In this study our aim was to investigate if there were bacteria or not in the radicular dentin of the adult periodontitis involved teeth.In the cases where bacteria were present in radicular dentin our aim was to observe the effects of systemic antibiotics,scaling and root planing on these bacteria.

MATERIAL AND METHODS

11 individuals having adult periodontitis participated in the study.Anterior teeth with 3rd degree of mobility and symmetrical horizontal and vertical defects were selected.

4 teeth from each patient,in total 44 teeth were extracted in order to investigate the individual effects of 2)scaling and root planing,3)systemic effect of Doxycycline and 4)their combined effects.The teeth were extracted at the first,14th and 28th days respectively(Fig.1).

None of these teeeth had any clinically detectable carious lesions or restorations.

Immediately after extraction the teeth were rinsed with a physiologic saline solution and were prepared for SEM evaluation(2). After these procedures the specimens were examined in a Leitz-Amray 1000 Scanning Electron Microscope.

210

THE STUDY PLAN

4 teeth from each patient

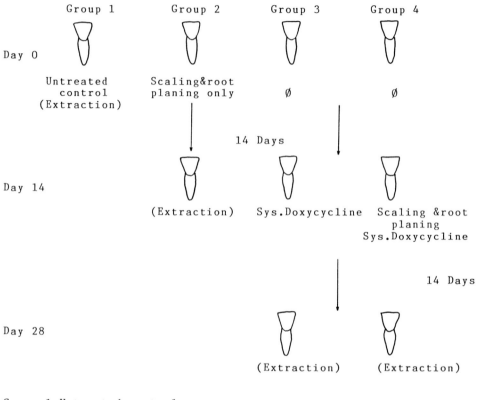

Group 1   Group 2   Group 3   Group 4

Day 0

Untreated   Scaling&root
control   planing only   Ø   Ø
(Extraction)

14 Days

Day 14

(Extraction)   Sys.Doxycycline   Scaling &root
planing
Sys.Doxycycline

14 Days

Day 28

(Extraction)   (Extraction)

Group 1:Untreated control
Group 2:Scaling & root planing only
Group 3:Systemic Doxycycline
Group 4:Scaling & R.planing+ Systemic Doxycycline

Fig.1. The Study Plan

RESULTS

In the control group,consisted of 11 untreated teeth,only 2 of
the roots showed few areas of resorption,dentinal tubules and
debris.Coccoid and rod-like structures were also found around
these orifices(Fig.2).

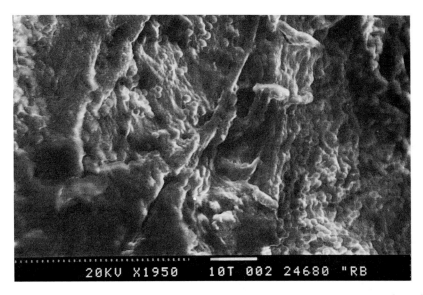

Fig.2:Resorption areas,dentinal tubules,debris,coccoid and
rod-like structures are seen on the control root surfaces.

In this control group no bacterial invasion was detected in
any of the dentinal tubules,beneath the cementum(Fig.3).

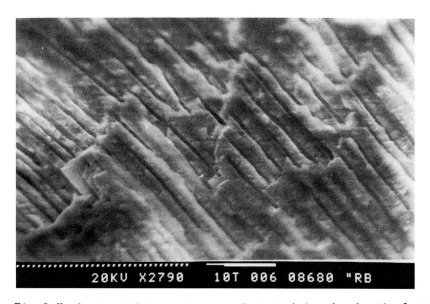

Fig.3:No bacterial invasion was detected in the dentinal tubules
in the control group.

212

The same results were found in the other three groups also(Fig4).

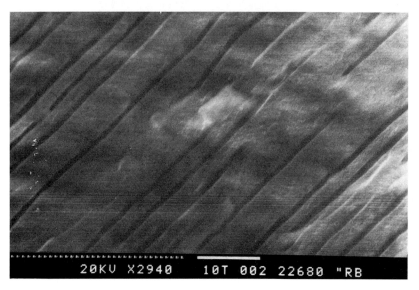

20KU X2940   10T 002 22680 "RB

Fig.4:There is no bacterial invasion in the dentinal tubules

In our study no bacterial invasion could be traced in the
dentinal tubules,but few bacteria were found in the limited
areas of cemental resorption.However,according to Saglie(7),
there some limitations in the SEM studies for bacterial identification.

REFERENCES
1. Adriens PA,De Boever JA,Loesche WJ (1988) J Periodontol.59:493
2. Adriens PA,Edward CA,De Boever JA,Loesche WJ(1988) J Periodontol
   59:222
3. Aleo JJ,Renzis De FA,Farber PA (1975) J Periodontol 46:639
4. Carranza FA,Saglie FR,Newman MG,Valentin PL (1983) J Periodontol
   54:598
5. Daly CG,Seymour GJ,Kieser JB,Corbet EF (1982) J Clin Periodontol
   9:266
6.Saglie FR,Carranza FA,Newman MG (1985) J Periodontol 56:619
7. Saglie FR (July-1990) Personal Comminication (in manuscript)

© 1991 Elsevier Science Publishers B.V.
Recent advances in periodontology Vol. II,
S.I. Gold, M. Midda and S. Mutlu, eds.

A STUDY OF MICROBES, ANTIMICROBIAL AGENTS SUSCEPTIBILITY AND RESISTANCE TESTING OF HUSBAND AND WIFE ORAL FLORA.

Prof. Dr. M. A. Soofi.
BDS (PB) DPD (UK) MICD (HON)
Chairman,
Department Dental Public Health,
College of Community Medicine
Lahore. (Pakistan).
Dr. Fakhar-ul-Islam. MBBS. DCP.
Dr. Mrs. Madiha Emran, MBBS
Dr. Emran Amir, MBBS
Services Hospitals, Lahore (Pakistan).

PURPOSE:

The purpose of this study is to compare the composition of cultivable micro-flora in the oral cavity of husband and wife for application of anti-microbial agents for control of periodontal diseases and to find out bacteriological agent responsible for causation of this disease by disc-method at 37°C for 48 hours in incubation.

The presence of a bacterial flora in the oral cavity is considered of importance and therefore its composition has been observed in two different close contact mouths. This information becomes interesting for detailed knowledge.

INTRODUCTION:

While dealing with clinical diagnosis, management and investigations of various types of periodontal cases, laboratory aids were sought for broad spectrum antibiotic coverage. Reports from laboratory of direct smear examination and culutre sensitivity test when received for treatment in my private surgery at Lahore, is different from the other life partner who have go close contact. Therefore, I decided to isolate such pairs for study. However, the present data is of isolation of common bacteria of clinically suspected cases of periodontitis and such observations were evolved during routine treatment and surgery.

OCCURANCE:

Viability and identification of the oral microbial flora between the husband and wife was studied using aerobic techniques. The 50 pairs were checked clinically for complaints of bleeding gums, watery mouth and shaky teeth. Specimen of pus from the 50 pairs were taken. All the patients were of average 40 years age.

No growth occurred in 3 cases. Growth of identical bacteria was observed in 21 pairs on culturing and direct bacteriological examination and 29 cases were found to have different flora in the husband and wife. Similarly some pairs with identical flora had different sensitivity to antibiotics.

INDIRECT SMEAR EXAMINATION:

Microbial flora, observed was mixed i.e. G+iv Cocci, Fusiformis and Vibrioes, and in cutlure was mainly of Staphylococcus pyogens, Streptococcus Pneumoniae and Actinomyces etc. The composition of the flora in all such cases, was similar to that which may be observed in dental plaque and that found in other studies.

MATERIAL AND METHODS:

Subjects of Periodontal patients (Husband & Wife)
Identification for Various microbes.

Tools a.   Bacteriology laboratory & Microbiologist.

        b.   Peri apical Radiographs.

        c.   Dental Unit, Chair & Examination Instruments like WHO Probe, Dental Mirror, and Tweezer.

SUBJECTS:

Bleeding and inflammed gingivae, moderate and advanced periodontal cases are common clinical conditions, which come across in our domicillary as well as teaching clinical practice. These alongwith many other clinical conditions are generally bacterial in origin and thus bacterial diagnosis becomes essential and these conditions need to be managed for antimicrobials. Recognition of various pathogens becomes essential for antimicrobial therapy so sensitivity and resistance testing is being done by the standard disc diffusion method.

The specimen samples were collected from 100 cases of (Husband and wife) clinically diagnosed advanced destructive periodontitis, moderate periodontitis and marginal gingivitis in our routine examination for planning the treatment of periodontal surgery. These patients were referred to this surgery from different parts of city and the province both by medical and dental practitioners. However, the present data is for isolation of common bacteria of clinically suspected cases of periodontitis and such observations are evolved during routine treatment and surgery.

MATERIAL AND METHODS:

Before examination of the oral cavity of each pair, a detailed record chart was filled, teeth were blasted with dry air and a sterile curette was used to take exudate from the sulcus of infected teeth. It was transferred to cotton swabs on wooden sticks prepared and sterilised by autoclaving and the sticks are kept in autoclaved test tubes for this process.

These swabs are then streaked all over the blood agar plate three times and are kept at room temperature after closing the upper lid for a few minutes and kept at 37oC for 24 hours and next day the colonies are isolated and bacterias are identified through type of colony and staining under microscope.

The antibiotic discs of various types are placed on the agar plate having a diameter of 9 - 10 cm. Each disc is pressed down gently to ensure even contact with medium to further 24 hours in incubation at 37oC and results are prepared.

RESULTS:

Direct smear results in 100 cases (50 pairs).
*	Gram +ve	65 cases
*	Fusiformis bacilli	19 cases
*	Gram -ve	1 cases
*	Only pus cells & epethial cells	15 cases

Culture and sensitivity test - 100 cases (50 pairs)

		male	female
*	Staphylococcus Pyogenes	20	30
*	Non-Haemolytic streptococcus	13	9
*	Haemolytic streptococcus	3	2
*	Strepto pneumoniae	4	4
*	Micrococci	4	1
*	Fusiformis bacilli	1	1
*	Haemolytic influenza	-	1
*	Escherichia Coli	1	-
*	Normal Flora	4	2

Types of microbes in 21 identical cases.
*	Staphylococcus pyogenes	14 cases
*	Streptococcus pnemoniae	4 cases
*	Staphylococcus aureus	1 cases
*	Non-haemolytic streptococcus	2 cases

Types of microbes in 29 non-identical cases
* Staphylococcus pyogene   18 cases
* Non-Haemolytic streptococcus 18 cases
* Escherichai coli.   4 cases
* Fusiformis bacilli,   2 cases
* Pathogene micrococci   5 cases
* Haemolytic influenza   1 cases
* Normal flora   3 cases

Types and No. of organisms in the two sexes.

		Male	Female
*	Staphylococcus Pyogene	30	20
*	Non-Haemolytic streptococcus	9	13
*	Haemolytic streptococcus	2	3
*	Streptococcus pneumoniae	4	4
*	Micrococci	1	4
*	Fusiformis bacilli	1	1
*	Haemolytic influenza	1	-
*	Escherichia coli	-	4
*	Normal flora	2	1
		-----	-----
		50	50

DISCUSSION:

All the cases had the periodontitis, resulting in the destruction of periodontal fibers and alveolar - bone loss as confirmed by the radiographs. The severity and rate of progression of disease varied not only from husband to wife but in certain cases from tooth to tooth in the same patient. The younger pairs also had the progression of the lesion supported by microbial results of the laboratory and radiographs. We have observed that he periodontal lesions were mostly localised to the molars and incisors which were involved in more advance disease. In certain cases the bone loss was accompanied by apical migration of the epithelial cells and then attachment in the anterior region.

The results of the laboratory has adequately demonstrated that the micro-organism cultured out of these cases were the aetiological agents. Certainly the dental plaque was the primary agent for implicating the periodontitis as observed (1) , (2), (3), (4).

The variation of the flora from mouth to mouth is different in our study and (5), (6) observed that the plaque flora varies from site to site within the same mouth as well as from individual to individual. Therefore, in our study a finite number of same species of bacteria were present in both the sexes. We found many gram+ve cocci in the direct smear and culture sensitivity examination in our study which confirms (1), (7),(8),(9),(3). The same has been observed in experimental gingivitis, where the predominant organisms were mostly gram+ve, (1),(7),(10). In our studies of most of the cases of long standing gingivitis and periodontitis, we have found gram-ve organisms in the sub-gingival sites taken out with the currette for testing. Similarly the studies of (8), (4), in which the longstanding gingivitis found with the microbial plaque having gram+ve approximately 25% of the organism were observed gram-ve, located primarily on the areas of the plaque in contrast with the tissues in the sub-gingival sites.

In our examination of the sub-gingival exudate associated with the destructive and advanced periodontitis, we have found the organisms like anaerobic gram-ve as (11) observed. The objective of these tests was to find out a treatment planning of in order to control the infection and inflammatory conditions for advance treatment, because this therapy i.e first to suppress or inhibit frowth of bacteria and then interference with surgery proves most successful. The potential pathogene on one hand are controlled due to proper concentrated use of anti-microbial agents against the specific organisms according to the lab: reports. This provides the better and longstanding results and the disease has been seccessfully treated. However, the disease have been first controlled by regular mechanical removal of supra-gingival and sub-gingival deposits though in certain cases this procedure becomes difficult and we do the ultra-sonic currettage. Consequently, the disease is controlled and chronic infection is eradicated.

Among such clinical cases of periodontism, samples and results show variation in the type of micro-organisms, inspite of the fact that husband and wife have close relations and transmission of the micro-organisms is very much possible. This demonstrates that the concept of droplet or cross infection is to be considered again. The micro-organisms flourish according to the type of environment. It depents upon the type of oral aptitude of the individual which provides the substrate to the bacteria. Saliva and its consistency provides the chance for initiation for the plaque and calculus formation, and the fluids secreted in various of food, the plaque the supragingival calculus, provide the chance to bacteria for irritation to the local tissues for production of enzyme and pocket formation. The plaque on tooth causes the gingival inflammation and stands for pocket formation and these pockets provide shelter to bacteria for advancing disease of periodontal domain.

CONCLUSION:

After having study the culture sensitivity reports of 50 couples the following observation were made: -

a.   21 couples out of 50 were those suffering from periodontal disease caused by identical organisms.

b.   29 couples out of 50 were those suffering from periodontal diseases caused by non-identical organisms.

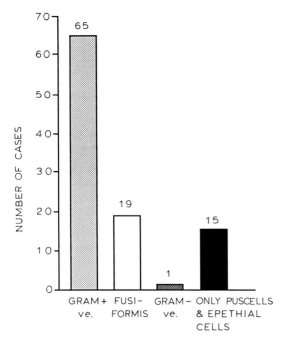

Figure 1. A study of oral flora in husband and wife.
Direct smear results in 100 cases (50 pairs)

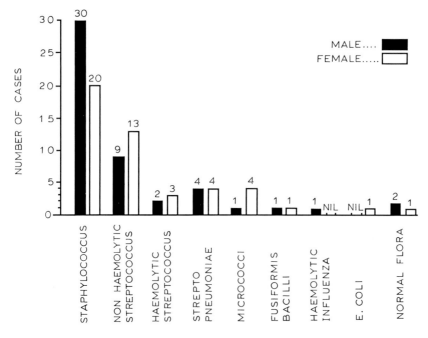

Figure 2. A study of oral flora in husband and wife.
Types and numbers of organisms in the two sexes.

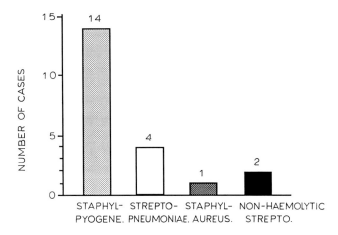

Figure 3. A study of oral flora in husband and wife.
Types of microbes in 21 identical cases.

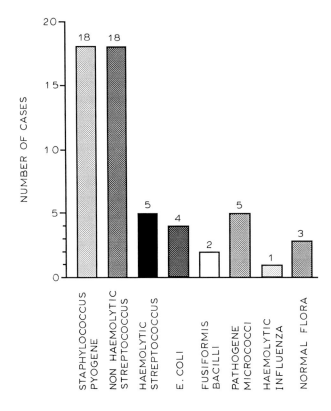

Figure 4. A study of oral flora in husband and wife.
Types of microbes in 29 non-identical cases.

This indicates that Staphylococcus is the microbes which is most commonly and easily transmitted from one person suffering from the periodontal diseases to the direct contact and other who is the closest and in direct contact.

Among the 29 couples who were suffering from periodontal disease a variety of organisms were seen to be the causative organisms.

REFERENCE:

1.   Loe H.Theilade E. and Jensed S.B.(1965). Experimental Gingivitis in man. J.Periodontal 36.177-187.

2.   Genco R.J.Evans R.T. and Ellison S.A.(1969). Dental Research in J.A.D.A. 78, 1016 - 1036.

3.   Socransky S.S. (1977), Microbiology of periodontal disease, present status and future consideration. J.Periodontal 48.

4.   Slots J.Mashimo P.Levine M.J.et al (1979) Periodontal Therapy in humans. Microbiological and clinical effects of a single course of periodontal scaling and root planning as an adjunct to tetracycline, J.Periodontal, 50, 495 - 509.

5.   Bowden G.H.Hardie J.M. and Slack G.L. (1975), Microbial variations in approximal dental plaque. Caries Res. 9,253 - 277.

6.   Moore W.E.C Holdeman L.V.Cato E.P.et al (1984) variation in periodontal floras. Infect Immun. 46, 720 - 726.

7.   Listagartem M.A.Mayo H.E. and Treamblay R. (1975) Development of Dental plaque on epoxy resin crowns in man. A light and electron-microscope study. J.Periodontal 46. 10-26.

8.   Listagartem M.A. (1976) Structure of the microbial flora associated with periodontal disease and health in man. A light electron-microscope study.J.Periodontal 47, 1 -18.

9.   Slots J. (1977a). The microflora in the healthy gingival sulcus in man. Scand J.Dent. Res. 85,247 - 254.

10.   Syed S. A. Loesche W. J. and Loe H. (1975), Bacteriology of Dental plaque in Experimental Gingivitis. II-Relationship between plaques score and flora. J.Dent. Rest. 54 - 72. abstract - 109.

11.   Slots J.(1977b). The predominant cultivable microflora of advanced periodontitis. Scand. J.Dent. Res. 85, 114 - 121.

© 1991 Elsevier Science Publishers B.V.
Recent advances in periodontology Vol. II,
S.I. Gold, M. Midda and S. Mutlu, eds.

CHANGES OF MICROFLORA IN EXPERIMENTAL ACUTE GINGIVAL LESION
EXPERIMENTAL STUDY ON CHANGES OF MICROFLORA IN ACUTE GINGIVAL
LESION

TAKASHI YAEGASHI,TERUYUKI YANAGAWA,ATSUSHI KUMAGAI,KEN KANNO AND
KAZUYUKI UYENO

Dept.of Periodontol.,School of Dent.,Iwate Med.Univ.,
1-3-27 Chuo-dori,Morioka-shi,Iwate-ken,Japan

INTRODUCTION

 Acute necrotizing ulcerative gingivitis (ANUG) is characterized
by necrosis which begins at the tips of the inter-dental
papillae. It is known that Spirochetes and Fusobacterium increase
in the lesion. However, the relationship between these microbes
and symptoms of this disease hasn't been clarified yet. Some
studies on this subject reported that the production of ANUG-like
lesions in animals was very difficult, and no right and strong
conclusion was obtained. We've indicated that these microbes have
significant relations with the clinical state of lesions, rather
than with pathogenic activities through the clinical cases and
experimental studies we observed.
 The present study was carried out to show the production of
ANUG-like lesions in animals and the change in the number of
microbes with the clinical states advancing.

MATERIAL AND METHODS

 Three adult beagle dogs were used in this experiment. The
gingiva of incisor and premolar site in both upper and lower jaws
of these dogs were selected as the experimental sites. In order
to produce ANUG-like lesions, two ways were used: one was the
application of the free gingival graft to denuded bones, and the
other was the application of arsenious acid salt to experimental
sites. Macroscopic, histologic and microbiologic examinations of
ANUG-like lesions were carried out before and seven days after
the production of the lesions. Particularly in microbiologic
investigations, we gave attention to two microbes: Spirochetes
and Fusobacterium, which have been reported in many studies to be
relevant to ANUG.

As for Spirochetes, after irrigation of the gingival surface, each sample was taken from the surface by one-minute contact of a sterile paper point with the lesion. Immediately the sample was put in a test tube containing three mililiters of phosphate buffered saline (PBS). After dispersion of the sample, one drop of the suspension was applied to a microscopic slide. The smears were methanol-fixed and Giemsa-stained. They were investigated by a light microscopy at a magnification of one thousand. In five microscopic fields at random, various types of Spirochetes were counted on each sample. The mean value of each sample was calculated and recorded. In order to observe the change of microflora, the healthy gingival sites were investigated before the production of lesions as control.

As for Fusobacterium, each sample was taken in a similar way to the Spirochetes's sample. Immediately the sample was put in a test tube containing three mililiters of ABCM-broth. Then the bacterial suspension was dispersed by a vortex mixer, and 0.03 mililiters of the undiluted solution were applied to a selective medium (modified FM culture medium) in order to isolate Fusobacterium species from the specimens. The solution was plated on the whole medium with a conlarge bar. The medium was the modified FM culture medium in order to isolate Fusobacterium species from the specimens. After anaerobic incubation for seven days at thirty seven degrees centigrade, the colony forming units grown (CFU), were counted, and some of the colonies were isolated for the further identification with a minitek system which includes about twenty biochemical character tests.

RESULTS

Fig.1 exhibits the macroscopic view after the production of lesions. These lesions were induced by bad local circulation of blood by the application of free gingival graft to denuded bones. The necrotic and ulcerous sites were observed in a part of the Fig.1. In the lesions induced by a strong chemical stimulus of arsenious acid salt, necrosis appeared more severely than in ones by free gingival graft. Sometimes a part of experimental gingiva fell off. The sample in Fig.2, the same one as Fig.1, was stained by hematoxyrin and eosin. A formation of necrosis and ulcer, a large number of neutrophil cells under the epithelial tissue were

obviously observed in the histological findings. The staining
method by A.S.Warthin and A.C.Starry was applied to a
histological specimen. Black colored sites which seemed just like
Spirochetes were observed in the lesions. Table 1 shows the
averages of Spirochetes in the smear samples. The results about
Fusobacterium are shown in Table 2. An increase tendency with
advancing lesions was observed in these results.

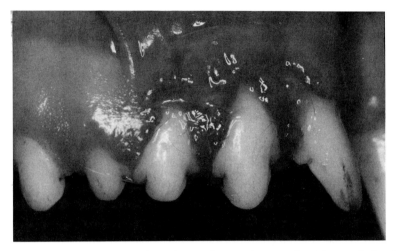

Fig.1 The macroscopic view after the production of lesions.

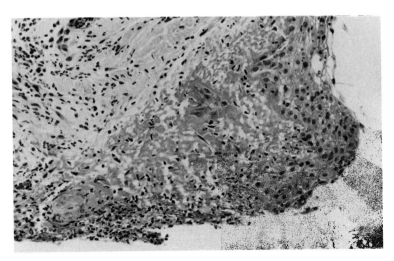

Fig.2 A formation of necrosis in histological specimen stained
by hematoxyrin and eosin.

TABLE 1   Spirochetes

	BEFORE	7 DAYS AFTER PRODUCTION OF THE LESION
AVERAGE	0.08	19.6
(range)	(0-0.4)	(3.2-92.4)
N=20		

TABLE 2   Fusobacterium

	BEFORE	7 DAYS AFTER PRODUCTION OF THE LESION
AVERAGE	0.24	18.24
(range)	(0-2)	(0-129)
N=25		

DISCUSSION

Necrotizing ulcerative lesions were induced by bad local circulation of blood or by severe chemical stimulus in this experiment. And the microbes, both Spirochetes and Fusobacterium, obviously increased in the lesions. This means that bad circulation and chemical stimulus can induce ANUG-like lesions, and also that as a result those microbes increase in the lesions. The results suggest that Spirochetes and Fusobacterium can be found in lesions because such a clinical state is suitable for their growth, not because the disease is induced by these microbes. In fact, they usually exist in dental debris. However, ANUG doesn't always appear in normal gingivae. We would like to make a further study of a relationship between microflora and host, by taking immunity into consideration.

ACKNOWLEDGEMENTS
We deeply thank Prof. Masaru Kaneko, Lect. Hisako Honda, and Clinical Technician Kunio Nakamura, department of microbiology of Iwate Medical University, for kind advice on bacteriological work.

© 1991 Elsevier Science Publishers B.V.
Recent advances in periodontology Vol. II,
S.I. Gold, M. Midda and S. Mutlu, eds.

PERIPHERAL BLOOD POLYMORPHONUCLEAR NEUTROPHIL (PMN) COUNT IN CAUCASIAN AND NEGRO PATIENTS WITH JUVENILE / POST-JUVENILE PERIODONTITIS (JP/PJP)

KADRIYE SATI, [+]JOHN S. BULMAN AND HUBERT N. NEWMAN

Depts. of Periodontology & [+]Community Dental Health, Institute of Dental Surgery, University of London, London (U.K.)

INTRODUCTION

It has been suggested that PMN dysfunction may underlie some forms of severe periodontitis, especially JP. It has also been hypothesized that borderline neutropenia may be associated with localized juvenile periodontitis (LJP) (1). Since haematological data concerning periodontitis patients seem to be scarce in the literature (1,2) the present study attempted to shed some light on the levels of circulating PMN in patients suffering from JP or PJP.

MATERIAL AND METHODS

The test group comprised otherwise healthy patients as follows: 31 caucasian male (CM), 43 caucasian female (CF), 36 negro male (NM) and 85 negro female (NF), all with JP or PJP, who attended the Eastman Dental Hospital for periodontal treatment. 50 CM, 100 CF, 18 NM and 127 NF healthy subjects were assessed as the control group. Patients aged between 13-25 years were classified as JP cases and between 26-58 years as PJP cases.

After the diagnosis the patients were referred to the haematology department for peripheral blood sampling in the morning. Samples were taken before any periodontal treatment had been initiated and differential PMN counts were performed.

Multiple regression analysis was performed using the Nanostat program marketed by Alpha Bridge Ltd., U.K.

RESULTS

The sample means for the data showed that, regardless of disease status,

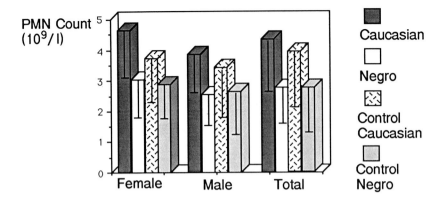

Fig. 1. PMN count data.

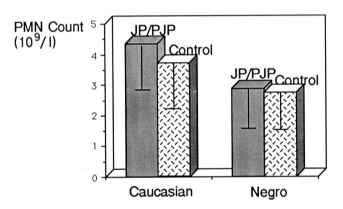

Fig. 2. PMN counts in caucasian and negro subjects.

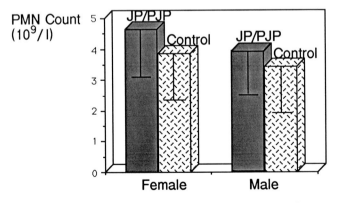

Fig. 3. Effect of sex on PMN counts in caucasians.

caucasians of both sexes had higher PMN counts than negroes. Again regardless of disease status, caucasian and negro females had higher PMN levels than caucasian and negro males. Test groups for females of both races and for caucasian males demonstrated higher PMN values than corresponding control groups.

Multiple regression analysis of the data indicated, with other factors held constant, that the difference between PMN levels in caucasians and negroes was highly significant ($p<.001$) (Fig. 2). A similar analysis on caucasian data alone indicated that the difference in PMN count between females and males was significant ($p<.05$) (Fig. 3). The data for women alone were further analysed and the difference between caucasians and negroes was again highly significant regardless of disease status ($p<.001$) (Fig. 4). When the contribution of disease in the caucasian group was assessed, higher PMN count for the test group was found to be at a borderline level of significance (Fig. 5). A similar effect was not demonstrable in the negro group.

CONCLUSIONS

In summary the findings suggest that:

1. Significantly higher PMN counts in caucasians compared with negroes may be due almost entirely to racial differences in such levels (3-5).

2. Higher PMN values for caucasian women regardless of disease status suggest sex-based differences as several studies have suggested (6,7).

3. The relatively small increase in PMN count in caucasian JP/PJP patients may indicate simply a response to infection.

4. Finally, the present study suggests that JP/PJP patients appear to possess an adequate number of circulating PMN.

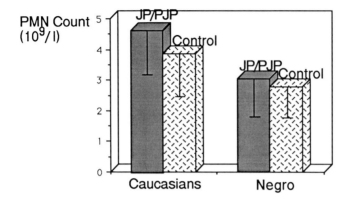

Fig. 4. Effect of race on PMN counts in females.

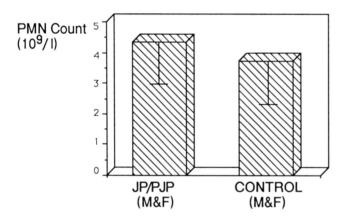

Fig. 5. Contribution of disease in caucasian group.

REFERENCES

1. Brightman V, Shenker B, Bogert M, et al (1989) J Dent Res 68:1228 (Abs.)
2. Karshan M (1951) J Periodontol 22:23-26
3. Broun Jr GO, Herbig FK, Hamilton JR (1966) New Engl J Med 275: 1410-1413
4. Kasili EG, Cardwell CL, Taylor JR (1969) East African Med J 46:676-679
5. Karayalcin G, Rosner F, Savitsky A (1972) NY State J Med 72:1815-1817
6. Heine H, Heine K, Schmidt H (1960) Acta Biol Med Germ 5:221-229
7. Bain B, England JM (1975) British Med J 1:306-309.

© 1991 Elsevier Science Publishers B.V.
Recent advances in periodontology Vol. II,
S.I. Gold, M. Midda and S. Mutlu, eds.

PERIODONTAL TREATMENT NEEDS ACCORDING TO PATIENT'S GENDER, BODY WEIGHT AND SMOKING

UROŠ SKALERIČ and MARIJA KOVAČ-KAVČIČ

Dept. of Oral Medicine and Periodontology, Faculty of Medicine, University of Ljubljana, Ljubljana, Yugoslavia

INTRODUCTION

Chronic inflammatory periodontal disease is an infectious process caused by bacteria and their products in dental plaque (1). The host response to the bacterial plaque challenge could be modified by several systemic factors and conditions(2). The research of different systemic conditions is necessary for better understanding the circumstances that we might expect for the progression of chronic inflammation in periodontal tissues. Therefor we decided to evaluate the periodontal conditions and treatment needs in a population of adult Ljubljana citizens according to their gender, smoking habit and body weight.

MATERIAL AND METHODS

Periodontal conditions of Ljubljana citizens being 45 yrs (N=244) and 55 yrs (N=237) old was assessed. In total 481 subjects, 232 males and 249 females were checked for periodontal treatment needs according to the Community Periodontal Index of Treatment Needs (CPITN) by Ainamo et al (3). Using CPITN methodology the periodontal status of all teeth of the participants was assessed.

Smoking habit was evaluated by questionnaire and subjects were devided into smoking and non-smoking group.

Body weight of the subjects was calculated from the ratio Q = body weight (g)/body height^2 (cm) according to Quetel Index (Q) (4). According to this Index citizens were devided in the normal or underweight group (Q=<2.56) and overweight group (Q=>2.56). Gender, smoking habit and body weight were compared between citizens with deep pockets (≥6 mm) needing complex periodontal treatment and subjects with mild or moderate periodontal inflammation needing only scaling and oral hygiene instruction. Statistical significance was evaluated by X^2 test.

RESULTS

Of 481 citizens participating in the survey 80 (32.9%) subjects in 45-yr-old group and 89 (37.5%) subjects in 55-yr -old group were found to need the complex periodontal treatment (CPT) including periodontal surgery, root scaling and oral hygiene instruction. Table I. shows that males in both age groups need CPT more frequently than females.

TABLE I.

COMPLEX PERIODONTAL TREATMENT(CPT) NEEDS OF 481 LJUBLJANA CITIZENS ACCORDING TO GENDER

Age(years)	Gender	CPT N (%)	Significance
45	m	53(41.7)	<0.01
	f	24(23.1)	
55	m	49(45.8)	<0.05
	f	40(30.8)	

Of all examined Ljubljana citizens 32.2% of the 45-yr-old group and 30.8% of the 55-yr-old group claimed to smoke cigarettes.
Evaluation of the smoking habit according to gender showed (Table II) that males smoke cigarettes more frequently than females in both age groups.

TABLE II.

NUMBER(N) AND PERCENTAGE(%) OF SMOKERS ACCORDING TO GENDER OF 481 LJUBLJANA CITIZENS

Age(years)	Gender	N(%) Smokers	Significance
45	m	50(39.6)	<0.01
	f	28(23.7)	
55	m	47(44.3)	<0.01
	f	25(19.2)	

When the CPT needs were evaluated according to smoking habit it was found that smokers need CPT more frequently than nonsmokers in both age groups (Table III). This difference is significant in 45-yr-old group.

TABLE III.

COMPLEX PERIODONTAL TREATMENT(CPT) NEEDS OF 481 LJUBLJANA
CITIZENS ACCORDING TO SMOKING HABIT

Age(years)	CPT	CPT N(%) Smokers	Nonsmokers	Significance
45	80	36(47.4%)	44(26.2%)	<0.01
55	89	30(44.7%)	59(34.7%)	NS

Evaluation of Ljubljana citizens body weight by Quetel Index(Q) showed that
57.8% of subjects in 45-yr-old group and 61.2% of subjects in 55-yr-old
group belong to overweight population.

Males were more frequently overweight than females in both age groups.
The difference was significant in 45-yr-old group (Table IV).

TABLE IV.

NUMBER(N) AND PERCENTAGE(%) OF 481 LJUBLJANA CITIZENS BEING
OVERWEIGHT (Q=>2.56)

Age(years)	Gender	Q N	%	Significance
45	m	91	(72.2)	<0.01
	f	50	(42.4)	
55	m	67	(63.2)	NS
	f	78	(59.5)	

When the CPT needs were assessed according to the subject body weight
we found that overweight citizens (Q=>2.56) need complex periodontal
treatment more frequently than citizens with normal and low body weight
(Q=<2.56) in both age groups. This difference was significant in 45-yr-old
groups (Table V).

TABLE V.

COMPLEX PERIODONTAL TREATMENT(CPT) NEEDS OF 481 LJUBLJANA
CITIZENS ACCORDING TO BODY WEIGHT(Q)

Age(years)	CPT	CPT N% Normal/Low weight (Q=<2.56)	Overweight (Q=>2.56)	Significance
45	80	23(29.0)	57(71.0)	<0.005
55	89	42(47.0)	47(53.0)	NS

The prevalence of periodontal disease and periodontal treatment needs in
the population of Ljubljana was found to be high and increasing with age(5).
Evaluation of complex periodontal treatment needs in 45-and 55-yr-old citizens
of Ljubljana according to their gender, smoking habit and body weight showed that males smoking cigarettes and being overweight have more frequently
deep periodontal pockets needing complex periodontal surgery treatment. The
results of this survey suggest that adult overweight cigarettes smoking males may represent a risk population for advanced inflammatory periodontal
disease.

ACKNOWLEDGEMENTS

The survey was financially supported by The Research Council of Slovenia,
Ljubljana, Yugoslavia.

REFERENCES

1. Löe H, Theilade E, Jensen SB(1965) J Periodontol 36:177-187

2. Pennel BM, Keagle JG(1977) J Periodontol 48:517-532

3. Ainamo J, Barmes DE, Beagrie BG, Cutress TN, Martin J, Sardo-Infirri
   J (1982) Int Dent J 32:281-291

4. Block G(1982) Am J Epidemiol 115:492-505

5. Skalerič U, Kovač-Kavčič M (1989) Community Dent Oral Epidemiol 17:304-306

© 1991 Elsevier Science Publishers B.V.
Recent advances in periodontology Vol. II,
S.I. Gold, M. Midda and S. Mutlu, eds.

POTENTIAL ROLE OF INTERLEUKIN-1 AND TUMOR NECROSIS FACTOR IN HUMAN PERIAPICAL AND MARGINAL PERIODONTITIS

TAMOTSU TSURUMACHI, OSAMU TAKEICHI, TSUYOSHI SAITO, *ICHIRO SAITO AND *ITARU MORO

Dept. of Endodont. and *Pathol., School of Dent., Nihon Univ., Tokyo, Japan

INTRODUCTION

Progressive destruction of alveolar bone is a major feature of periapical and marginal periodontitis. The identification and characterization of local factors have expanded the knowledge of cellular mechanisms and interactions in resorptive bone diseases. Recent investigations have revealed that Interleukin-1 (IL-1) and tumor necrosis factor (TNF) are analogous to osteoclast activating factor and promote bone resorption. These findings have suggested the possibility that IL-1 and TNF may play a significant role in initiation and development of periapical and periodontal deseases. To elucidate the mechanisms of tissues breakdown in periodontitis, we measured levels of IL-1 and TNF in the inflammatory exudate such as periapical exudate (PE) and crevicular fluid (CF) of patients with periodontal disease by ELISA.

It has been reported that a large number of cells are present in PE and CF of patients with periodontal disease. The great majority (>95%) of these cells are polymorphonuclear leukocytes (PMNs). However, the functional ability of these cells is only partly understood. The purpose of the present study is to see whether these PMNs, which share a number of commom properties with macrophages (such as being phagocytic, and having a common progenitor cell and similar receptors and antigens on their cell surface), would be capable of producing IL-1 and TNF. We have used reverse-transcriptase polymerase chain reaction (RT-PCR) to provide a rapid, accurate method for detection of cytokine expression in the cells from inflammatory exudates.

MATERIALS AND METHODS

Patients and Samples : Eighteen patients with periapical periodontitis and seven patients with generalized moderate to severe marginal periodontitis, ranging in age from 25 to 54 years , were selected from the Department of Endodontics at Nihon University Dental Hospital. Patients received a complete dental examination which included medical history, clinical symptoms, measurements of periodontal clinical indexes, periapical radiographic features, and properties of exudates. All patients were subjected to this study utilizing a capillary tube.

Preparation of cells : PE and CF were centrifuged at 400 g for 10 min. The cells were washed three times with PBS. The total cell numbers were counted and cell viability was determined using the Trypan blue dye exclusion test. The mean number of cells recovered from the washing was $1 \times 10^5 - 1 \times 10^6$ /ml with a mean viability of 87.5%. Differential cell counts were determined on slides stained with Wright's stain. The cells were distinguished as PMNs, macrophages, and lymphocytes.

Isolation of peripheral blood (PB) - cells : Peripheral blood was isolated by venipuncture and the erythrocytes were sedimented by adding Dextran (Sigma, St. Louis, MO.) to a final concentration of 3 % (v/v). The leukocyte - rich plasma was aspirated after centrifugation, and the pellet was suspended in buffered isotonic ammonium chloride for 10 min. at 4 °C.

Induction of cytokines from cells in PB-cells : The cell suspensions that were prepared as described above were cultured in 24-well Nunc plates (Denmark) in a humidified 5% CO_2 in air incubator at 37 °C. Each well contained 1 ml of cells (1×10^6 cells/ml) with or without different concentrations of LPS (0 - 200 μg/ml), con A (0 - 100 μg/ml), and zymosan (0 - 1000 μg/ml). The cells were cultured for different lengths of time (0 - 48 h.) and then centrifuged at 400 g for 10 min. At the end of each culture period, cells and the cell-free supernatant were stored at -20 °C until the cytokines were assayed.

Enzyme Linked Immunosorbent Assay (ELISA) for the quantitation of IL-1α,β, and TNF : Ninety-six-well microplates were coated with 50μl of monoclonal antibody for IL-1α (Genzyme Co, Boston) at 4°C overnight. The wells were blocked with 100μl of 1% BSA-PBS at room temperature for 2 h, washed with PBS-Tween 10 times, and 50μl of culture supernatants or purified IL-1α (standard solution) were added. After over night incubation at room temperature, the wells were washed as above, 50 μl of rabbit anti-IL-1α antibodies was added and they were incubated at room temperature for 2 h. The wells were washed and 50 μl of horseradish peroxidase - labelled goat anti-IgG (Vector) was added and they were incubated at room temperature for 2 h. After the wells were washed, 100 μl of o-Phenylenediamine substrate was added and then absorbance was measured at 490 nm.

RNA isolation : The RNA was isolated from the cell by lysing 1 X 10^6 pelleted cells in 200 μl of ice-cold lysis solution containing 4 M guanidine thiocyanate, 25mM sodium citrate (pH 7.0), 0.1 M 2-mercaptoethanol, and 0.5% (wt/vol) sarcosyl. After the nuclei and cellular debris were removed by centrifugation at 2,000 g for 20 min, the supernatants were extracted three times with an equal volume of 1:1 (vol/vol) phenol and chloroform, and one additional time with an equal volume of chloroform alone. The RNA was precipitated from solution in 70% ethanol, 0.4 M NaCl at -20°C.

Amplification method : We used RT-PCR for assaying the cytokine expressions of small number of cells in PE and CF. For each sample, a 10μl aliquot of the amplified products were fractionated by 1.7% agarose gel electrophoresis, and were visualized by UV fluorescence after staining with ethidium bromide.

Oligonucleotides used for amplification : Oligonucleotides were synthesized using a DNA synthesizer (model 391 PCR-MATE; Applied Biosystems, Inc., Foster City, CA) (Table.1). The 5' primers spanned the junction of the first two exons, or 3'primers spanned the junction of next two exons. Primers were purified by column chromatography using Sephadex G50 (Pharmacia) equilibrated with distilled water.

RESULTS AND DISCUSSION

ELISA was used for measuring levels of IL-1α, IL-1β and TNF in inflammatory exudates such as PE and CF. Both of IL-1 α and IL-1 β were detected in PE and CF, whereas TNF was not detected (Fig 1). The levels of IL-1α and IL-1β were not associated with the clinical findings. However, the average level of IL-1β was higher than that of IL-1α in the inflamatory exudates. This result suggested that IL-1 may play a critical role in inflammatory reaction. This experiment demonstrated that both PE and CF contained IL-1α and IL-1β. However, whether the PMNs in PE and CF have possibility of cytokine production are still not clear. Therefore, we examined these functions of peripheral blood (PB)-PMN stimulated with various mitogens. We found a significant production of IL-1α and IL-1β by PB-PMN. However, These IL-1α and IL-1β were higher levels in the supernatants of peripheral blood lymphocytes (PBL) and peripheral blood macrophages (PB-Mϕ) than in PB-PMNs. In addition, time course study of IL-1 produced by PB-PMN showed IL-1 α in late culture period (24h) and IL-1 β in the early culture period (6-12h). TNF was not detected in the supernatants of PB-PMN with this ELISA, whereas PBL and PB-Mϕ indicated high levels of TNF.

Fig 1   IL-1 production in PE and CF

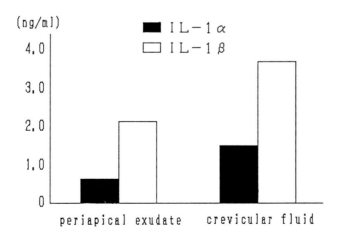

To detect IL-1α, IL-1β and TNF expression of the cells from PE and CF, we have used RT-PCR, since these samples have contained a small number of cells. We found significant reactivity of these cytokines expressions by PE and CF. However, the expression of TNF was significantly less than IL-1α and IL-1β. The cells from PE and CF showed no difference in cytokine expressions. These results suggest that the cells from marginal inflammatory site may be same as periapical lesion in termes of their ability to produce these cytokines. In this context, ELISA study did not detect TNF by stimulated PB-PMN in contrast to PBL and PB-Mφ. However, RT-PCR assay showed that PB-, PE-, and CF-PMNs isolated with Ficoll-Hypaque contained transcripts for TNF. This data suggests that PMNs are capable of synthesizing a small amount of TNF mRNA transcripts.

Taken together, these data indicate that IL-1α , IL-1β, and TNF delivered by PMNs may be another direct mediator of periodontal disease, since Mφ has been reported to express a wide range of cytokines in these tissues. The findings that PE - and CF-PMNs express multiple cytokines, and produce them under these conditions in vivo, will have important biological ramifications.

Table 1   Sequences of primers

	5' primer	3' primer
IL-1 α	GTCTCTGAATCAGAAATCCTTCTCTC	CATGTCAAATTTCACTGCTTCATCC
IL-1 β	CAGCTGGAGAGTGTAGA	CTTCAGTGAAGTTTATTTC
TNF	CAGAGGGAAGAGTTCCCCAG	CCTTGGTCTGGTAGGAGACG

REFFERENCES
1. Skapski H., Lehner L. (1976) J. Periodontal Res. 11:19-24
2. Charon J. A., Luger T. A., Mergenhagen S. E., Oppenheim J. J. (1982) Infection and Immunity38:1190-1195
3. Jandinski J. J., Leung C., Macedo B., Rynar J., Deasey M. (1987) J. Leukocyte Biol. 42:601
4. Hattori N., Tsurumachi T., Saito I.,Komiyama K., Mezawa S., Saito T.(1988) Recent advances in clinical periodontology 649-652
5. Goh K., Furusawa S., Kawa Y., Negishi-Okitsu S., Mizoguchi M. (1989) Int. Arch. Allergy Appl. Immunol. 88:297-303
6. Erlich H. A. (1989) J. Clinical Immunology 9:437-446

© 1991 Elsevier Science Publishers B.V.
Recent advances in periodontology Vol. II,
S.I. Gold, M. Midda and S. Mutlu, eds.

IMAGE ANALYZABLE RESEARCH ON THE RADIOGRAPH OF THE ALVEOLAR BONE ON THE
OCCLUSAL TRAUMATISM

TAKASHI MIYATA, HISAO ARAKI, KITETSU SHIN AND KATSUMI IKEDA*

Post-Doctoral Institute of Clinical Dentistry, School of Dentistry, Meikai
University, 5-1-3 Toyooka Iruma Saitama, 358 Japan

*Department of Periodontics, School of Dentistry, Meikai University, 1-1
Keyakidai Sakado Saitama, 350-02 Japan

INTRODUCTION

This study was to investigate the relationship between occlusal contact
and morphological alveolar resorption analyzed from the dental X-ray film
referring to mandibular molars showing premature contact in the intercuspal
position.

The measurements of occlusal contact were carried out to determine the
Occlusal Contact Area(OCA)area and Luminosity Grade 1(LG1)area, using an
image analyzer system which can measure the difference in luminosity each
of its images from bite resistration in the intercuspal position.

MATERIAL AND METHODS

The subjects

The subjects were 16 patients who were selected because they have premature contact in the intercuspal position, alveolar resorption, no missing
teeth, no prothodontic treatment, no TMJ dysfunction, no loose tooth with mobility over 2 degrees, no post history of occlusal adjustment and interdental
separation over 110μm.

And the cases were 16 teeth including 12 first molars and 4 second molars.

Observation method on the shape of alveolar resorption

According to the method of Kawasaki, on X-ray film was prepared, the image
of which then was analyzed using the image analyzer (the Schonic-GA system). The image of alveolar resorption in the inter alveolar septum and
interdental septum was prepared by modification with concentration at the
alveolar bone. From the binary modificated image, images of alveolar resorption were divided into three types, the Type I resorption have the mesial or
distal top of interalveolar septum, Type II have the mesial and distal top of
interalveolar septum and Type III have interdental septum.

Measurement of the Occlusal contact positions and occlusal contact area

After sufficient trainning of the patients for stable occlusion in the
intercuspal position, using the bite-checker (GC Co.) and the bite regist-

ration tray (Coe Co.),maxillomandibular registration in the intercuspal
position was applied 3 times each to every patients.

The analyses of the occlusal examinations were carried out by measuring
the number of dots using the image analyzer system (Image-PC system) which
consists of the image analyzer (IMAGE PC;edec Co.), a CCD camera (WV-CD1;
National Co.) and a personal computer (PC-9801F;NEC Co.).

Measurement of OCA and LG1

The degree of the occlusal contacts were distingishied with its luminosity grades on OCA and LG1. The OCA area is a part wherat the contact area of
the maxillomandibular teeth is clearly obserbed at the luminosity level of
17 to 63 in this system. The LG1 area is a part whereat the maxillomandibular resistration is completely broken due to tight contact of the superi-
or and inferior teeth,noted at a luminosity level of 49 to 63 in this
system at an interocclusal distance of about 36 μm.

Observation method of the occlusal contact position

The occlusal contact position were recorded using our own classified
chart of occlusal contact position (Fig.1,Table 1).

Further,Wilcoxson's test was employed for the statistical processing in
this study.

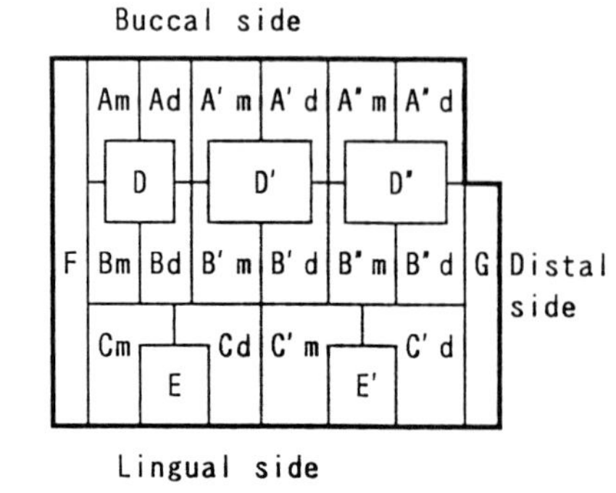

TABLE 1
CLASSIFICATION OF OCCLUSAL CONTACT
POSITIONS

Buccal side

Fig.1.Classification of occlusal
contact position

A :Outer inclines of mesiobuccal cusp
A' :Outer inclines of distobuccal cusp
A* :Outer inclines of distal cusp
B :Inner inclines of mesiobuccal cusp
B' :Inner inclines of distobuccal cusp
B* :Inner inclines of distal cusp
C :Inner inclines of mesiolingual cusp
C' :Inner inclines of distolingual cusp
D :Top of mesiobuccal cusp
D' :Top of distobuccal cusp
D* :Top of distal cusp
E :Top of mesiolingual cusp
E' :Top of distolingual cusp
F :Mesial marginal ridge
G :Distal marginal ridge
 ※ Mesial inclines of A,B,C:m
    Distal inclines of A,B,C:d

RESULTS

The relationship between the morphological alveolar resorption and the mesiodistal distribution

The OCA and LG1 areas in the intercuspal position showed a trend of distributions corresponding with the side of alveolar resorption in Type Ⅰ. In Type Ⅱ and Ⅲ, a trend of distribution in the distal area which however was not significant statistically (Tables 2,3).

TABLE 2
ALVEOLAR RESORPTION AND MESIODISTAL
DISTRIBUTION IN OCA AREA   (%)

Alveolar resorption	No.	Mesial	Distal	Test
Ⅰ	6	50.5	49.5	
	7	15.1	84.9	NS
	10	0.0	100.0	P<0.07
	12	7.1	92.9	
Ⅱ	5	47.2	52.8	
	8	10.8	89.2	NS
	14	36.7	63.3	P<0.07
	15	26.7	73.3	
Ⅲ	1	35.1	64.9	
	2	0.0	100.0	
	3	54.9	45.1	
	4	52.3	47.7	NS
	9	49.1	50.9	P<0.21
	11	41.6	58.4	
	13	55.9	44.1	
	16	31.6	68.4	

Wilcoxson test
NS:Not significant

TABLE 3
ALVEOLAR RESORPTION AND MESIODISTAL
DISTRIBUTION IN LG1 AREA   (%)

Alveolar resorption	No.	Mesial	Distal	Test
Ⅰ	6	54.3	45.7	
	7	9.0	91.0	NS
	10	0.0	100.0	P<0.07
	12	2.9	97.1	
Ⅱ	5	60.4	39.6	
	8	9.1	90.9	NS
	14	37.2	62.8	P<0.15
	15	22.5	77.5	
Ⅲ	1	33.6	66.4	
	2	0.0	100.0	
	3	88.2	11.8	
	4	39.5	60.5	NS
	9	59.7	40.3	P<0.32
	11	41.0	59.0	
	13	56.4	43.6	
	16	35.3	64.7	

Wilcoxson test
NS:Not significant

The relationship between morphological alveolar resoption and baccalo-lingual distribution

In Type Ⅱ, there was a tendency of distribution on the outer and inner inclines of the buccal cusp, inner inclines of the lingual cusp and distal marginal ridge, in Type Ⅲ on the outer and inner inclines of the buccal cusp and inner inclines of the lingual cusp (P<0.05)(Tables 4,5).

240

The relationship between the outer or inner inclines and the alvolar resorption

there was a tendency that the distribution of the OCA and LG1 areas to the outer or inner inclines in the inter cuspal posotion showed no statistically significant defference in Type I and II,but in Type III distribution to the inner inclines was noted (P<0.05)

TABLE 4
ALVEOLAR RESORPTION AND BACCALO-
LINGUAL DISTRIBUTION IN OCA AREA(%)

Posi-tion	Alveolar Resorption		
	I(n=4)	II(n=4)	III(n=8)
A	23.5±17.9	27.9±17.1	27.7±12.9
B	10.9±12.4	36.3±29.8	37.4±20.5
C	33.0±14.8	24.1±16.9	22.0±14.8
D	10.9±18.9	0.0± 0.0	0.7± 1.7
F	2.7± 4.7	1.6± 1.6	1.6± 1.6
G	17.2±16.1	10.2± 7.0	8.2± 9.5

Mean±SD.
n=number of cases.
A:outer inclines of buccal cusp.
B:inner inclines of buccal cusp.
C:inner inclines of lingual cusp.
D:top of buccal cusp.
F:mesial marginal ridge.
G:distal marginal ridge.

TABLE 5
ALVEOLAR RESORPTION AND BACCALO-
LINGUAL DISTRIBUTION IN LG1 AREA(%)

Posi-tion	Alveolar Resorption		
	I(n=4)	II(n=4)	III(n=8)
A	25.1±18.8	23.6±20.2	24.6±12.4
B	12.6±13.0	40.9±32.5	37.1±19.9
C	32.1±18.8	23.6±16.1	24.4±19.8
D	6.6±11.4	0.0± 0.0	0.7± 2.0
F	1.2± 2.0	0.2± 0.3	9.1±11.4
G	22.5±24.7	11.9± 9.3	4.1± 7.5

Mean±SD.
n=number of cases.
A:outer inclines of buccal cusp.
B:inner inclines of buccal cusp.
C:inner inclines of lingual cusp.
D:top of buccal cusp.
F:mesial marginal ridge.
G:distal marginal ridge.

CONCLUSION

A study was carried on the cases,wherein one of the reasons why alveolar resorption was caused is considerd to be premature contact(occlusal trauma), in view of the occlusal contact area and their position.

It was suggested that uneven distribution of occlusal contact is participated in alveolar resorption.

REFERENCES

1. Araki H,Shin K,Ando E,Miyata T,Maeda S,Kanai A,Ikeda K (1988) J Jap Ass Periodont 30:844-859
2. Araki H (1990) J Jap Ass Periodont 32:587-602
3. Glickman I,Smulow J B (1967) J Periodontol 38:280-293
4. Glickman I,Roeber F W,Brion M,Pameijier J H N (1970) J Periodontol 41:30 -35

© 1991 Elsevier Science Publishers B.V.
Recent advances in periodontology Vol. II,
S.I. Gold, M. Midda and S. Mutlu, eds.

CANINE PLATFORM FOR POSTERIOR TOOTH ERUPTION AS AN ADJUNCT IN PERIODONTAL THERAPY

AVINOAM YAFFE, NIRA HOCHMAN, JACOB EHRLICH

Department of Prosthodontics, Hebrew University-Hadassah School of Dental Medicine, P.O. Box 1127, 91010 Jerusalem (Israel)

INTRODUCTION

Periodontal disease is prevalent all over the world[1-2]. Irrespective of its etiology, periodontal disease has severe consequences, including attachment loss and mutilation of the dentition. Advanced periodontal disease is characterized by loss of attachment, adverse crown-to-root ratios, and various osseous defects giving rise to reduced posterior support, drifting and shifting of teeth accompanied by tooth mobility, thereby increasing the load on the anterior teeth leading to flaring. Lack of or inappropriate treatment may result in loss of teeth. Several periodontal non-surgical[3-5] and surgical[6-8] treatment approaches for this condition have been described.

The use of orthodontics in periodontal treatment is well documented[9-10]. Several researchers have described the beneficial effects of extruding the teeth on the alveolar bone. Ingber (11) found a reduction of probing depth following such treatment. Creating conditions to allow posterior tooth eruption may be useful for treating deep bite associated with gingival impingement[12]. This approach has also been employed in patients with posterior bite collapse, loss of occlusal vertical dimension, and flared maxillary anterior teeth[13]. Forced or active eruption leads to interesting changes in the attachment appartus. This treatment should only be carried out under control and the maintenance of good oral hygeine is essential[3-4]. In such cases, the bony defects can generally be corrected by levelling off and the crown-to-root ratio can be improved.

The modified Hawley appliance is in common use for the treatment of advanced periodontal disease[3,4,14]. However, patients may find the removable appliance esthetically or phonetically unacceptable. Inaddition, the difficulty in controlling plaque may cause periodontal tissue irritation and aggravate periodontal inflammation. The Hawley appliance does not allow maxillary tooth eruption. The appliance must be worn all the time, requiring full patient cooperation.

This paper describes a modified approach for tooth eruption that can serve as an adjunct in periodontal therapy.

MATERIALS AND METHODS

Forty patients with moderate to advanced periodontal disease, ranging from 32 to 58 years in age, were included in this study. All the subjects had natural dentition, several had crown restorations, and a few had one or two teeth missing. The patients were screened for periodontal and occlusal problems by taking full sets of X-rays, and noting probing depth fremitus and tooth mobility[15]. The first stage of therapy included scaling, root planing, curettage and oral care instructions. In the second stage, a new occlusal vertical dimension was established by using a canine platform (the application of acid-etch composite resin material on the lingual incline surfaces of the maxillary canines (Fig. 1)). In patients with increased canine overjet, composite resin material may be applied to incisal labial aspect of the mandibular canines and it should be examined periodically for possible wear or damage.

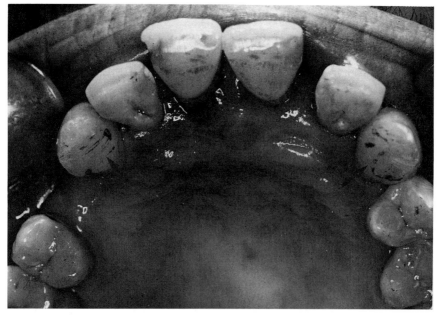

Fig. 1. Application of composite resin on the lingual incline of the maxillary canine surfaces (indicated by arrows).

In centric occlusion, only the labial incisal aspect of the mandibular canines is in contact with the platform while the posterior teeth and the incisors remain entirely free, thereby avoiding direct trauma to the soft tissues and ensuring occlusal rest. The posterior clearance should be minimal in order to allow posterior tooth eruption and to prevent lateral tongue thrusting. The tooth eruption and its newly established position is due to biological tissue reactions without the application of force. Scaling, root planing and occlusal adjustment is carried out regularly.

RESULTS

The active phase of canine platform treatment lasting between 3 and 14 months and the ensuing tooth eruption reduced the probing depths and tooth mobility in forty patients. The amount of tooth eruption varied in different locations, and the use of selective grinding allowed additional eruption of selected teeth. Periodontal status was assessed both clinically and radiographically. Limited surgery was carried out in eleven cases. The subjective response was positive with no complaints regarding mastication, esthetics or phonetics. Only a few patients reported minor discomfort during the first two weeks, and correction and adjustment was required in several cases. After the completion of active treatment, the canine platform was left in place for additional support and guidance in most cases, while it was removed in other patients.

DISCUSSION

This study demonstrates the applicability of the canine paltform as an adjunct in periodontal treatment. This method avoids many of the inconveniences associated with Hawley appliance, and since it does not involve esthetic and phonetic effects, it is universally acceptable to patients. Its major advantage is that it allows eruption of both maxillary and mandibular posterior teeth. The canine platform is an easy, simple, inexpensive chair-side procedure which utilizes physiological forces and biological tissue reactions. The canine platform method may be used both for improving the periodontal condition and in cases of deep or locked bite requiring an increased vertical dimension. Using support on the canines only is based on the assumption that the masticatory muscles exert less force on the anterior than on the posterior teeth[16], and, according to Storey[17], occluding the anterior teeth suppresses the activity of the elevator muscles.

REFERENCES

1. Waerhaug J (1966) In: Romfjorf SP, Ken DS, Ash MM (eds) World Workshop in Periodontics. Ann Arbor, MI, University of Michigan, p. 179

2. Loe H, Anerud A, Boysen H, Smith M (1978) J Periodontol 49:607

3. Amsterdam M (1977-1980) Graduate lecture program: Periondontal Prosthesis University of Pennsylvania.

4. Amsterdam M (December 1974) Alpha Omega (scientific issue)

5. Badersten A, Nilveus R, Egerlberg J (1984) J Clin Periodontol 11: 63

6. Waerhaug J (1971) J Dent Res 50:219

7. Caffesse R (1980) Dental Clin N. Amer 24:751

8. Isidor F, Karring T (1986) J Periodont Res 21:462

9. Brown JS (1973) J Periodont 44:742

10. Kraal JH, Digiancinto JJ, Dail RA, Lemmerman K, Peden JW (1980) J Prosthet Dent 43:156

11. Ingber J (1974) J Periodont 45:199

12. Marks MH, Corn H (1989) Atlas of Adult Orthodontics. Lea and Febiger, Philadelphia, PN

13. Marks MH, Corn H (1977) Alpha Omega 10:54

14. Ehrlich J, Brayer L (1973) Quintessence International 4:59

15. Goldman HH, Cohen DW (ed) (1980) Periodontal Therapy. CV Mosby Co, St. Louis.

16. Okesson JP (1989) Mangement of Temporomandibular Disorders and Occlusion. CV msoby Co, St Louis, p 112

17. Storey AT (1982) Neurophysiological Aspects of TM Disorders. President, American Dental Association, Chicago

© 1991 Elsevier Science Publishers B.V.
Recent advances in periodontology Vol. II,
S.I. Gold, M. Midda and S. Mutlu, eds.

RADIOGRAPHIC ASPECTS OF PERIODONTAL DISEASE

ERDOĞAN TURGUT, D.D.S., M.S.
Professor of Oral Diagnosis/Radiology, Hacettepe University
Faculty of Dentistry, Ankara, Turkey

The diagnostic quality of a radiograph is affected by its density, contrast and sharpness. Density is the degree of blackness present in the processed film. Contrast is the gradation of the differences in film density in different areas of a radiography. Sharpness refers to the ability of a film to reproduce the sharp outlines of an object.

A high electric potential of about 90kv and a low exposure time give the most satisfactory density and contrast for the interpretation of periodantal disease.[1]

The optimum radiographic technique must be employed to gain the maximum value from radiography. The bisecting-angle technique is based on directing the central beam perpendicular to an imaginary plane that bisects the angle formed by the plane of the film and the long axis of the teeth. If the bisecting-angle technique is used, dimentional distortion (elongation or forshortening) is unavoidable.

The long-cone paralleling technique is advisable for more accurate radiographs from the standpoint of periodontal disease. In this technique the plane of the film lies parallel to the long axis of the teeth and the central beam is directed perpendicular to the film and the object.

In addition, the bite-wing series provide much-needed information related to crestal bone involvement in periodental disease.

The xeroradiographic image is superior to conventional radiographs for visualization of soft tissue and calculus deposits.[2]

Radiographs have some limitations in the interpretation of periodontal disease. First of all, relationship between soft and hard tissue are not demonstrated on the radiograph. For this reason, the depth of the periodontal pockets can only be determined radiographically by the use of opaque media such as metal probes, silver or gutta-percha points.

Images of defects on the vestibular or lingual side of the teeth are not reliably shown on radiographs since the bone over the roots in these areas is relatively thin so that the contrast between defect and normal adjacent bone is very slight. Also, the density of the root superimposed on the image of the defect tends to obscure the bone height.[3]

In addition, tooth mobility is not always reflected on radiographs.

Whatever the limitations, radiographs have an important role in the assesment of irregularities in the crest of the interproximal bone.

Normal alveolar bone crest lies about 1 to 1 1/2 mm below adjacent cementoenamel junctions. Between the interior teeth, the alveolar crest is pointed and well corticated. Between the posterior teeth, the alveolar crest is parallel to a line between the adjacent cementoenamel junctions.

In the incipient stage of periodontal disease, a triangular widening of the periodontal space at the crest of interproximal bone can be recognized radiographically. This is called triangulation. Triangulation is an early sign of possible alveolar bone loss.[1]

In horizontal bone loss, which may be classified as localized or generalized, both the buccal and lingual plates of bone and the intervening interdental bone have been resorbed. Generalized horizontal bone loss suggests a systemic factor such as diabetes mellitus.[5] When there is greater bone loss on the proximal of one tooth than on the adjacent tooth, the bone level is not parallel to a line joining the cementoenamel junctions.

Such V-shaped destruction is called vertical bone loss.

In advanced periodontal disease, the entire bony support of the involved tooth may be completely destroyed and the tooth appear to be floating in a radiolucency.

On the other hand, increased bone condensation of an alveolar bone crest of normal height also demonstrates incipient peridontal diseaese.

Radiographs are of value in locating irritants which may be possible local etiologic factors of periodontal disease such as calculus, overhanging restorations, rough carious margins, ill-fitted crowns, open contacts and migration of teeth.[6]

In fact, radiographic examination plays an integral role in establishing a prognosis and in evaluating the healing process rather than in diagnosing periodontal disease.

REFERENCES

1. Wuehrmann A.H., Manson-Hing L.R. (1969) Dental radiology ed 2, The CV Mosby Co., St Louis, pp 290-299.

2. Gratt B.M., Sicles E.A., Armitage G.C., (1980), Use of dental xeroradiographs in periodontics. J Periodontol 51:1-4

3. Roth H, (1965), Some speculations as to predictable fenestrations prior to mucogingival surgery. J Am Soc Periodontol 3:29-31

4. Goaz WG White CW (1982) Oral radiology the CV Mosby Co., St Louis p 356

5. Sonis ST, Fazio RC, Fang L (1984) Principles and practice of oral medicine WB Saunders Co., Philadelphia p 159

6. Micthell D.E., Standish S.M., Fast T.B. (1969) Oral diagnosis/Oral medicine, Lea and Febiger, Philadelphia p 144

© 1991 Elsevier Science Publishers B.V.
Recent advances in periodontology Vol. II,
S.I. Gold, M. Midda and S. Mutlu, eds.

SELF-PERFORMED SUBGINGIVAL IRRIGATION: AN EFFECTIVE METHOD OF
TREATING ISOLATED DEEP PERIODONTAL POCKETS

YUVAL ZUBERY and HAIM TAL
Department of Periodontology, The Maurice and Gabriela Goldschleger
School of Dental Medicine, Tel Aviv University, Israel

INTRODUCTION

The effect of subgingival irrigation, as a monotherapy with and
without preceding scaling and root planing, was studied extensively
with conflicting results (1-8). Wieder et al. (7) reported a
significant reduction in periodontitis as measured by bleeding
index and pocket depth, following subgingival irrigation. Braatz
et al. (8) reported no additional effect on clinical measurements
using daily irrigation performed by the patient over 24 weeks.
However, the positive effect of irrigation on the subgingival flora
has been shown in many studies (1-3,6,8). This effect is probably
achieved by the combination of both the flushing effect on the
loosely adherent subgingival flora and the antibacterial properties
of the solution used. The purpose of this retrospective study was
to evaluate the healing response of isolated deep periodontal
pockets to self-performed subgingival irrigation (SSI) with 0.2%
chlorhexidine gluconate solution.

MATERIAL AND METHODS

Fifteen periodontally involved sites with bone loss exceeding 40%
and probing depth not less than 6 mm from 10 patients suffering
from localized advanced periodontitis were treated at Tel Aviv University, School of Dental Medicine during the years 1986-1990.

After initial examination and diagnosis, patients were instructed
in oral hygiene; scaling and root planing were performed under
local anesthesia.

Patients were re-evaluated 2-3 months later. Sites which did not
respond favorably to the initial treatment were selected for SSI
treatment. Probing depth was recorded and radiographs were taken
using the parallel cone technique. Patients were then instructed
in the SSI technique and were seen once a month for evaluation of
their compliance. On the third month and every 3 months thereafter, re-evaluation, including probing depth measurement and
radiographic examination were performed.

The SSI technique was performed twice daily by using a blunt 23G needle mounted on a 5 mL disposable syringe filled with 0.2% chlorhexidine gluconate solution. The needle was then inserted into the pocket until it encountered resistance, 0.5-1 mL of the solution was then injected into the pocket (Fig. 1).

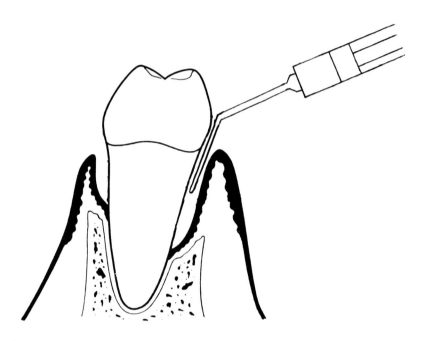

Fig. 1. Illustration of the SSI technique

The radiographic bone support was analyzed using a Schei ruler which measures the percentage of root length supported by bone. Results were analyzed by the paired Student's t-test.

RESULTS

Decrease in probing depth was the most impressive observation; in most cases probing depth was reduced to 4 mm or less. Average decrease was 3.53 ± 2.13 mm and was statistically significant, $p < 0.01$ (Fig. 2). The radiographic comparison showed remarkable increase in percencentage of bone support. The average increase of bone support was $16.7\% \pm 4.91\%$ and was statistically significant, $p < 0.01$ (Fig. 3). There was a tendency to gain more bone support in defects which initially presented more bone loss.

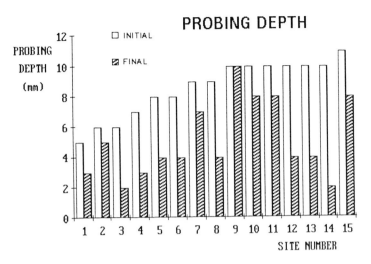

Fig. 2. Initial and final probing depth measurements

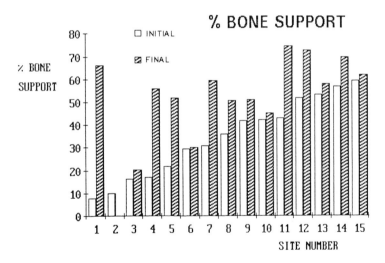

Fig. 3. Initial and final percentage of bone support

DISCUSSION

The effect of subgingival irrigation on periodontal status is not
evident from previous studies since these studies did not examine
the long-term results of changes in clinical parameters used by the
clinician, i.e., probing depth measurements and analysis of radiographs. This technique is limited to isolated deep periodontal
pockets mostly in anterior teeth since it requires good patient
dexterity. This may account for the lack of effect of subgingival

irrigation in the study of Braatz et al. (8). There is no study, however, that measures bone level changes in sites treated by SSI. The use of the parallel cone technique in this study and the analysis of radiographs using the Schei ruler minimized the possible measurement error (9).

Results indicate that a significant reduction of probing depth of 3.53 ± 2.13 mm can be achieved using this technique; gain of bone support as measured on radiographs averaged $16.7\% \pm 4.91\%$. There is a tendency toward more gain of bone support after therapy in sites with less initial bone support. The indications for the use of SSI are isolated deep periodontal pockets, esthetic considerations, refractory sites, "hopeless" teeth, cases in which periodontal surgery is contra-indicated, patients unwilling to undergo periodontal surgery, and furcation involved teeth and areas inaccessible to other oral hygiene measures.

CONCLUSIONS

Easy to handle and safe technique, significant reduction of probing depth (3.53 ± 2.13 mm, $p < 0.01$), significant gain of bone support ($16.7\% \pm 4.91\%$, $p < 0.01$), and gain of bone support increases with increasing bone loss.

REFERENCES

1. Listgarten MA, Gronberg D, Schwimer C, Vito A, Gaffar A (1989) J Periodontol 60(1):4-11

2. Greenstein G (1987) J Periodontol 58(12):827-836

3. Mazza JE, Newman MG, Sims TN (1981) J Clin Periodontol 8:203-212

4. Soh LL, Newman HN, Straham JD (1982) J Clin Periodontol 9:66-74

5. Nylund K, Egelberg J (1990) J Clin Periodontol 17:90-95

6. Schmid E, Kornman KS, Tinanoff N (1985) J Periodontol 56:330-333

7. Wieder SG, Newman HN, Straham JD (1983) J Clin Periodontol 10:172-181

8. Braatz L, Garret S, Claffey N, Egelberg J (1985) J Clin Periodontol 12:630-638

9. Kelly GP, Cain RJ, Knowles JW, Nissle RR, Burgett FG, Shick RA Ramfjord SP (1975) J Periodontol 46:381-386

© 1991 Elsevier Science Publishers B.V.
Recent advances in periodontology Vol. II,
S.I. Gold, M. Midda and S. Mutlu, eds.

SUBEPITHELIAL CONNECTIVE TISSUE GRAFT IN PERIODONTAL SURGERY.
INDICATION FOR ROOT COVERAGE, ESTHETIC PURPOSE, AND IN TREAT-
MENT OF OSSEOUS LESIONS: THE SANDWICH TECHNIQUE

ROBERT AZZI
Enseignant en Parodontologie Université Paris 7, France

This article describes the use of subepithelial tissue
graft to correct mucogingival problems as well as obtaining a
full coverage of any kind of recessions, using a particular
flap design and a specific suture. The donor site is a distal
wedge and is a closed wound. This technique can be associated
with a normal flap surgery while treating a periodontal pocket
and in this case, the donor site will be the connective tissue
taken from the thinning of the palatal flap.

The free gingival graft was used initially by Bjorn[1] and
Nabers[2] to correct mucogingival problems and gingival recessions.
GRUPE and WARREN[3] treated the isolated gingival cleft by the
lateral sliding flap. This technique gives the best results
when there is a narrow root dehiscence and an adjacent tissue
donor site, keratinized and wide enough to serve as a pedicle
graft.

The survival of the graft on wide denuded root surfaces of
maxillary teeth has not been predictable. Bernimoulin et al[4]
proposed a two-stage procedure. Initial placement of keratinized gingiva was followed by a second procedure in which the
graft was pulled coronally; the percentage of root coverage was
43.9%. This technique was expounded by Maynard[5] and others, and
had 36.1% root coverage. Matter[6], Guinard and Caffesse[7] obtained
35.7% root coverage. The tissue often retracted within a short
period of time, leaving a portion of the root still exposed.
The free gingival autograft has been used to cover denuded
roots associated with localized gingival recession since the
first report on the application of the technique was published
by Sullivan and Atkins[8] in 1968. Miller (1982-1985)[9-10] reported
89.4% root coverage and advocates that the graft procedure be
preceded by root planing and saturated citric acid application
to the affected root and the use of a thick butt-jointed free
gingival graft. Holbrook and Ochsenbein[11] obtained 44% root
coverage using thick, stretched free gingival grafts, as a
one-stage procedure to cover recessions.

A successful technique using a subepithelial connective tissue graft was recently described by Langer and Langer[12], Ratzke[13] and Nelson[14]. The purpose of this paper is to describe the Sandwich Technique, using the subepithelial connective tissue graft to correct mucogingival problems and to gain total root coverage with no use of citric acid, just root planing while treating a periodontal disease; thus attaining two goals in one surgical procedure.

Surgical technique :

An envelope type split-thickness flap surgery is performed. An intrasulcular incision is made around the collar of the teeth and across the interdental papilla at the level of the cemento-enamel junction. The split-thickness flap is dissected, far behind the mucogingival line to allow us the possibility of pulling it coronally. Care is taken not to perforate the periosteum or the flap. Where the flap has to be pulled coronally, the part of the papilla that is in contact with the flap has to be disepithelialized. There are no vertical releasing incisions to avoid disturbing the blood supply; root planing is performed, and occasionally reduction of root convexities. No citric acid is applied.

Donor site :

A second surgical site is created at the retromolar tuberosity area. A distal wedge is performed with a thinning of the flap of the palatal aspect. The "harvested" tissue is trimmed and cut as required and all adipose tissue is removed. Some of the band of epithelium, which is taken with the donor connective tissue, is allowed to remain on that portion which will be covering the denuded root and that is not covered by the flap. In the case of a normal flap surgery to treat periodontal disease and correct mucogingival problems, the donor site will be the connective tissue gained from the thinning of the palatal flap. Immediately after taking the graft material, the distal wedge and the flap are sutured, and there is a healing by primary intention.

Recipient site :

The epithelial connective graft is placed over the denuded roots. The partial-thickness recipient flap is positioned coronally so that it covers as much of the graft as possible

and, using a 4.0 silk suture, is sutured to the grafted material to make one of the flap and the graft. An 0 suture goes
inside the flap through the grafted material, comes out of the
flap and is sutured. Then the partial-thickness flap and connective tissue graft is sutured in position. There is no need for
periodontal dressing and the patient is instructed to use
Chlorexedine mouthwashes several times a day, to exercise good
plaque control and to stop smoking. (The worst results were
with heavy smokers).

Discussion :

The most important thing about this technique is that its
purpose is two-fold : the correction of the mucogingival problems and the treatment of the periodontal disease during the
same surgical procedure. In fact, connective tissue graft is
routinely used for different purposes: full coverage is obtained
in the case of mucogingival recessions. The correction of recessions around the crowns is easily obtained,thus assuring an
esthetic appearance. It gives the best results in creating a
nice collagenic collar around teeth with a thin or inexistent
gingiva. Creation of papilla and ridge augmentation, horizon-
tally and vertically, lasts with time. Wound healing is improved
over implanted biomaterials in infra-bony defects, when papilla
are thin or when the two flap margins do not closely approximate . In conclusion, this simple technique which we have been
routinely using for over eight years in periodontal surgery for
plastic remodeling, prosthetic considerations and treatment of
periodontal defects during the same procedure, has proven
valuable and has given us excellent results so far, except in
the case of smokers.

Fig.1

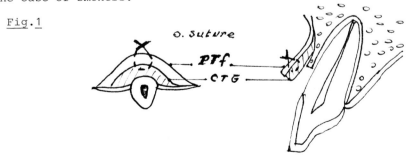

PTF: Partial-thickness Flap
CTG: Connective Tissue Graft

254

Fig. 2

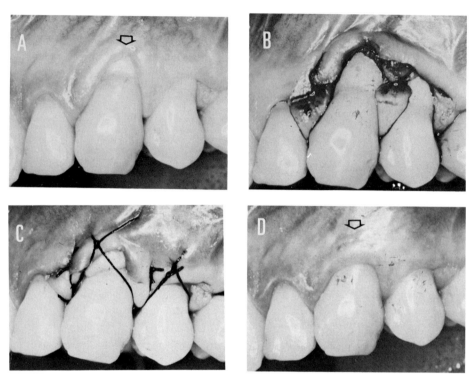

A. Wide recession on the canine. There is no keratinized gingiva.
(Arrow). B. Incisions are made intrasulcularly and across the
interdental papilla to elevate a PTF. C. The connective tissue
graft is secured to the PTF and sutured in position. D.Results
after three months show total root coverage and a wide zone of
keratinized gingiva. (Arrow).

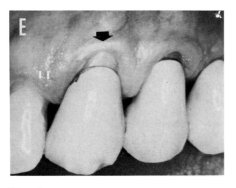 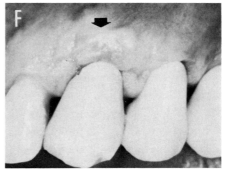

Fig.3

E: Recession of the canine. There is no attached gingiva.

F: Three months post operative result. Correction of the recession and creation of wide and thick keratinized gingiva.

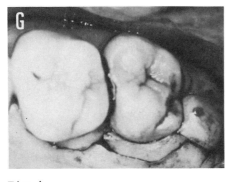 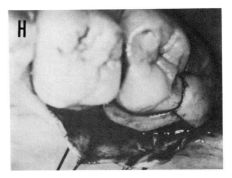

Fig.4

G: A distal wedge is performed

H: Thinning of the flap on the palatal aspect.

References

1. BJORN, H: Free transplantation of gingiva propria. Sveriges Tandlakerforbunds Tidning 55:684. 1963.

2. NABERS.J.H: Free gingival grafts. Periodontics 4:243. 1966.

3. GRUPPE, H. and WARREN,R.: Repair of gingival defects by a sliding flap operation. J.Periodontal 27:92. 1956.

4. BERNIMOULIN, J. LUSCHER.B. and MUHLEMANN.H.R: Coronally repositioned periodontal flap. J. Clin. Periodontol 2:1.1975

5. MAYNARD, J.G: Coronal positioning of a previously placed autogenous gingival graft. J. Periodontol 48:151. 1977.

6. MATTER, J: Free gingival graft and coronaly repositioned flap.

7. GUINARD,E.A. and CAFFESSE.R.G: Treatment of localized gingival recessions. Part III; Comparison of results obtained with lateral sliding and coronally repositioned flaps. J. Periodontol. 49: 457. 1978.

8. SULLIVAN,H.C. and ATKINS,J.H: Free autogenous gingival graft grafts. Part III. Utilisation of grafts in the treatment of gingival recessions. Periodontics 6:152. 1968.

9. MILLER,P.D. Jr: Root coverage using a free soft tissue autograft following citric acid application. Int. J. Perio Rest. Dent. 2(1): 65. 1982.

10. MILLER,P.D.Jr. Root coverage using a free soft tissue autograft following citric acid application III. A successful and predictable procedure in areas of deep and wide recession. Int. J. Periodontol Rest. Dent. 5(2):14. 1985.

11. HOLBROOK,T. and OCHSENBEIN,C: Complete coverage of the denuded root surface with a one-stage gingival graft. Int.J. Periodontol. Rest. Dent. 3:9. 1983.

12. LANGER,B. and LANGER,L: Subepithelial connective tissue graft technique for root coverage. J.Periodontol. 56:12.1985

13. RATZKE,P.B: Covering localized areas of root exposure employing the envelope technique. J.Periodontol. 56:7. 1985.

14. NELSON,S.W: The sub-pedicle connective tissue graft. A bilaminar reconstructive procedure for the coverage of denuded root surfaces. J. Periodontol. 58:2. 1987.

© 1991 Elsevier Science Publishers B.V.
Recent advances in periodontology Vol. II,
S.I. Gold, M. Midda and S. Mutlu, eds.

TREATMENT OF GINGIVAL DEFECTS BY SUBEPITHELIAL CONNECTIVE TISSUE GRAFTS : NEW PROPOSALS IN PERIODONTAL SURGERY AND IMPLANTOLOGY

RAPHAEL SERFATY, JOEL ITIC and MARC MONGEOT

Department of Periodontology, University of Paris 7, Paris (France)

INTRODUCTION

Introduced at first to increase the width of attached gingiva (1), connective tissue grafts gave us access to more predictible and long lasting results when used as subepithelial connective tissue grafts (S.E.C.T.G.) for root coverage (2),(3),(4).

Our proposals for new applications are partly suggested by these authors. These new approaches are applied with a follow up of five to eight years, giving us reproducible, esthetical and long lasting results (5).

The clinical analysis of the gingiva was investigated after S.E.C.T.G., when this protocole is applied (6),(7),(8) :
- in guided tissue regeneration
- in cases of root dischromic problems combined with poor and thin gingiva
- with partially keratinized grafts
- for the treatment of gingival recessions after cementation of fixed crowns and bridge-work
- for implanted biomaterials coverage
- for the management of operatory errors
- in plastic surgery
- in repositioned flaps or in apically, coronally or laterally repositioned flaps
- during crown lengthening
- during apical surgery
- in implantology at various stages
- for esthetical frenectomy
- for the treatment of gingival clefts after orthodontic treatments
- for the regeneration of papilla

- for lingual gingival grafts and
- for root coverage (9)

MATERIAL AND METHODS

Though root coverage was not the aim of all surgeries (recessions treated in the context of global treatment, during flaps, G.T.R. or apical surgery), 245 recessions (49 % situated on mandibulary teeth, 51 % on maxillary teeth) of 1 to 8 mm, concerning 100 patients (67 females, 33 males), were treated by S.E.C.T.G., with a follow up of 1 to 5 years.

A gentle mechanical treatment of root surfaces was completed by tetracycline Hcl solution of 100 mg/ml, pH 1.9, for 3 minutes.

RESULTS

Our results are summarized in the following comparative table:

Study	Cases	Root coverage %		
1) Classical grafts				
HOLBROOK-OCHSENBEIN 1983	50 cases	95.5 % R<3 mm	80.6 % 3 to 5 mm	76.6 % R>5 mm
MILLER 1985	100 cases	100 % R<3 mm	86.6 % 3 to 5 mm	100 % R>5 mm
2) S.E.C.T.G.				
RAETZKE 1985	12 cases	80 % coverage for all cases 100 % coverage in 42 % cases		
LANGER 1985	56 cases	Percentage of coverage not recorded		
NELSON 1986	29 cases	100 % R<3mm	92 % 3 to 6mm	88 % 7 to 10mm
JOURNEE 1989	22 cases	100 % R<3 mm	94 % 3 to 6 mm	58 % R>6 mm
SERFATY 1990	245 cases	100 % 1 to 3 mm 27 cases	96 % 4 to 6 mm 140 cases	69 % 7 to 8mm 78 cases

R = recession

Our results confirm those of previous studies.

In this study, 60 % of the recessions ⩾ 7 mm, only have a one year follow up, however these recessions need more observation.

The protocoles of Holbrook-Ochsenbein (10) and Miller (11) do not give us constant results.

Recession measurements are not standardized in these studies and the follow up varies from 3 months to 5 years.

The esthetical aspect needs more than 3 months for the stabilisation (contraction and densification).

The creeping attachment is constant and progresses 1 to 3 mm or more from the third to the sixth month.

The attached gingiva, sometimes looks like a connective tissue covered by mucosa (12), in other cases, it looks like a keratinized gingiva.

An histological study seems to be necessary.

NEW APPLICATIONS

In this short article, it is not possible to describe all of these protocoles, however we can emphasize some important aspects.

During flap surgeries, S.E.C.T.G. allows in one surgical step the treatment of root surfaces, bony defects and mucogingival problems : just before suturing the flaps, the connective tissue graft is secured in a good position.

Esthetical frenectomy consists in placing a connective tissue graft under the flap containing the frenum : after healing, no scars occur and the frenum after 2 or 3 months have migrated apically.

With this approach, we have also treated gingival clefts and bucco-sinusal communications.

In implantology, there are great possibilities to improve the gingival situation creating an adequate attached gingiva.

CONCLUSIONS

This approach provides a double-blood supply (underlying periosteum and overlying flap) which could explain the great potential of healing.

This work demonstrates the great versatility of connective tissue, when used as subepithelial graft.

This technique allows in one surgical step the treatment of root surfaces, bony defects and mucogingival problems.

Clinically, "the attached gingiva" created is healthy,

functional and esthetic.

Root coverage obtained confirms previous results attained by RAETZKE, LANGER and NELSON.

The creeping attachment seems to be faster than usual with no difference between upper and lower jaw.

Post operative probing depths have ranged from 1 to 3 mm in all cases, with no recurrence of recession.

This approach shows long lasting results, stable over 5 to 8 years.

REFERENCES

1. Edel A (1974) Clinical evaluation of free connective tissue grafts used to increase the width of keratinized gingiva J. Clin. Periodont. 1 : 185-196

2. Raetzke PB (1985) Covering localized areas of root exposure employing the "envelope" technic J. Periodontol. 56 : 397

3. Langer B and Langer L (1985) Subepithelial connective tissue graft for root coverage J. Periodontol. 56 : 715-720

4. Nelson SW (1986) The subpedicle connective tissue graft. A bilaminar reconstructive procedure for the coverage of denuded root surfaces J. Periodontol. 58 : 95-102

5. Serfaty R and Itic J (1990) Subepithelial connective tissue grafts : new applications in periodontal surgery and implantology IADR, 235, Bern, Sept. 1990 To be published J. Dent. Res. Special issue, 1991

6. Nguyen V (1990) Les greffes conjonctives, approche des protocoles et applications aux différentes disciplines en odontologie Thesis, Dir. Serfaty R, Paris 7

7. Serfaty and Itic J (1990) Proposition pour de nouvelles applications des greffes de conjonctif enfoui en odontologie L'inf. Dent., accepted for publication, July

8. Serfaty R (1990) Les greffes conjonctives L'inf. Dent. 72 (23) : 2075

9. Serfaty R and Itic J (1990) Le recouvrement des dénudations radiculaires : apport des greffes conjonctives J. de la Douleur 7-9

10. Hollbrook T and Ochsenbein C (1983) Complete coverage of the denuded root surface with a one-stage gingival graft Int. J. Periodontol. Rest. Dent. 3 : 9

11. Miller P (1982) Root coverage using a free soft tissue autogenous graft following citric acid application I. Technique. Int. J. Periodontol. Rest. Dent. 2 : 65

12. Ouhayoun JP, Goffaux JC, Sawaf HM, Etienne D and Forest N (1988) Greffes gingivales à partir de greffons conjonctifs et epithélio-conjonctifs : étude clin. et histol. chez l'homme J. de Parodontol. Vol. 7 N° 1 : 7-18

© 1991 Elsevier Science Publishers B.V.
Recent advances in periodontology Vol. II,
S.I. Gold, M. Midda and S. Mutlu, eds.

HISTOLOGICAL RESEARCH INTO TRANSPLANT OF TOOTH GERMS

GIAMPIERO MASSEI, Via Bardonecchia 29, 10139 TORINO, ITALY

JANTIEN DUNS, Via Bardonecchia 29, 10139 TORINO, ITALY

CESARE PIAGGIO, Via Orzali 215/A, 55100 LUCCA, ITALY

ENRICO CARBESI, Ospedale Martini, 10139 TORINO, ITALY

In the transplant of dental germs both the technique and the attention paid during the operation are determining factors for a successful long term result.

A successful operation will feature the following clinical aspects: a normal colour of the tooth, (healthy gingiva), shallow sulcus, well formed alveolar bone and normal root formation with normal periodontal space and the presence of a lamina dura on the X-ray.

When this clinical aspects are present we have a good prognosis and the transplanted tooth will be considered like any other tooth on the dental arch.

The formation of a normal periodontal ligament is a constant feature of transplanted dental germs, whereas in the transplant of teeth it is easier to find areas of ankylosis.

Various factors which determine successful transplant:

1) Source of transplant:

any germs may be used for autotransplant.

The mostly used germs are the following: third molars, bicuspids, lower incisors, supernumerary teeth, germs which cannot erupt and the ones contained in follicular cysts.

2) Receiving site:

asuitable site must have a sufficient alveolar bone support and   adherent gingiva.

3) Stage of root development of transplant:

the primary objective will be to obtain the maximum development of both the root and the ligament.

One must therefore perform the transplant in the most favourable conditions, that is the presence of a 3-6 mm root.

4) Surgical technique:

The surgeon must avoid surgical traumata through a delicate manipulation of the tissues and a minimal manipulation of the transplant itself.

At first one proceeds with the removal of the germ from the donor site.

Having, then, ascertained its shape and size one replaces the germ in the donor site and proceeds with the preparation of the alveolar site.

EVOLUTION OF AN AUTOTRANSPLANT

The transplant is followed by normal healing with re-formation of the ligament, revascularization of the pulp and growth of the root.

Successive X-rays will show a formation of the lamina dura and a normal periodontal space.

Later radiological checks show that the root grows again normally even if a little shorter.

Generally this reduction is not over 2-3 mm, that is 10% of the normal final length of the tooth.

A thinning or a distortion of the root or the obliteration of the pulp chamber and the root canal may be observed.

These variations are a response to the trauma undergone during the operation.

REGENERATION OF BOTH PERIODONTAL LIGAMENT AND PULP IN TRANSPLANTED GERMS

We have examined 10 block sections of germ transplants in a retromolar area where a third molar had previously been extracted from.

The sample was taken from 4 to 450 days after the implant.

Samples were immersed in formalin for 1-3 days, mildly decalcified with picric acid, then enclosed in paraffin.

The said samples then sectioned in 5-6 micron slices and coloured with eosin haematoxillin and some with Mallory threecromic.

Towards the 4th post-operative day the periodontal ligament begins to be richly vascularized and features a gradual regeneration and cell replacement.

The proliferation of connective tissue continues and evolves in a normal bond between bone and cementum.

Towards the 25th day areas of demineralization in the cementum can be observed. It is not possible to avoid this type of reaction even if the greatest care was ensured during the operation in order not to damage either the pulp or the root. This type of resorption is reversible and, at a later stage, the small gaps will be filled with cementum which acquires a normal appearance.

If there are any areas of the root subjected to trauma during the operation the cementum will not grow and there will not be an adequate bond with the bone.

Nevertheless the degree of resorption found after careful surgical operation has never endangered the success of a transplant. In the long term a physiologically incorporated transplant will feature a normal size periodontal space and the growth of the lamina dura. From the second post-operative day the odontoblastic layer shows areas of detachment of neodentin and an inflammatory infiltrate with associated hyperemia (Northway et al.).

There will be a period – from 3 to 5 days – of relative nutritional reduction until vascularization develops again.

Together with revascularization in many cases a reinnervation develops. In other instances reinnervation is absent and one only has a revascularization process. In the formation of dentin following the transplant an increase in the growth of non-tubular dentin was observed.

Nevertheless, after about 3 months, the growth of tubular dentin re-established itself. The pulp tissue tends to appear normal in the middle and third apical part of the root. Beginning from the end of the third month the crown portion of the pulp may be mixed with osteodentin or with a connective tissue rich with collagenous fibres.

During this period there is a transformation of odontoblastic layers into fibroblastic type cells. These changes result from an initial lack of vascularization. With the subsequent re-establishement of the blood flow the growth processes of both pulp and root become normal.

REFERENCES

1. Agnew, R.G. and Fong, C.C.: Histological Studies on Experimental Transplan-
    tation of Teeth, Oral Surg. 1: 18, 1956

2. Andreasen, J.O. Hjorting-Hansen E. and Jolst O./ A Clinical and Radiogra-
    phic Study of Seventy-Six Autotransplanted Third Molars, Scand. J. Dent.
    Res. 78: 512-523, 1970

3. Bolton, R./ Autogenous Transplantation and Replantation of Teeth: Report on
    60 Treated Patients Brit.J. Oral Surg. 12: 147-165, 1974

4. Massei, G.P./ Transplant of Dental Germs and Formation of Periodontal
    Ligament. 4th Congress Panamerican Association of Periodontology Buenos
    Aires 26-29 Nov. 1986

5. Massei, G.P./ Reformation of Periodontal Ligament in Transplant of Dental
    Germs. 4th Congress Italian Association of Parodontology Catania 5-6 June
    1987

6. Northway, W.M./Autogenetic Tooth Transplantation, Am. J. Orthod. 77
    n° 2 Feb. 80

7. Slagsvold, O. and Bjercke, B./ Autotransplantation of Premolars with partly
    Formed Roots, A Radiographic Study of Root Growth, Am. J. Orthod. 66:
    335-336, 1974

8. Urbani, G./ Autotransplant of Germs in the HUman, Stomatologia Mediterranea
    8th year n° 3 July-September 1988

© 1991 Elsevier Science Publishers B.V.
Recent advances in periodontology Vol. II,
S.I. Gold, M. Midda and S. Mutlu, eds.

GINGIVA OF KIDNEY TRANSPLANTED PATIENTS BEFORE AND AFTER PERIODONTAL TREATMENT WHO WERE MEDICATED BY CYCLOSPORIN A (CyA).

SELÇUK YILMAZ, ÜLKÜ NOYAN, OKTAY ARDA*
M.U. Dental Faculty, Periodontology Department.
*İ.U. Cerrahpaşa Medical Faculty Histology and Embryology Department.
İstanbul (Turkey).

INTRODUCTION

Clinical applications of CyA started since 1978 (1). The exact mechanism of CyA's immunosuppressive action is not fully clear. CyA preferred specifically among the other immunosuppressive drugs in postoperative immunosuppression of the organ transplanted patients, because of it's nonmyelotoxic character. The side effects of CyA are nephrotoxicity, hepatotoxicity (2), hirsutism (3) and gingival hyperplasia (GH) (4). The short interval of CyA's application in clinic couldn't explain the etiology of GH by clinical and histopathological studies. Scientific data up to date only points out the histopathological changes observed in patients who display GH.

The primary objective of our study is to give a comparative ultrastructural description of the morphological changes that we observed in organ transplanted patients' gingiva who did or didn't display GH following CyA therapy.

The second objective is to review and compare the ultrastructural morphology of post operative condition of gingiva following periodontal surgical treatment with the ones who didn't show GH.

MATERIAL AND METHOD

Following kidney transplantations, all the patients had CyA, azathioprine and corticosteroid medication. The gingival biopsy specimens of the patients who didn't display GH formed the 1st. group. Pre and post surgical gingival biopsy specimens of the ones who displayed GH assembled the 2nd and 3rd. groups respectively. There were 5 patients in each group.

The specimens prefixed overnight in 4% glutaraldehyde mixed in Milloning phosphate buffer at pH 7.3 and 0-4oC. After rinsing with the same buffer, they post fixed for 1 h in 1% osmium tetroxide mixed in the same buffer, pH and temperature. They dehydrated in ethanol, passed through propylene oxide and embedded in Araldit. The blocs cut on a REICHERT O-UM 3 Ultramicrotome. Sections placed on naked copper grids and stained with uranyl acetate and lead citrate. Observations carried out with a CARL ZEISS EM 10-A electron microscope.

RESULTS

Group 1

The interstitial spaces of the epithelium widened moderately and desmosomes reduced. Fig. 1. Cell/fiber proportion in the connective tissue appeared to be normal. The most prominent morphological change was in mast cell granules (MCG). Among the normal ones some displayed centrally accumulated electron dense material Fig. 2 and a few was in crystalline form. This may resulted from cellular immunosuppression (5) and/or CyA's direct effect on mast cells (MC) (6).

266

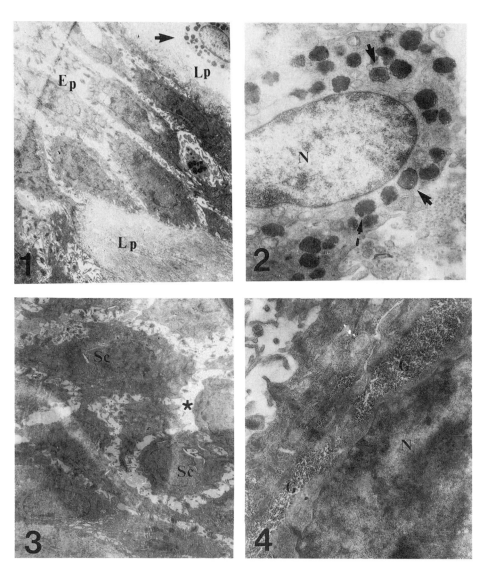

Fig. 1. Epithelium (Ep), Mast cell (->), Lamina propria (Lp),
Fig. 2. Mast cell nucleus (N), Normal granules (-->), Granules with
centrally accumulated electron dense material (->),
Fig. 3. Interstitial space (*), Spinal cell (Sc)
Fig. 4. Nucleus of spinal cell (N), Glycogen (G),

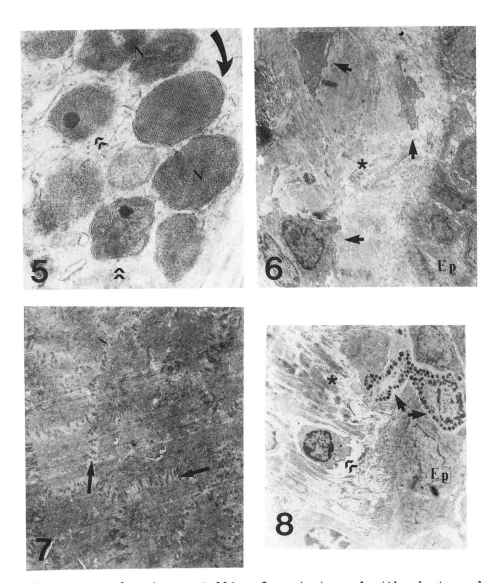

Fig. 5. Granule; in crystalline form (->), and with electron dense core (>>), Normal MCG (N)

Fig. 6. Epithelium (Ep), Fibroblast (->), Connective tissue matrix and fibirs (*)

Fig. 7. Interstitial spaces and spinal cell junctions (->)

Fig. 8. Epithelium (Ep), Mast cell (->), Connective tissue and fibers of lamina propria (*), fibroblast (>>).

Group 2

Increase in widening of interstitial spaces and destruction of epithelial attachments suggested the initiation of edema. Fig. 3. In a patient's epithelial cells, there were accumulations of glycogen alpha particles Fig. 4. This may be due to corticosteroid stimulation (7). Highly activated plasma cells markedly increased. CyA inhibits cellular immune system (5). Somewhat unaffected B-cells may permit patients to maintain humoral response to potential pathogens while avoiding the effects of T-cell system (8). There is no observation of GH in edentulous mouths (9) or after extraction of the teeth the hyperplastic tissue that surrounds the teeth replaces itself to normal mucosa (10). This again points out the triggering effects of antigens as far as humoral immune response concerned.

MC were very closely located next to B-cells. Electron dense core and crystalline forms of MCG increased remarkably Fig. 5. Again this may resulted from cellular immunosuppression (5) and/or direct effect of CyA on MC.

There were supplementary vascularization and increased fibroblastic activity Fig. 6. This immunosuppression permits antigens to trigger humoral immune response. Onset of inflammation provokes the increased activity of fibroblasts.

Group 3

The epithelium was morphologically normal. Destruction of desmosomes and presence of edema vanished Fig. 7. Connective tissue returned to it's normal status. The number of plasma cells decreased. These changes suggested the successful result of surgical treatment. Yet there were many MC located near epithelium. They were morphologically similar as seen in group two Fig. 8. This points out the ready humoral defense and recurrence of GH.

ACKNOWLEDGMENT

Archives of our specimens and electron micrographs, statistics and word processing carried out by an IBM P/S 2 70 model computer kindly donated by IBM Turkey.

REFERENCES

1. Calne RY et-al (1978) Lancet 23-30:1323-1327
2. Bennett WM, Norman DJ (1989) An Rev Med 37:215-224
3. Goldman MH, et-al (1985) Surg Clin North Am 65:637-659
4. Friskopp J, Klintmalm G (1986) Swed Dent J 10:85-92
5. American Hospital Formulary Service -Drug Information. Bethesda, MD, American Society of Hospital Pharmacists (1985) pp 826-828, pp 1731-1737, pp 612-613
6. Pedersen H et-al (1985) Allergy 40:103-107
7. Haynes RC, Murad F (1983) In: Gilman AG, Goodman JS, Gilman A (eds) The Pharmacological Basis of Therapeutics. Macmillian Pub C Inc, London, pp 1470-1489
8. Daley TD, Wysocki GP (1984) J Periodontol 55:708-712
9. Wysocki GP, et-al (1983) Oral Surg 55:274-278
10. Rateitschak-Plüss EM, et-al (1983) 10:237-246

© 1991 Elsevier Science Publishers B.V.
Recent advances in periodontology Vol. II,
S.I. Gold, M. Midda and S. Mutlu, eds.

APPLICATION OF ADHESIVE RESIN-BONDED BRIDGES WITH NATURAL TEETH PONTICS IN PERIODONTALLY INVOLVED ANTERIOR DENTITIONS

ORHUN BENGİSU

Department of Periodontology,Dental Faculty, Ege University, Bornova-İzmir(Turkey)

INTRODUCTION

If there is a hopeless tooth requiring extraction in a periodontally involved anterior dentition, the patient often faces the problem of replacing it with a conventional bridge. In most of the cases, the remaining anterior teeth have also considerable amount of attachment loss and are quite mobile. In that case, there are mainly two alternatives; one is the extraction of the remaining mobile incisors and construction of a bridge between canines and the other is the construction of an extended fixed partial denture in order to permanently splint the mobile teeth while replacing the missing one(s). The former situation is physiologically and psychologically debilitating to many patients, while the latter is expensive, time consuming, requires great amount of irreversible tooth preparation and may cause problems especially if used to preserve teeth with a poor prognosis. A third alternative now exists involving the construction of a cast metal resin-bonded lingual plate(splint) on which the patient's periodontally condemned natural tooth is bonded as pontic after extraction, endodontic obturation and preparation for resin bonding to the cast metal framework. Thus, the remaining mobile teeth are both preserved and stabilized as well as the extraction site is restored with the original natural tooth.

The advantages of this technique over conventional bridges are technique simplicity, ease of application, conservation of natural tooth structure, reduced cost and improved esthetics. Besides, since the tooth modifications, impressions and restoration margins are supragingival, the entire procedure is kinder to the periodontal tissues and allows easy plaque elimination. This flexible method also provides for the possible loss of periodontally compromised teeth in an existing prosthesis. If one of the abutment teeth which are resin bonded to the lingual plate do not respond to periodontal and/or endodontic treatment, they do not need to be removed, instead, gingivally submerged part of the condemned tooth is surgically removed and the apical surface recontoured. Endodontic access may be acomplished incisally or through preconstructed lingual access openings on metal.

Case Presentations

The following photographs highlight several cases, in which the problems of tooth loss and mobility are solved with the application of this technique. The patients had reported that a marked improvement in comfort due to loss of mobility has happened and an excellent esthetics was provided.

Case No.1 : The lower anterior dentition was so badly periodontally involved that extraction of all incisors had been recommended. Actually, bone support was minimal and the teeth were extremely mobile(Fig.1). After a meticulous debridement, only tooth 41 was extracted and the remaining anterior teeth were prepared for resin bonding(Fig.2). The apical surface of the root was recontoured to give it a pontic shape and the root canal was cleaned and later obturated with a composite material through an apical access. After then it was bonded to the cast metal lingual plate(Fig.3). After acid etching of teeth, the adhesive bridge is bonded to the teeth with the help of Panavia Ex(Fig.4).

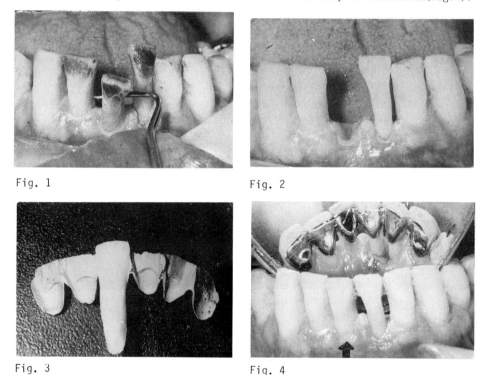

Fig. 1

Fig. 2

Fig. 3

Fig. 4

Figs. 1, 2, 3, 4. Clinical presentation of Case No. 1

Case No.2 : A 32 year old woman had extensive bone loss and very high mobility in her lower incisors. During the flap operation, tooth 41, which had no remaining support was extracted. After healing, teeth which were still mobile were prepared for the adhesive bridge(Fig.5). After construction of the cast-metal lingual plate, first the extracted tooth was bonded into place (it was now a resin-bonded bridge)(Fig.6), and then the bridge was bonded to the teeth(Fig.7) The metal framework was invisible and the esthetic harmony was exceptional that it was hard to obtain with a conventional bridge.

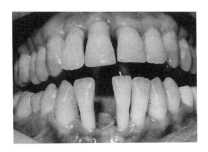

Fig. 5

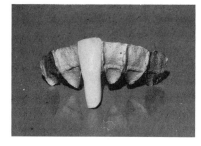

Fig. 6

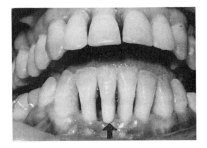

Fig. 7

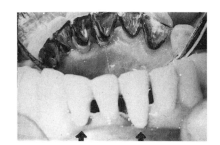

Fig. 8

Figs. 5, 6, 7. Case No. 2   Fig. 8. Case No. 3

Case No.3 : Tooth 31 and 42 were the patient's extracted natural teeth which served as pontics in this resin-bonded adhesive fixed partial denture (FPD)(Fig8)

Case No.4 : A 42 year old woman had severe bone loss and a periodontal abcess on tooth 41 (Fig.9). During the flap operation, this tooth was extracted (Fig.10) After healing, a resin bonded adhesive bridge, with tooth 41 as the natural pontic was fabricated and bonded to the fairly mobile anterior teeth (Fig.11) Should a conventional bridge have been constructed in this case, a great deal of tooth preparation and maybe multiple pulpectomies would have been necessary, or the remaining anterior teeth would have been extracted.

Case No.5 : The patient had lost tooth 21 and the remaining anterior teeth had considerable attachment loss and multiple diastemas due to pathologic tooth migrations (Fig.12). This tooth was replaced into its original place by an adhesive FPD, but the diastemas persisted (Fig.13). They were later closed with visible-light cured composite resin (Fig.14). A satisfactory esthetics was thus obtained and the patient was more pleased as both his natural tooth was preserved and the diastemas were closed.

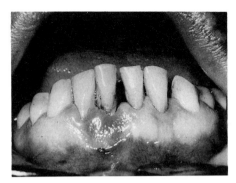

Fig. 9 Case 4.Preoperative view

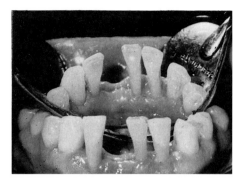

Fig. 10 Case 4.Postoperative view

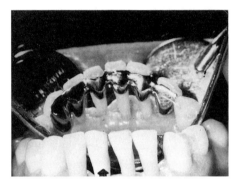

Fig. 11 Case 4.Splint bonded into place

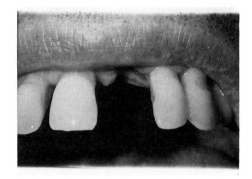

Fig. 12 Case 5.Pre-treatment view

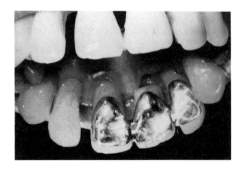

Fig. 13 Case 5.Adhesive bridge bonded

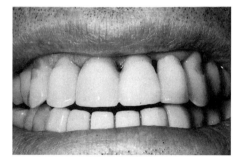

Fig. 14 Case 5.Diastemas were closed

* References available upon request from the author.

© 1991 Elsevier Science Publishers B.V.
Recent advances in periodontology Vol. II,
S.I. Gold, M. Midda and S. Mutlu, eds.

RELATIONS BETWEEN MOTIVES OF CONSULTATION AND LEVEL OF HYGIENE

FRANÇOIS ALCOUFFE

Department of Periodontology, School of Dental Surgery, PARIS 7 University. (France).

INTRODUCTION

It is a well-accepted fact that patient compliance is one of the keys to therapeutic succes in periodontology. Nevertheless most individuals fail to perform adequate home care.For this reason, screening of patients based on Rotter's survey has been carried out by various authors. Rotter identified two distinct types of patient personalities :"internals" and "externals". Internals see themselves as being in control of what happens to them.One could say: "motivated".Contrastingly externals do not respond as well to preventive dentistry.Rotter, considered a patient's personality to be firmly established and suggested scoring it prior to tratment.But most of these procedures are time and personnel consuming. The present study was undertaken with the aim of setting up an immediate "behavior forecast" based on the motives of consultation.

In others words, can a patient's chief complaint be a reliable predictor for his prophylactic behavior?

MATERIAL AND METHODS

147 adult patients (89 females and 58 males) consulting in private practice in an urban community.Plaque indices were recorded according to O' Leary (1972) and grouped in ten classes: from O % to 10 % :Class O, from 11% to 20% Class 1 ,etc,up to Class 9 which ranges from 91 to 100 %.

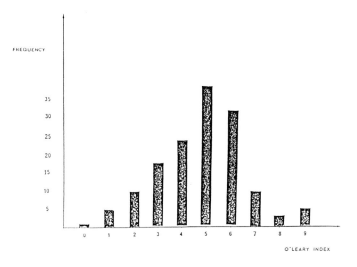

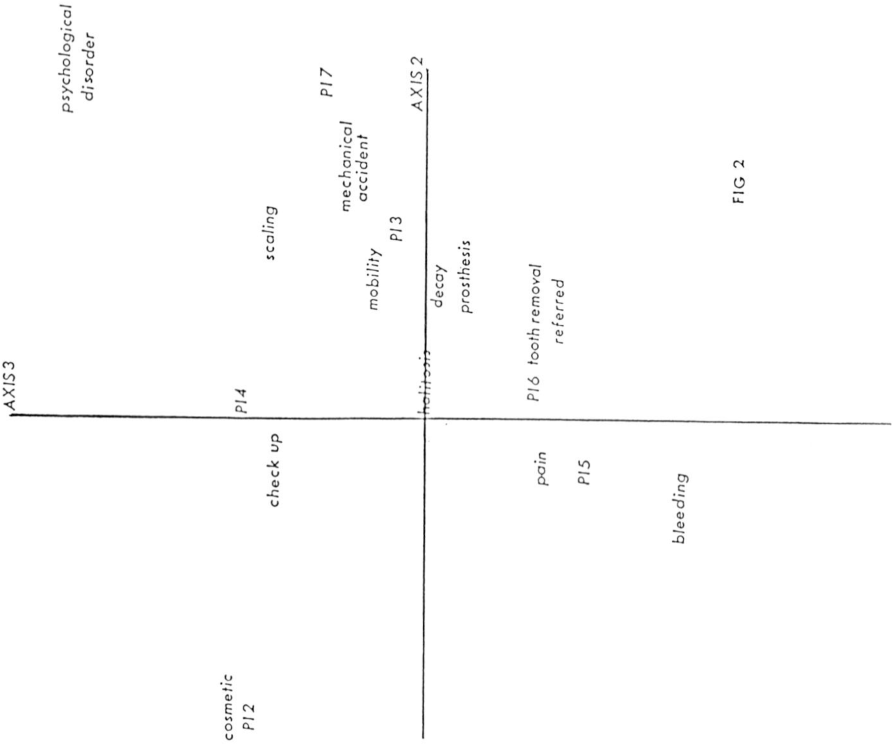

FIG 1

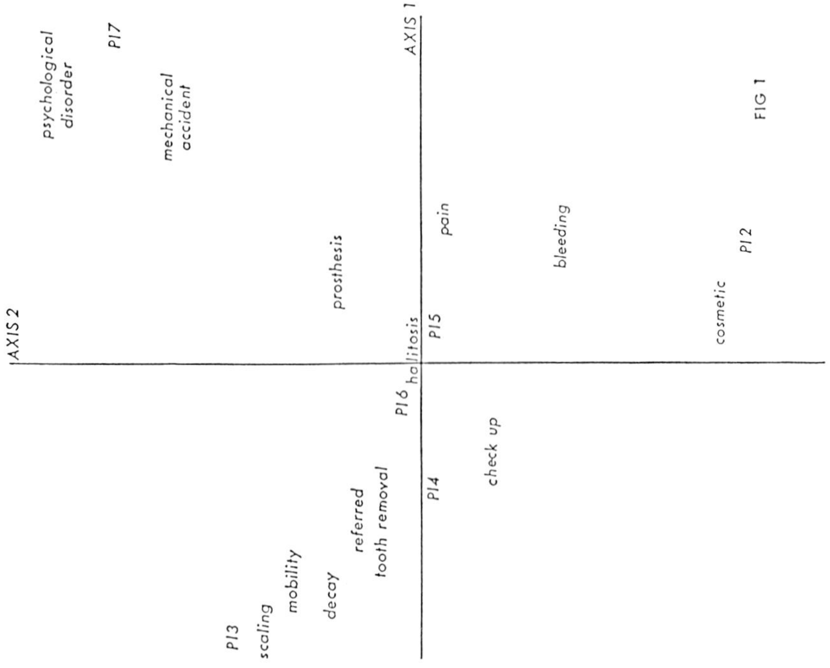

AXIS 2

AXIS 1

psychological disorder

P17

mechanical accident

prosthesis

pain

P13
scaling
mobility
decay
referred
tooth removal

P14

P16 hallitosis

P15

check up

bleeding

cosmetic

P12

FIG 2

AXIS 3

AXIS 2

psychological disorder

scaling

mechanical accident

P17

mobility

P13

decay

prosthesis

P14

check up

halitosis

P16 tooth removal

referred

pain

P15

bleeding

cosmetic

P12

The patient's different motives of consultation were classified by extrapolation of Rotter's concept.The external motives were considered as urgengy motives ,usually subjected to events.

External motives:

10*pain of any kind

11 mechanical accident (tooth breaking, loss of filling,etc...)

12 gum bleeding or exsudate

13 halitosis

14 tooth mobility

15 decay (with food impaction)

16 any irreversible pathology leading to tooth removal

In contrast to external motives, internal motives, were rather considered as linked to preventive behavior.

Internal motives:

20*cosmetic preoccupations

21 request for prosthesis

22 check up

23 scaling or cleaning

Patients who belonged to neither of the above categories and who consulted for miscellanous reasons were labelled 'others'.

Others:

30* referred patients

31 patients with psychological disorders.(* means : arbitrary code).

RESULTS

The statistical analysis was carried out using a factorial analysis of correspondence It showed a proportion of cumulated variance of 84.62% explained by the three first axis: 35.31% for the first axis,27.61% for the second axis and 21.70% for the third axis.

The matching of the index classes with the motives was based upon these 3 axes.

(1) Study of axes 1 and 2. (fig.1) Axis 1 shows contrasting behavior patterns between subjects whose indices were respectively PI 3 andPI 7.On the right side of axis 1 it appears clearly that there is positive correlation betweenPI 7 (poor hygiene) and mechanical accident, whereas,on the left, PI 3 (good hygiene) is essentially associated with scaling.Axis 2 is simply the reproduction of the data as delivered by the computer in a two dimensional space.Nevertheless, a correlation between PI 2 and cosmetic problems is noticeable.

(2) Study of axes 2 and 3. (fig 2) Axis 2 (above mentioned). Axis 3 shows contrastinG patterns between subjects whose indices were PI 4 (check up motives)andPI 5 (pain and bleeding).

DISCUSSION

To our knowledge, the current literature on the comparison between motives of consultation and level of hygiene is scarce .Given the present controversy concerning the clinical response to oral hygiene , one might of course wonder whether studies on oral hygiene are at all relevant? Still, the strong positive correlation between plaque and disease makes hygiene the main goal at the community level (Pilot 1984). Our data tend to indicate positive correlations :

(1) emergency behavior_poor hygiene.

(2) preventive behavior_good hygiene.These results have to be confirmed by further investigations with other patient samples (of different socio-economic levels, for instance) But they do appear rather logical: people of a prophylactic behavior are consistent with themselves and behave similarly at home and at the dental office.

CONCLUSION

In conclusion, one cannot be sure of the mental mechanisms which lead to consultation but whithin the limits of this study, good hygiene is associated with prophylactic behavior ,whereas poor hygiene is associated with emergency behavior.

It appears that the borderline between the two groups is around 50% plaque index according toO'Leary.

REFERENCES

1.ROTTER, J.B. (1966). Generalized expectancies for internal versus external control of reinforcement.
PsychologicalMonographs. 8O=1-28.

2. O'LEARY ,T.J.,,DRAKE ,R.B. ,and NAYLOR,J.E. (1972). The plaque control record.
Journal of Periodontology. 43=38-4O.

3. PILOT, T. (1984).Implementation of preventive periodontal programmes at the community level in public health aspects of periodontal disease.
Ed Quintessence. p255.

© 1991 Elsevier Science Publishers B.V.
Recent advances in periodontology Vol. II,
S.I. Gold, M. Midda and S. Mutlu, eds.

CPITN-BASED TREATMENT OF PERIODONTITIS IN AMERICAN VETERANS

ROY S. FELDMAN (1,2)

CECILLE A. FELDMAN (2,3)

ANN E. ESHENAUR-SPOLARICH (1,4)

Veterans Affairs Medical Center (1); School of Dental Medicine, University of
Pennsylvania, Philadelphia, PA (2); University of Medicine and Dentistry of New
Jersey, Newark, NJ (3); Thomas Jefferson University, Philadelphia, PA (4)
(USA).

INTRODUCTION

Periodontal disease in adult populations is increasingly important as a
major cause of dental morbidity (1). As part of the study "Periodontitis in
the Aging Veteran: Effect and Cost of Unmet Needs", a longitudinal
investigation of disease and its progression, we have monitored periodontal
treatment need and actual therapy according to an objective numerical model,
the Community Periodontal Index of Treatment Needs (2). This numerical scoring
system was designed for use in comprehensive dental care systems for adult
populations with history of high caries prevalence and extensive restorative
treatment, a characteristic of patients actively maintained on the roles of the
Philadelphia Veterans Affairs Medical Center, a tertiary care urban hospital
with emphasis on outpatient programs. We assessed periodontal disease by
recording of periodontal pocket formation (3), scored as the worst finding of
all teeth in a sextant. We referred patients for sextant-specific treatment to
hygienists and periodontists. On the basis of this model of clinical disease,
treatment of lesions is not mandatory, as individual providers prescribe
therapy, but assignment of patients to providers was accomplished by CPITN.

This protocol is designed to economize in the collection of data and to
maximize the applicability of these data to comparable populations. These data
will allow us to establish measure of clinical outcome as a basis for
comparison of these treatment protocols over time, and to establish cost
assessments on the basis of the personnel employed and the facilities used (4).

METHODS

Patient Recruitment

Service-connected eligible veteran patients presenting to this medical center for dental treatment were enrolled in this protocol if at least twenty teeth were present, the patient was likely to return for follow-up visits and informed consent was obtained. We enrolled patients in three therapeutic protocols: treatment directed by CPITN; by periodontist or by dental hygienist. All delegation of patients to study protocol was by random assignment, without regard for medical, psychiatric or periodontal status.

Data Collection Technique

All baseline data were obtained by trained examiners who were not health care personnel responsible for treatment. Except for initial full mouth radiographic survey, all baseline data were maintained separate from treatment records. Periodontal charting was recorded for four sites per tooth: mesial, buccal, distal and lingual, using a AMFLEX II 23/ Probe 2 12 No. ZM21857 periodontal probe*. Caries was determined on coronal and radicular surfaces with the explorer and recorded as virgin or recurrent, and association with a previous restoration was recorded.

Patient Treatment Assignment and Recording

CPITN recordings of pocket depth for the most severe pocket per sextant were used to assign sextant-specific health care providers. Scores of 1,2 and 3 were referred to the dental hygienist for therapy, and score of 4 was referred to periodontist as "complex treatment" (2). Treatment for the CPITN sextants was unrestricted, in that providers were at liberty to treat according to their training, proficiency and clinical privileges. Treatment experience over 20 study months was recorded by health care provider, by sextant, by procedure and at ten minute intervals. In all, two clinical periodontists and seven dental hygienists were monitored. All data were recorded in Optical Scan format and prepared for analysis (5).

* GC International, Scottsdale, AZ USA

Figure 1.   CPITN Scoring System

CPITN SCORE	DIAGNOSTIC FEATURES	RECOMMENDED THERAPY
0	Healthy Tissues	None
1	Bleeding on gentle probing	Education "self-care"
2	Calculus, ≤3mm	Education and prophylaxis
3	At least one pocket 4-5mm	Education and prophylaxis and root scaling/planing
4	At least one pocket ≥6mm	Education and prophylaxis and deep scaling and surgery (prn)
X	<2 teeth functioning	Excluded

RESULTS

At baseline, the mean age of these volunteer patients was 57.0 years; not surprisingly, all but two were male. Charting at baseline indicated mean pocket depth was 2.64mm and mean attachment loss was 3.47mm. Disease extent was assessed at 87% sites with loss of attachment $\geq$ 2mm; of these 98% were assessed $\geq$ 4mm, 84% $\geq$ 6mm and 44% $\geq$ 8mm. These assessments suggest greater age-related periodontal pathology as compared to similar US populations (1, 5). Data on caries and restoration history indicated 24.9 Decayed, Filled coronal surfaces and 1.1 Decayed, Filled root surfaces, suggesting extensive experience of this group with restorative dentistry and confirmed the greater exposure to dentistry of this group compared to other US adults (5).

CPITN recordings for the deepest periodontal pocket recordings are presented according to pocket severity, by number of patients and number of sextants:

Table 1.   CPITN Scoring (N=50 Veteran Patients at Baseline)

Score	X	1	2	3	4
No. Patients	7	19	5	49	27
No. Sextants	9	47	10	156	75

During 20 study months, treatment data were gathered for the providers according to sextant, procedure and referral pattern. Provided services included universal scaling and root planing by the periodontists over multiple visits, in addition to hygienist therapy. Patient management is presented by referral pattern and sextant treated:

Table 2.   Patient Referral Pattern and Sextants Treated (20 Months)

Treatment by:	Dental Hygienist	Dentist	Both DH + DDS
No. Patients	10	7	33*
No. Sextants	102	47	278*
% Sextants	46.4%	30.4%	23.1%

* $p < 0.05$ by one-tailed x^2

Significantly more sextants were treated by both providers, a reflection of multiple treatment visits for management of disease referred between hygienist and periodontist.

We recorded sextant-specific treatment by provider to indicate therapeutic interventions over the study months:

Table 3.   Workload Recorded by CPITN and Provider (Sextants Treated)

CPITN Score	Oral Hygiene		Scaling/Root Planing		Surgery
	DH	DDS	DH	DDS	DDS
4	35	28	35	73	19
3	106	9	85	55	10
1,2	88	22	124	22	4
Total	288		394		33

Hygienist-treated patients, appropriately, receive the majority of oral hygiene instruction and prophylaxes, and surgery was restricted to the dentist. Of interest, the number of sextants scored 3 and 4 that were treated by scaling and root planing did not differ between the two health care providers. These data indicate that 25% of sites scored by CPITN for complex treatment have received periodontal surgery as compared to 6% of sites with lesser disease severity that have received surgery. Total sextants treated indicate workload of 14.3 sextants/ patient treated over 20 study months by both providers.

DISCUSSION

This population offers an interesting model for the analysis of dental care delivery systems as high disease prevalence and no fee-for-service barriers allow for investigation of novel and potentially valuable treatment protocols (4,5). Maintenance of patients is in-built, as is appropriate for longitudinal investigation (6). Estimation of treatment need for specific populations is hampered by lack of a universally accepted methodology, a "missing link" in the information required for manpower planning (7). In this protocol, we have chosen an available objective measurement scale, and insured that disease management was primarily directed at control of etiologic factors (1). Certainly, we are aware of the caution necessary in the estimation of disease from composite periodontal indexes (8). Abrogation of an epidemiologic measure for treatment planning of individual disease manifestation is not intended by this protocol.

While fully 54% of patients were referred to periodontist after baseline recordings, our observations suggest that therapy proceeded with self-restriction of periodontal surgery to 40% of sextants referred to periodontist, and one-half our patients identified by CPITN as surgical candidates received surgical treatments. Periodontal treatment may be directed by objective criteria and based on broad scale epidemiologic indicators, if treatment providers are at liberty to assess further disease indexes and to formulate individual plans for therapy. When compared to actual treatment experience, assignment to therapy based on objective criteria seems to support conventional practice treatment patterns in the management of periodontal disease by periodontist or dental hygienist. Referral patterns between providers after CPITN assignment also appear consistent with many facets of typical practice, irrespective of treatment philosophy.

SUMMARY

Workload analysis of these clinical variables suggest that assignment of patients to health care providers on the basis of CPITN provided a useful management protocol for periodontal therapy. The workload described during 20 study months suggests that the nature of services provided does not seem to be restricted by use of the objective scale of assignment to treat, and periodontist and hygienist were likely to treat each patient in this protocol. Findings include specialist utilization for surgical therapy in less than half the identified sites and universal conservative management of disease by scaling and root planing, irrespective of provider. The use of the CPITN as an objective numerical system for assignment to health care providers may offer effective and economical management protocol for periodontal patients with identified severity of disease.

ACKNOWLEDGEMENTS

The authors wish to acknowledge the dilligent clinical assistance of Ms. Nora Cotrell and Trudy Johnson and the capable technical support of Ms. Shirley Bethea. This program was supported by the Health Services Research and Development Program of the US Department of Veterans Affairs, No. IIR 85-113.

REFERENCES

1. Williams RC (1990) NEJM 322:373-382
2. Ainamo J, Barmes D, Beagrie G, Cutress T, Martin J, Sardo-Infirri J (1983) Int Dent J 32:281-291
3. Bergstrom J, Eliasson S (1989) J Clin Periodontol 16:588-592
4. Antczak-Boukoms AA, Weinstein MC (1987) J Dent Res 66: 1630-1635
5. Brunelle JA, Miller-Chisholm AJ, Loe H (1988) Oral Health of United States Adults. The National Survey of Oral Health in U.S. Employed Adults and Seniors: 1985-1986. Regional Findings. USDHHS, PHS, NIH Pub. No. 88-2869
6. Feldman RS, Alman JE, Chauncey HH (1986) J Clin Periodont 13:505-510
7. Oliver RC, Brown LJ, Loe H (1989) J Periodont 60:371-380
8. Carlos JP, Wolfe MD, Kingman A (1986) J Clin Periodontol 13:500-505

© 1991 Elsevier Science Publishers B.V.
Recent advances in periodontology Vol. II,
S.I. Gold, M. Midda and S. Mutlu, eds.

CLINICAL AND MICROBIOLOGICAL COMPARISONS OF FOUR DIFFERENT CHEMICAL AGENTS WITH SUBGINGIVAL IRRIGATION

UTKU ONAN (*), FUNDA KARAER(*), ERHAN FIRATLI(*), GÜLDEN IŞIK(*), ERGENE BUGET(**), NEZAHAT GÜRLER(**)

(*)Dept.of Periodontol. Faculty of Dentistry
(**)Dept.of Microbiol.Istanbul Faculty of Medicine
Univ.Istanbul 34390 Çapa,Istanbul,Turkey

INTRODUCTION

The role of plaque in the etiology of periodontal diseases was demonstrated by many studies using the experimental gingivitis model and widely established.These studies also demonstrated the reversibility of gingivitis by plaque control.

For many years chemical agents in conjunction with or even instead of mechanical plaque control have been tested by several methods.These agents were used by brushing, flossing, rinsing and supra-subgingival irrigation methods.Many investigators demonstrated that rinses or irrigation at the gingival margin did not reach more than 3 mm depth intrasulcularly, so subgingival irrigation gains more attention novadays(1).

This double blind placebo controlled study was planned to evaluate the clinical and microbiological effects of subgingival irrigation with 0.2 % Chlorhexidine(Chx) digluconate, Listerine antiseptic(LA),Sanguinarine(Sng), Tetracycline HCl(Tet) and saline solution(SS) on experimental gingivitis model.

MATERIALS AND METHODS

50 voluntary dental students were selected according to the following criteria:
Approximal periodontal pockets between 2-4 mm, medically fit, including no recent history of drug therahy, voluntary agreement of students to participate in the study.
The patients were divided into 5 groups;

Group 1:Irrigated with Chx,

Group 2:Irrigated with Sng,

Group 3:Irrigated with LA,

Group 4:Irrigated with Tet,

Group 5:Irrigated with SS.

Each experimental, randomly selected quadrant was assessed using

the following parameters:1)Plaque index(2), 2)Bleeding at probing,
3)Pocket depth(at baseline).

After the initial clinical and microbiological parameters were
recorded, all patients were instructed in oral hygiene and subjected to a single episode of supragingival instrumentation.There
was no further instrumentation during the remainder of the study.
The study groups performed excellent toothcleaning for a period of
2 weeks.After they were asked to refrain from all oral hygiene
measures, at the third day the clinical parameters were recorded
and the randomly selected quadrants of the 5 groups were irrigated
by a syringe with the needle inserted to about half the depth of
the pocket by the same operator.The quadrants were irrigated every
third day to give a total exposure of 15 days.Clinical parameters
were measured every third day and bacterial samples were taken at
day 18.

Microbiological Sampling

Samples of the subgingival microflora were taken at day 18.Bac-
terial samples were taken from the pockets using upward strokes of
a no 7/8 Gracey curette.The material thus retrieved was dispersed
in 100 ml of sterile saline containing 1% Gelatin.A drop of solution was placed on a glasslide, covered with a coverslip and
examined by darkfield optics at a magnification of X1000.The
percentage of spirochetes, motile rods and other nonmotile
organisms was calculated(3).

Statistical Analysis

The values were detected by a computer.ANOVA was performed to all
results.The t-test with paired observations was carried out on the
clinical scores for intra and student t test was carried out for
inter group comparisons.

RESULTS

Clinical results were summarized in Table 1.Chx group yielded
significantly lower PI scores than the other groups (p 0.001).The
Listerine and Tetracycline group yielded lower PI scores than the
Saline group but they were not statistically significant.The
Listerine and Tetracycline groups yielded very significantly fewer
gingival sites which bled on probing.Also Chx group yielded
significantly fewer gingival sites which bled on probing.Sangui-
narine group was not statistically significant in both plaque

accumulation and bleeding on probing.

Microbiological Findings

The dark field microscopic counts schowed marked reduction in the
percentage of motile organisms (spirochetes and motile rods)in Chx,
LA and Tet groups.There were also a marked reduction in the percentage of nonmotile organisms in these groups.In the sterile physiological saline solution, these percentages showed increased amounts.
The post treatment sites of Chx, Listerine, Tetracycline and to a
lesser extend Sanguinarine were all similar in the morphological
appearance of their flora.Sites underwent a shift in colonisation
from one where spirochetes of all sizes abounded, together with
fusiforms, rods,filamentous organisms and motile bacteria, to one
where there was a generalised reduction in all cell numbers Chx, LA
and Tet irrigations were clearly associated with a reduction in
motile cell numbers.Only minimal effects were seen with Sng and SS
irrigation.

DISCUSSION

Failure of hygienic efforts to eliminate gingival inflammation
may have been accounted forby limited generation into pockets by
brushing, flossing or rinsing.In the sites which have been equal to
or more than 3 mm probing pocket depth supragingival antimicrobial
rinses and irrigators were unable to elicite a noticable clinical
effects.This may have been due to an osmotic gradient created by
gingival crevicular fluids that prevented solutions from influencing pockets(3).

The clinical results of the present study have shown that the
subgingival irrigation with 0.2 %Chx led to a decrease in the mean
PI significantly.Both LA and Tet groups yielded lower PI scores
the saline group but they were not statistically significant.These
findings were inagreement with previous studies(4,5).The results of
BP scores have shown that LA and Tet groups yielded very significantly fewer gingival sites which bled on probing.The differences
and contraversary between PI and BP values might be due to ;
1.Listerine and tetracycline may effect the compoition of sub-
ginival flora but not the amount of bacterial accumulation.The
binding of Chx to bacterial cell membrane inhibits the cellular

adhesion between bacteria and host tissues and the plaque accu-
mulation(5), but we failed to find literatures about the other anti-
septics`mechanisms.These are also inagreement with our microbio-
logical findings.The better results of Listerine and Tetracycline
groups on bleeding at probing may be due to their effects on the
inflammatory changes of the host tissues.

We conclude that Chx,Listerine and Tetracycline led to a decrease
in inflammatory responses and Chx inhibits the plaque accumulation
better than the other chemicals.

TABLE 1

Plaque Index(PI) and Bleeding at Probing(BP) values(Mean+SD) of
Chlorhexidine(Chx),Sanguinarine(Sng),Listerine(LA),Tetracycline HCl
(Tet) and Sterile Saline(SS) groups.

PI	1.Control	2.Control	3.Control	4.Control	5.Control	6.Control
Chx	1.42+0.37	1.28+0.52	1.31+0.52	1.24+0.47	1.16+0.49	1.08+0.55
Sng	1.01+0.59	1.48+0.49	1.38+0.40	1.47+0.42	1.70+0.53	1.53+0.55
LA	0.73+0.48	1.17+0.22	1.16+0.41	1.28+0.47	1.35+0.41	1.31+0.40
Tet	0.47+0.31	1.11+0.53	1.21+0.75	1.42+0.45	1.56+0.47	1.55+0.34
SS	0.99+0.74	1.59+0.68	1.79+0.39	1.63+0.36	1.68+0.23	2.11+0.46

BP	1.Control	2.Control	3.Control	4.Control	5.Control	6.Control
Chx	0.30+0.16	0.35+0.19	0.39+0.23	0.38+0.23	0.40+0.23	0.34+0.24
Sng	0.30+0.19	0.38+0.20	0.45+0.20	0.40+0.28	0.53+0.21	0.46+0.24
LA	0.30+0.27	0.20+0.24	0.20+0.22	0.21+0.23	0.23+0.25	0.25+0.28
Tet	0.34+0.19	0.29+0.21	0.29+0.21	0.32+0.19	0.32+0.18	0.35+0.18
SS	0.23+0.11	0.55+0.39	0.58+0.26	0.63+0.26	0.63+0.30	0.65+0.29

REFERENCES

1.Flotra L,Gjermo P,Rolla G, Waerhaug J (1972) Scand J Dent Res
  80:10

2.Silness J,Löe H (1964) Acta Odont Scand 22:121-155

3.Hardy JH, Newman HN,Strahan JD (1982) J Clin Periodontol 9:57

4.Gordon JM, Lamster B, Seiger MC (1985) J Clin Periodontol 12:697

5.Hull PS (1980) J Clin Periodontol 7:431

6.Hugo WB, Longworth AR (1968) J Pharm Pharmacol 17:28

© 1991 Elsevier Science Publishers B.V.
Recent advances in periodontology Vol. II,
S.I. Gold, M. Midda and S. Mutlu, eds.

THE ACCESSIBILITY AND EFFECTIVENESS OF A NEWLY-DESIGNED ULTRASONIC SCALER TIP
FOR FURCATION AREAS

SHIGERU ODA, HSUING-TSO WENG, DIEGO ANTONIO BORGESE and ISAO ISHIKAWA

Department of Periodontology, School of Dentistry
Tokyo Medical and Dental University
1-5-45, Yushima Bunkyo-ku, Tokyo (Japan)

INTRODUCTION

When periodontitis advances around multi-rooted teeth, the treatment for
furcation areas frequently becomes the key to success in periodontal therapy.
However, it is not easy to arrest periodontal damage of furcation areas, since
the complexity of their morphology makes effective plaque control difficult(1-
3). Therefore, there was a need for a new instrument with the capacity to
effectively remove soft bacterial plaque from multi-rooted teeth in the
treatment of furcation involvements. This study was undertaken to investigate
the accessibility and effectiveness of the newly-designed tip in furcation areas
"in vitro"(4) and "in vivo".

MATERIAL AND METHODS
Newly-designed furcation tip and ultrasonic device

The end of the tip was designed to be spherical of 0.8mm in diameter, to
protect the root surfaces and soft tissues from injury and improve contact with
the root surfaces. The tip was also to have a spiral shape with a radius
curvature of about 9mm. Two types, clockwise and counterclockwise, were
ordered. The ENAC-OE3 multi-function ultrasonic system* was selected
for this experiment. The setting of the system was maintained at graduation 5
throughout the experiment.

Methods

Experiment 1. One hundred-twenty molars were randomly divided into three
groups, each group consisting of 20 upper and 20 lower teeth. The teeth of each
group were instrumented with either the furcation tip, a conventional ultrasonic
scaler tip(ST-08 type) or Gracey curettes**. The roots of each tooth were
dissected 2mm apical from the dome of the furcation. The furcation area of each
molar was coated with a black felt-tipped marker, according to the method
described by Heins and Canter(1). Each tooth was set at the location of the

---

*Osada Electronics Co., Ltd., Tokyo, Japan.
**Hu-Friedy Manufacturing Co., Chicago, IL

first molar in an artificial jaw model* and then instrumented until the operator determined that a smooth, hard surface had been obtained. The dome surface of the furcation was photographed using a stereomicroscope at magnification 5 from each tooth.

A reticular grid divided into 1mm squares was placed over the photograph to quantify the amount of total furcation areas and the remaining colored areas. The incidence of colored areas remaining on the teeth was calculated as a percentage from the total furcation area in each case. After photographing, replica models were prepared to be observed under scanning electron microscopy**.

The Kruskal Wallis one-way analysis of variance was used to determine the significant differences among the three groups.

Experiment 2. Ten furcation involved molars which had been previously diagnosed to require extraction were used. Each tooth was instrumented with the furcation tip and the time required for the instrumentation of each tooth was recorded. After extraction, the incidence of the residual visual calculus and disclosed plaque on the teeth was assessed from the photographs as a percentage of the total furcation areas, as in Experiment 1. The teeth were then observed under scanning electron microscopy.

RESULTS

Experiment 1

The mean percentages of remaining colored areas in the upper molars were 15.1, 50.1 and 61.1 for the furcation tip, conventional ultrasonic scaler tip and Gracey curettes, respectively(Table 1). For lower molars, the mean percentages of remaining marker were 16.7, 44.1 and 39.5 in the same order as shown in Table 1. These measurements indicated that the furcation tip had a superior effect to remove the marker from upper and lower furcation areas, in comparison to other scalers ($p < 0.01$).

SEM observation revealed that the end of the furcation tip could reach the furthest into the furcation areas and produce a smoother surfaces. In few instances, the tip created an irregular surface including scattered small depressions. SEM of areas treated with the conventional ultrasonic scaler tip showed that the entrance of the furcation was shaved deeply. The hand scaler also made a depression at the entrance but a smooth surface as a whole.

Experiment 2

The mean percentages of residual calculus were 26.9 and 21.8 respectively to

---

*Nissin Co., Ltd., Kyoto. Japan.
**JSM-T20, JEOL Ltd., Tokyo, Japan.

upper and lower molars(Table 2). The means of residual plaque were 35.5% and 24.4%, respectively, as shown in Table 2. The mean time required for the instrumentation were 224 and 210 seconds, respectively, as shown in Table 2. The mean values of residual calculus and plaque of lower molars were lower than for upper molars.

SEM observation revealed that the dome of the furcation was capable of instrumentation with the furcation tip, produced a comparatively smooth surface with few scratches. SEM of the areas which were not instrumented into the furcation areas were indicated by the evidence of residual calculus on the dome of the furcation.

TABLE 1

THE MEAN PERCENTAGE OF THE REMAINING COLORED AREAS

	Newly-designed furcation tip	Conventional ultrasonic tip	Gracey curettes
Upper molars (n=60)	$15.1\pm7.6^{a,b}$	50.3 ± 11.6^{a}	61.1 ± 10.8^{b}
Lower molars (n=60)	$16.7\pm7.9^{c,d}$	44.1 ± 17.1^{c}	39.5 ± 13.1^{d}

Mean ±standard deviation

n:number of teeth

a,b,c,d:significant difference(p<0.01)

TABLE 2

THE MEAN PERCENTAGE OF RESIDUAL CALCULUS, PLAQUE AND
THE TIME REQUIRED FOR INSTRUMENTATION

	Residual calculus(%)	Residual plaque(%)	Time required for instrumentation (sec.)
Upper molars (n=6)	26.9 ± 18.7	35.5 ± 21.4	224 ± 74.1
Lower molars (n=4)	21.8 ± 8.3	24.4 ± 7.0	210 ± 38.8

Mean±standard deviation

n=number of teeth

DISCUSSION

The percentage of the areas with marker remaining for the new furcation tip in the case of upper molars was smaller than that of lower molars, in spite of the added difficulty in the instrumentation of upper molars tri-furcated structure. The results we obtained with the method used for experiment 2, with respect to the percentages of residual calculus in both, upper and lower molars were lower than those reported by Matia et al(5). Then, both the percentage of residual calculus and plaque in upper molars were higher than for lower molars "in vivo". This results have suggested that there are various factors, such as proximity and fusion of the roots, long root trunks, closed contact with adjacent tooth, which make scaling and root planing difficult.

In conclusion, the newly-designed furcation tip improved the instrumentation of furcation areas in these experiments. However, the use of this tip must be further investigated "in vivo" with respect to the efficiency in clinical practice.

REFERENCES

1. Heins PJ, Canter SR (1968) The furca involvement: A classification of bony deformities. Periodontics 6:84-86

2. Bower RC (1979) Furcation morphology relative to periodontal treatment. Furcation root surface anatomy. J Periodontol 50:336-374

3. Waerhaug J (1980) The furcation problem. Etiology, pathogenesis, diagnosis, therapy and prognosis. J Clin Periodontol 7:73-95

4. Oda S, Ishikawa I (1989) In vitro effectiveness of a newly-designed ultrasonic tip for furcation areas. J Periodontol 60:634-639

5. Matia JI, Bissada NF, Maybury JE, Ricchetti P (1986) Efficiency of scaling of the molar furcation area with and without surgical access. Int J Periodontics Restorative Dent 6(6)25-35

© 1991 Elsevier Science Publishers B.V.
Recent advances in periodontology Vol. II,
S.I. Gold, M. Midda and S. Mutlu, eds.

ULTRASTRUCTURAL COMPARISON OF GINGIVAL HYPERPLASIA (GH) DUE TO PHENYTOIN (PHT) AND CYCLOSPORIN-A (CyA).

ÜLKÜ NOYAN, SELÇUK YILMAZ, OKTAY ARDA*
M.U. Dental Faculty, Periodontology Department.
*İ.U. Cerrahpaşa Medical Faculty Histology and Embryology Department. İstanbul (Turkey).

INTRODUCTION

Fibrous gingival hyperplasia may occur due to iatrogenic, hereditary, or idiopathic factors. The most frequent one is iatrogenic factor (1). PHT is an anticonvulsive drug generally used in epileptic patients. It has the highest incidence of GH among the other drugs. GH is a well known side effect of this drug in some patients (2).

Another drug that is causing GH is CyA. It is an immunosuppressive drug and used in organ transplanted patients also in autoimmune diseases such as Behçet, psoriasis and type I diabetes mellitus (3). It preferred frequently, because of it's nonmyelotoxic and reversible action on T-Lymphocytes (1).

Although these two drugs have different chemical composition and activity, The clinically similar side effect of them is GH. We aimed to compare ultrastructurally the morphological differences of the GH caused by them.

MATERIAL AND METHOD

All the patients displayed GH. First group, formed from epileptic patients who medicated with PHT. Second group formed from patients who had CyA, azathioprine and corticosteroid medication after kidney transplantations. There were 5 patients in each group.

The specimens prefixed overnight in 4% glutaraldehyde mixed in Milloning phosphate buffer at pH 7.3 and 0-4°C. After rinsing with the same buffer, they post fixed for 1 h in 1% osmium tetroxide mixed in the same buffer, pH and temperature. They dehydrated in ethanol, passed through propylene oxide and embedded in Araldit. Sections placed on naked copper grids and stained with uranyl acetate and lead citrate. Observations carried out with a CARL ZEISS EM 10-A and EM 9S electron microscopes.

RESULTS

First group (PHT)

The fiber/ground substance proportion was higher in the latter Abundant cells and collagen fiber bundles scattered in this distended matrix of connective tissue. There were many MC closely located next to plasma cells and fibroblasts Fig. 1. Most of the mast cells degranulated Fig. 1, 2. In some others there were unusually large granules showing uniform structure. Fig. 3. In general the structure of MC granules were nearly normal when compared with second group. Frequently there were granules in fibroblasts resembling MC granules Fig. 1, 4. We agree with Angelopoulos (4) in that; PHT has a direct effect on the gingival MC. It results degranulation and release of histamine, heparin, hyaluronic acid in to connective tissue matrix. Fibroblasts phagocytose some of these granules (5), and stimulated to produce

292

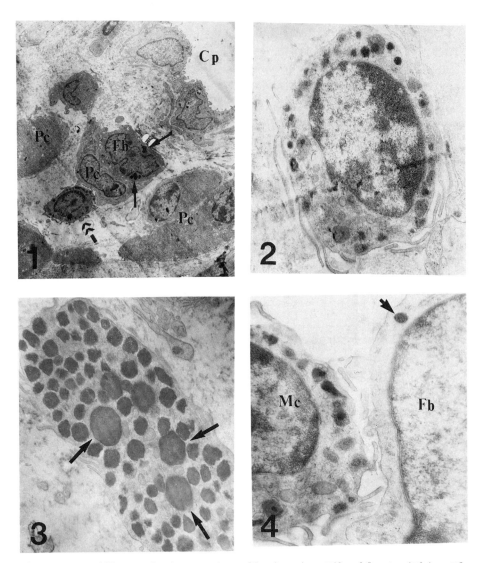

Fig. 1. Capillary (Cp), Mast cell (->>), Fibroblast (Fb), Plasma
cell (Pc), Granule that look like MCG (->),
Fig. 2. Degranulated Mast cell
Fig. 3. Unusually large granule showing uniform structure (->)
Fig. 4. Mast cell (MC), Fibroblast (Fb), Granule that look like MCG
(->),

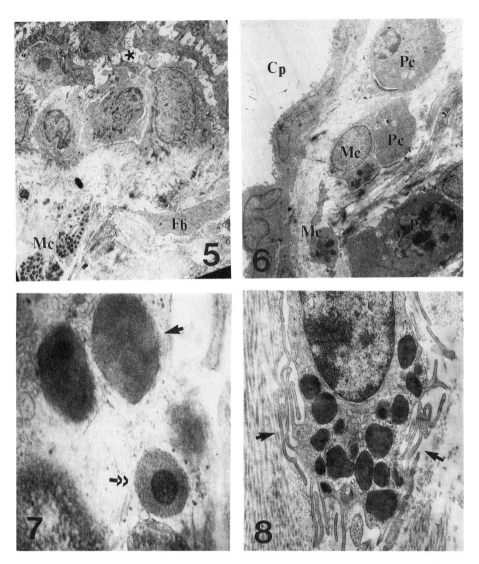

Fig. 5. Increased interstitial spaces (*), Mast cell (MC), Fibroblast (Fb),
Fig. 6. Capillary (Cp), Plasma cell (Pc), Mast cell (MC)
Fig. 7. Crystalloid (->) and electron dense (->>) core granule
Fig. 8. Microvilli (->), Collagen (Cl)

the increased connective tissue matrix and fibers. The above reaction amplified with the influence of local irritating factors.

Second group (CyA)

Increased interstitial spaces and destruction of desmosomes were indications of edema Fig 5. There were many fibroblasts, plasma cells and MC in the connective tissue Fig. 5, 6. In contrast to the first group, the ratio of fiber/ground substance increased in fibers with multiplied population of cells, resulting the GH. Fibroblasts were more activated in this group because CyA suppressed the T-Cell system including the lymphokines that are cytotoxic for fibroblasts (6) and gingival irritants gained potential for GH according to the sensitivity of individual. Somewhat unaffected B-cells may permit patients to maintain humoral response to potential pathogens while avoiding the effects of T-cell system (7). Mainly CyA inhibits cellular immune system. The immunosuppression action of CyA may result from specific and reversible inhibition of T-lymphocytes in the resting and first gap, postmitotic or presynthetic phase of the cell cycle. It particularly inhibits T_4 cells and some of T suppressor, T cytotoxic and interleukin-2 producing T cells. It also inhibits production or release of lymphokines or both, including interleukin-1 and interleukin-2 (8). There is no observation of GH in edentulous mouths (9) or in mucosa left behind from the hyperplastic tissue surrounding the extracted teeth (10), which again points out the triggering effects of antigens as far as humoral immune response concerned.

MC granules have changed their morphology strikingly. There were many crystalloid and electron dense core granules present next to normal ones Fig. 7. Increased microvilli of MC pointed out additional cellular interaction of the cell with connective tissue matrix Fig. 8. We think that MC granule release mechanism inhibited because of CyA action (11) and/or cellular immunosuppression characteristic of the drug (7).

These drugs have different modes of action on the fibroblasts and MC of the gingival connective tissue. They induced clinically similar GH, but we concluded that ultrastructure of GH that they cause is different.

ACKNOWLEDGMENT

Archives of our specimens and electron micrographs, statistics and word processing carried out by an IBM P/S 2 70 model computer kindly donated by IBM Turkey.

REFERENCES

1. Wysocki P, et-al (1983) Oral Surg 55:274-278
2. Parlar A (1988) A.Ü.Diş Hek Fak Derg 15:9-12
3. Rostock MH, Fry HR, Turner JE (1986) 57:294-299
4. Angelopoulos AP (1975) J Can Dent Assoc 41:103-106
5. Takeda Y (1985) Virchows Arch [Pathol Anat] 406:197-201
6. Wahl SM, Gately CL (1983) J Immunol 130:1226-1231
7. American Hospital Formulary Service -Drug Information. Bethesda, MD, American Society of Hospital Pharmacists (1985) pp 826-828,pp 1731-1737, pp 612-613.)
8. Daley TD, Wysocki GP (1984) J Periodontal 55:708-712)
9. Wysocki GP, et-al (1983) Oral Surg 55:274-278
10. Rateitschak-Plüss EM, et-al (1983) 10:237-246
11. Pedersen C et-al (1985) Allergy 40:103-107

© 1991 Elsevier Science Publishers B.V.
Recent advances in periodontology Vol. II,
S.I. Gold, M. Midda and S. Mutlu, eds.

TOOTHPASTE CONCENTRATION CHANGES DURING BRUSHING PERIOD AND OTHER FINDINGS ON BRUSHING HABITS

GÜL ATILLA   ŞÜKRÜ KANDEMİR

Ege University, Faculty of Dentistry, Department of Periodontology
Bornova-35100, İzmir / TURKEY

INTRODUCTION

It has been determined that bacterial plaque can not be controlled a long time through chemical means and even if this were possible, each subject would need a toothbrush and toothpase in order to make the white appearance last on the teeth while at the same time removing plaque (14, 15, 18). Studies have also shown that a brushing that will both eliminate the bacterial plaque and rub the toothpaste over the teeth should be carried out twice a day and for approximately 2 minutes using an amount of paste which is in accordance with pellicle formation of the subject (1, 9, 18).

Various agents are added to the paste to give it caries preventive and plaque controlling features along with its abrasive and polishing properties, and by emphasising these features the producers have been selling their products. On the other hand, studies have also shown that abrasive materials and other ingredients in the paste reduce the function of these chemical agents or destroy them completely (2, 16). Another problem is that as the paste is diluted by saliva during brushing, paste concentration in the mouth diminishes rapidly and a part of it is spat out. For this reason, the following study has been arranged to determine how much of the paste is diluted by saliva during brushing and what percentage of it is spat out over how long period.

MATERIAL AND METHODS

100 subjects, who had applied to the Periodontology Clinic of the Faculty of Dentistry of Ege University took part in ourstudy. In the choice of the patients, we preferred those who had not previously been treated in our clinics and who had at least 20 teeth in their mouths.

In the first appointment, we asked them to bring their tooth brushes and toothpastes. In the second appointment, the subjects were requested to brush their teeth as they usually did and they were observed carefully. How long the brushing procedure lasted, how much paste was used and how many times the toothpaste was spat out were all recorded. It was also determined that how often they changed their brushes, from whom they learned to brush their teeth and whether they used interdental cleaning devices or not.

The slurry was collected in porcelain cups from 10 subjects each time it was spat out during brushing in order to determine how much toothpaste was diluted by saliva during brushing. At this stage of the experiment each of the subjects used the same kind of toothpaste which contained a certain amount of solid matter. The weight of saliva in the porcelain cups was determined, and thereafter the cups were heated to $800^{o}C$ and thus the amount of solid matter in the slurry was obtained.

RESULTS

In this study, it was determined that all subjects generally spat out toothpaste 3 times; only 11 of them spat 4 times during brushing. It was established that the subjects used approximately 850 ± 210 mg tootpaste, and they took approximately 68.3 ± 7.6 seconds to brush their teeth. They spat for a second time after approximately 18.73 ± 6.4 seconds and for a third time after approximately 10.26 ± 1.7 seconds. Paste concentrations in slurry obtained on the firs, second and third occasions, and the approximate amount of paste in them are shown in Fig. 1 and Fig. 2.

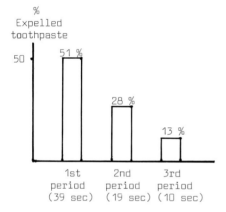

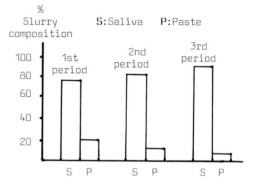

Fig. 1 : The mean expelled tooth-paste and spit out time during brushing.

Fig. 2 : The mean percentage composition ($\pm$ SD) of toothpaste slurries during toothbrushing.

Along with these findings, subjects were also asked how often they changed their brushes. The following answers were given : 23 % changed brushes every 1-3 months, 37 % every 3 to 6 months and 40 % after 6 months to 2 years. Our next observation was that 67 % of the subjects learned to brush their teeth from their parents and only the remaining 33 % had learned from TV or from a dentist. In our study, it was also found that 14 % of the subjects used interdental cleaning devices along with a brush.

DISCUSSION

Research which has been carried out to prevent the caries chemically by fluoride pastes has proved that they do not give the desired results compared with fluoride rinses (5, 6, 10). Researchers have also observed that the caries reduced 20-40 % when fluoride was applied topically and that this rate was between 0-20 % when it was applied with toothpaste. Topically applied rinses lasted 1-2 minutes and the amount of fluoride uptaken was 225 ppm/day. In our opinion, the main reason for this effect is that fluoride reacts quickly with paste components and that no free fluorine ions remain in the paste. Research has shown that fluorine ions should be free in order to be effective (8, 17). In some of the pastes produced in Turkey, Bostancı et.al. (3) could not find free fluorine ions while in some others they found them at low levels.

Bacterioides melaninogenicus which is a suspected periodonto-pathogen, will only die after 8 hours in 700 ppm fluorine solution (20). According to our findings indeterminate fluorine ion concentration in the paste falls to around 20 %, bacause paste is diluted by saliva after 39 seconds. Kandemir et.al.(12) prepared a solution of toothpaste and applied it to cultures of Str.Mutans, which is a primary etiologic agent of caries for 18 hours and observed that the acid producing effect of this bacteria was not inhibited. The findings of this study showed that fluorine in low concentrations in the mouth can not be effective over a short period. In account with the toxisity of fluorine, its concentration in commercially produced toothpastes is kept to between 1000 and 1500 ppm. According to our findings, the concentration of the toothpaste in saliva in which the amount of free fluorine ions are in any case indeterminate, falls to 20 % within 35 seconds, which is the first spitting out period. At the end of 68 seconds which is the mean brushing time in this study, this level dropped to 7 %. Similar cases were also observed in Duke's and Forward's studies (4). In previous studies, it has been shown that as the fluorine concentration is reduced and the application period is shortened, the amount of fluorine which enters the enamel decreases and the resistance against caries also diminishes (11, 19). According to our estimates, another reason why the expected effect is not observed when fluorine is added to the paste is that fluorine concentrations rapidly diminishes in the oral enviroment.

As the toothpaste is diluted by saliva during brushing and a part of it is ejected after a short time, an agent which will inhibit plaque chemically must be selected so as to be effective in a short time or so as to retain to the plaque or tooth surfaces in order to have a high substantivity.

The brushing period of the subjects was below the desired period and most of them used their brushes for extended periods i.e. between 3 months-2 years. However it is widely accepted that if the brushing period is kept longer and the brush is changed more often a better mechanical cleaning can be obtained (7). In this study 67 % of the subjects had been learned how to brush from their families. A similar finding was also observed in Kandemir's study (13). Thus, it has been shown that first of all the families should be educated in tooth brushing.

REFERENCES

1. Addy M, Griffiths G, Dummer P, Kingdom A and Shaw WC (1987) The distribution of plaque and gingivitis and the influence of toothbrushing hand in a group of South Wales 11-12 year old children. J Clin Periodontol 14:564-572

2. Addy M, Willis L and Moran J (1983) Effect of toothpaste rinses compared with chlorhexidine on plaque formation during a 4-day period. J Clin Periodontol 10:89-90

3. Bostancı H, Yılmaz T, Arpak N (1986) Potantiometric investigation of fluorine ions in toothpastes. J Faculty of Dentistry of Ankara University, 13:73-78

4. Duke SA, Forward GC (1982) The conditions occuring in vivo when brushing with toothpastes ä Dent J 152:52-54

5. Ericsson Y (1980) Fluorides state of art. J Den Res 59:2131-2136

6 FDI Technical Report No:20 (1984) The prevention of dental caries and periodontal disease. Int Dent J 34:141-158

7. Glaze PM and Wade AB (1986) Toothbrush age and wear as it relates to plaque control. J Clin Periodontol 13:52-56

8. Hellwege KD (1984) Die Praxis der zahnmedizinisschen prophylaxe. Dr.Alfred Hüthing Verlag Heidelberg pp90-110

9. Hodges CA, Bianco JG, Cancro LP, Lever D, Lever R and Edgewater NJ (1981) The removal of dental plaque under timed intervals of toothbrushing. J Dent Res 60:425

10. Horowitz AM (1983) Effective oral health education and promotion programs to prevent dental caries. Int Dent J 33:171-180

11. Iıjima Y, Koolourides T (1988) Mineral density and fluoride content of in vitro remineralized lesions. J Dent Res 67:577-581

12. Kandemir Ş, Kandemir S, Tokbaş A (1989) The antibacterial activity of toothpastes produced in Turkey. Presented in the 1st Congress of the Academy of Military Medicine of Gülhane.

13. Kandemir Ş (1989) The value of preventive dentistry in the dental treatmens of Turkey. Presented in the 1st Preventive Dentistry Symposium prepared by Ankara University

14. Kitchin PC and Robinson HBG (1948) How abrasive need a dentifrice. J Dent Res 27:501

15. McCauley HB, Sheehy MJ, Scott DB, Keyes PN and Panale SJ and Dale PP (1946) Clinical efficacy of powder and paste dentifrices. J Am Dent Assoc 33:993

16. Moran J and Addy M (1984) The antibacterial properties of some commercially available toothpastes in vitro. Br Dent J 156:175-178

17. Oktay I, Saydam G and Doğan F (1988) The investigation of the factors which effect the high or low substantivity of fluorids on enamel. Textbook notes of the faculty of Dentistry of İstanbul University. pp 1-20

18. Robinson HBG (1969) Individuallizing dentifrice:The Dents Responsibility. J Am Dent Assoc 79:633

19. Saxegaard E and Rolla G (1989) On the mechanism of caries inhibition caused by topical fluoride application. Caries Res 23:106-107 (Abstract)

20. Yoon NA and Newman MG (1980) Antimicrobial effect of fluorides on Bacterioides melaninogenicus subspecies and Bacterioides araccharolyticus. J Clin Periodontol 7:489-494

© 1991 Elsevier Science Publishers B.V.
Recent advances in periodontology Vol. II,
S.I. Gold, M. Midda and S. Mutlu, eds.

CLINICAL,RADIOGRAPHICAL AND SCANNING ELECTRON MICROSCOPICAL
INVESTIGATION OF THE BONE STRUCTURE BY BIOAPATITE IMPLANTATION
PERFORMED IN HUMAN BEINGS "EXTRACTION SITE"

A Case Report

PEKER SANDALLI(I) VİLDAN GÖKSOY(I) TÜRKAN ERBENGİ(2)

1- Dept. of Periodont. Faculty of Dentistry

2- Dept. of Histology and Embriology, Istanbul Faculty of
Medicine Univ. Istanbul 34390 Çapa-Istanbul TUKEY

INTRODUCTION

Although such materials as plaster of Paris,dentin,sclera,
cement, cartilage, duramater and periodontal paste have been used
as bone graft, graft materials of ceramic origin are of u'most
importance among them. A great number of investigators have
used ceramic since 1970's both on animals and on particularly the periodontal defects of human beings. [1,2] These materials,
which may be of different chemical and morphological structures,
have found field of application under various forms with the
advancement of technology.

Bioapatite, one of the substances, which has became the subject of our case, is a synthetic bone graft material, which is
prepared by precipitation from a boiling aqueous solution. [3]Cal-
cium phoshate crystals are white aggregates of 5000 A°length and
500 A°width and their crystal structures are different from the other graft materials. Their surfaces are of a smooth structure with
microgranules. Moreover, they have a parallel grain structure.
Their rate of porosity is 74%.

There have been very few studies so far which have examined under electron microscopy the osteogenesis and ultrastructural cons-
tructure of the Bioapatite graft material. [4,5,6,2] Studies on Bio-
patite bone graft material by Benqué et al, under light microscopy
have been found remarkable.[7]

In this case report, in order to maintain alveolar crest reconstruction attempts have been made to examine the X-rays at 3,6,9,12 and
15 months of Bioapatite bone graft material was used in the extraction cavity of 2 teeth extracted due to an extensive periapical lesion. Furthermore a reentry procedure was attempted in this region
at 15 months and the relation of the obtained material with the bone was evaluated by scanning electron microscopy (SEM).

CASE REPORT

Our patients, who as been the subject of our case, is a boy 14 years old who applied to the Faculty of Dentistry of the Istanbul University in 1987. The reason why he refered to the Faculty was that
his maxillary first and second incisor were looseened and he complained of pain. He also added that a swelling occurred occassionally
on the vestibular side of these teeth and that there was a discharge
of suppuration. Upon examination it was confirmed by the radiographs
obtained (with panoramic, occlusal and periapical radiograms) and
vitality tests that the teeth were devitalized. The avarage pocket
depth of these teeth was 6mm and their degree of mobility was 3 and
2 for maxillary left first and second incisors respectively.

In his history, it was seen that C.T.had an injury when he was 3,
with resultant that his primary teeth were fused with his permanent
teeth germs,causing a prolonged and slowly devoloping periapical lesion to be formed.

Extraction was indicated due to the fact that these teeth were
nonhealthy periodontally, that there was a periapical lesion and that
their normal morphological periodontal environment was deteriorated.
After the teeth were extracted and the lesion removed, bone graft
was indicated to prevent the depression in alveolar processus due to
the fact that extraction cavitywas too large, and that there was a
large bone loss in the vestibule. Not entire but a smaller portion
of the lesion volume was filled with Bioapatite bone graft. The reason why it was not completely filled is that this material is swollen with blood, thus causing its bulk to be enlarged. After flaps
were approximated and sutured, that same day, radiographs of this
same region were obtained. Later, the patient was followed and X-rays
at 3,6,9,12 and 15 months were taken. At 15 months, the region in
which Bioapatite was used, was done reentry with the consent of the
patient. When it was clinically examined after the reflection of the
flap, it was seen that bone tissue had devoloped around nonresorbed
synthetic apatite crystals but that no fibrous tissue was encountered
with. The newly formed bone was of a harder bone. Furthermore it could not be penetrated with probe **(Fig 1).** The fact that these particles could be visualized clearly even at 15 **months.** confirms that they
were not resorbed and that, although they were replaced in large
portions, smaller apatite particles were confronted with is a clear
characteristics of semi-resorbability of this substance. From the
region which was opened, material was obtained to examine the

ralation between synthetic apatite particles and the bone. In this region was replaced by Bioapatite material again. This material which was taken was followed under SEM. The sample is seen same as that in Fig 2 under original 1000 magnification. The axes of the apatite crystals were either flat, round or oval-like shaped. As the material obtained was tortuous, occasional fissures appear in the form of dark shadows between crystals aggregates.

In the radiographic, there is a denser, radiopaque difference of vision between the radiographic appearance when the Bioapatite was first implantated and that at 15 months. The reason for this is that the collagenous structure around crystal aggregates is ossified.

DISCUSSION

In this case, the clinic, radiographic and histologic findings obtained after 15 months seem to be conformity with the investigations effected previously on this subject.
Benqué et al, examined under light microscopy the Bioapatite material replaced into periodontal defects in man and in the exraction cavity in the pigs. As no inflammatory reaction was appeared around Bioapatite crystals, they also establish how compatible this substance was with the tissues.[7]
In our case, we were confronted with a bone clinically harder than normal bone, and no collagenous tissue was encountered with under microscopy.

Ogilvie et al who examined under TEM the ultrastructural construction of osteogensis which resulted 6 to 12 months after Bioapatite implantation into the intraosseous periodontal lesions in man reported that apatite crystals were round or oval-like in shape.[2] These findings show conformity with ours.

Again, Frank and co-workers examined under TEM and SEM the ultrastructure of the Bioapatite bone graft replaced on normal periodontium tissue after 6 and 12 months. It was observed that at 6 months a fibrous connective tissue developed round Hydroxylapatite (HA) crystals. At 12 months bone formation was entirely completed and covered by periostum.[4] We assume that osteogenesis was completed at approximately 12 months in our case as well.

Microscopic findings of the researchers confirm that Bioapatite crystals have the ability to induce bone formation and showed a perfect biocompatibility.

Sandallı et al who observed this biocompatibility clinically applied Bioapatite bone graft on 6 patients who had intraosseous defect. When examined clinically and radiographically it was obser_ved that there was a decrease in pocket depth, a reduction in tooth movement, and ossification at X-rays.[8]

In conclusion, we agree that Bioapatite bone graft is a biomaterial with a perfect biocompatibility feature, which is used in the treatment of bone defects in man. Our investigations regarding this matter, however still continues.

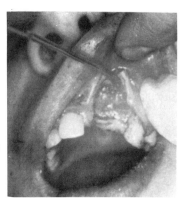

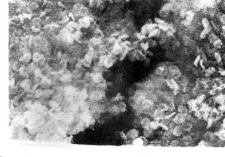

Fig: 1 Reentry appearance in 15th months.

Fig:2 Appearance on SEM with original 1000 magnification

REFERENCES

1- Bhaskar, S.N., Brady, J.M., Getter, L., Grower,M.F., Driskell, T.D (1971) Oral Surg 32:336

2- Ogilvie, A., Frank, R.M., Benqué, E.P., Gineste, M., Heughebaert, M., Hemmerle, J. (1987) J. Periodont. Res 22:270

3- Trombe,J.C (1972) Contribution a I étude de la de Composition et de la reactivité de certaines apatites hydroxylées ou fluorées, alcalinoterreusses. Thése d' Etat, University Paul Sabatier, Toulouse

4.Frank,R.M.,Gineste,M.,Benque ,E.P.,Hemmerle,J.,Duffort,J.F., Heughebaert,M.(1987)J.Biol. Buccale.15:125

5.Jarcho,M.,Kay,J.P.,Gumaer,K.I.,Doremus,RH.,Drobeck,H.P.(1977) J.Bioengineering.I:79

6.Misiek,D.J.,Carr,R.F.(1984)J.Oral Maxillfac.Sur.42:150

7.Benqué,E.P.,Gineste,M.,Heughebaert,M.(1985)J.Biol Buccale.13:271

8.Sandallı,P.,Yıldıran,B.Göksoy,V.(1987) Turkish Periodontology Association 18th Scientific Congress Antalya-TURKEY

© 1991 Elsevier Science Publishers B.V.
Recent advances in periodontology Vol. II,
S.I. Gold, M. Midda and S. Mutlu, eds.

PLURYFUNCTION FIXTURE AS FOR SINGLE CROWN BRIDGES AND MONODIREC-
TIONALY MAGNETICAL PROTHESYS:CLINICAL SOLUTIONS

MARIO MANCINI(1) BARIŞ TUNALI(2)

(1)Italian Association Implantology Research, Via Guerrieri 3,
00153 Rome (Italy)
(2)Department of Periodontology, Faculty of Dentistry, University
of Istanbul (Turkey)

INTRODUCTION

In implantology, a great number of studies have been carried out
so far both on the meterials utilized and on the technical procedures. At present, all the studies and developments are progressively
directed at obtaining conditions, which ara closest to the natural
conditions orally by employing perfect materials and particularly
those biologically accepted by the organism. At the present time implants made of titanium, which are intended to be inserted intraosse-
ously are in practice. The following characteristies are required to
be found in such an implant:
-No chance of mobility
-No transperency in peri-implantar region
-0,2mm of bone loss during the first 5 years
-No symptomatology
-%55 of success in the first 5 years and %80 of success in the first
10 years (1).
The reasons for failure in an implant may be listed os follows:
-Surgical misakes
-Suprastructural problems
-Fracture of the implant
-Loss of the natural elements (2).

MATERIAL AND METHODS

This study is based on morphologic, psychologic,functional and
esthetic factors.This implant is o screw implant of titanium and has
arisen from mechanical, chemical, biological approaches as well as
those rinected at the clinics of implantology. The advantages of a
screw implant may be listed as follows:
-Unless the inplant is sustained to microtraumas and occlusal compressions, there will always be osteogenesis produced around the
implant
-Even if there is an intraosseous sulcus with a diameter larger than

that of the implant, it still allows osteıgenesis to immobilize the
implant
-The peri-implantar tissue produced around the implant may only be
produced when a prosthesis is çonstructed on the implant (3).
This system contains only two instruments for placement of titanium
fixture:
1)calibrated willer of titanium-nitrurate of diameter 3,3 mm developed in the orthopedical field. The drilling has an optimal effect of
two sizes with a relative profendity of 11 mm and 16mm correspondence length and 3,7 mm correspondence diameter of the fixture.
2)The triangle digital allows the screw to be finely inserted in to
the site.
    This implant system has two phases:
1)Surgery
    a)Reflection of the flap b)drilling C7inserting implant d)Suturing
    In this tecnique, an incision is carried out at the apex of the
alveolar crest, but at a line deeger than the vestibule of the crest
to reflect the flap. Such a flap may be said to have the following
advantages:
-Complete exposure of the alveolar crest
-There will be no such problem as the filling of soft tissue debri-
dements into the socket to be drilled
-Allows the route of the drill to be çompletely arranged during
perforation
-Avoids apical migration of the epithelium
-Protects the implant against the external medium by covering iten-
kineyş postoperatively (3).
2)Prosthodontic solutions
    We can start the second phase 180 days after the surgical inter-eııt
vent. For single crown and fixed bridges we use the telescoping abutments that are parallelable directly in mouth because they have a
spherical ending of 2,8mm in diameter with a 5mm high conic cap 12,5°
which is covered over it. In this system, this telescoping abutment
ıs screwed and cemented 10mm deep inside the fixture, that gives anç
excellent prosthetic stability. After insertion and fixing the wel-
ded abutments inside the implants inthe oral cavity, the single
crown or fixed bridge will be built over this structure.
    Furthermore, monodiretional magnetical circuit prostheses may al-
so be applied in this system. This biocompatible magnetical circuit
is used as attraction part in a removable mucosupport prosthesis

actioned on a truss contromagnetical splint fixed over the the implants.

RESULTS

Finally this system proves to be an economical, multifunctional, easly applicable and practical system.

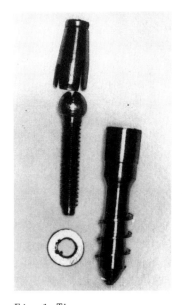

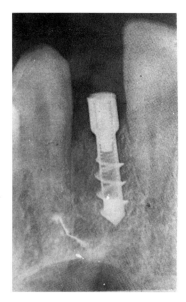

Fig.1.The appearance
of the screw implant

Fig.2.The radiographical
image of the implant inserted
in to the bone

REFERENCES

1. Cordioli GP(1990) In:Implantological Experiences of the School of Dentistry of Padua Univertity. 8th I.R.C.O.I. World Congress of Oral Implantology, Modena.
2.Leghissa G(1990)In:Failures in my clinical practice:When and why. XX International Meeting on Dental Implants and Transplants, Bologna
3.Mancini M, Mancini E (1986)In:Vite sepolta autofilettante con moncone regolabile e parasllelizzante in bocca. New Implant 85 s.r.l, Roma.

© 1991 Elsevier Science Publishers B.V.
Recent advances in periodontology Vol. II,
S.I. Gold, M. Midda and S. Mutlu, eds.

SUBPERIOSTEAL IMPLANT FOR EDENTULOUS UPPER JAW, TREATED WITH
GRAFT RECONSTRUCTION AND VESTIBULOPLASTY

DR. DR. YALÇIN İSMAİL GÜRKAN, ORAL SURGEON
Private Clinic: Halâskârgazi cad. 289A/3, 80260 Osmanbey, Istanbul,
(Turkey)

INTRODUCTION

   We operated on E.P., a 44-year old woman, to find a solution
for the extensive resorption of her maxilla and to free her
from her psychological crisis, caused by a lack of retention
of several upper complete dentures, made by different dentists.

CASE HISTORY

   E.P. was first operated on for this purpose in 1980 at the
Department of Oral Surgery, University of New York, N.Y., U.S.A.
In this Clinic a transplantation of an autogenous graft, had
been carried out, to reconstruct her maxillary alveolar crest.

   During the following year E.P. suffered severely from nasal
exudate and pain in her maxilla. She was therefore referred
to the Clinic of Maxillo-Facial Surgery, University of Duesseldorf,
West Germany. On the 31th of July 1981, E.P. underwent surgery
once more in this Clinic.

   According to their operation-report, the cartilage graft had
become dislocated submucously into the upper lip causing a
jutting into the anterior nasal spine. Dorsally it was extending
towards the nasal septum. The graft was removed totally. The
nasal perforation was sutured through mobilising the inferior
nasal and septal mucosae. The anterior nasal spine was resected. The
anterior part of the upper vestibule was deepened via vestibuloplasty. The flabby ridge in the same area was excised. As a result
the vestibule was considered to be deep enough, to carry a complete
denture satisfactorily.

MATERIAL AND METHODS
Findings

   On the 31th of May 1983, the patient was referred to my Clinic
with the following complaints: The anterior half of the maxilla
was extensively resorbed resulting in three oral perforations, one
into the left antrum and two into the nasal cavity. Contents

of the mouth were consequently pouring out through the nose.In figure 1 the plaster-model of the free lying maxilla is seen.

First operation

On 13.6.1983,I operated on the patient under local anesthesia and absolute sterile conditions.The incision was passed through the peak of the alveolar crest,between both the tuber maxillae.A second incision was laid on the midline,extending 2cm bucally.The palatal and the bucco-labial mucoperiosteal flaps were loosened,the first as far as the soft palate border,the latter extending 2-3cm upwards.An alginate (sterilised with ultraviolet-rays) impression was taken from the free maxillary bone[2,3].Then the incision was temporarily sutured.

Planing and construction of the implant

The cobalt-chrom implant was planned and produced in our own dental laboratory,according to the following principles[1,2,3]:
1) Framework parts,underlying the incision-lines,were avoided as far as possible, 2)the framework was nowhere constructed wider than 2.8mm (for modelling,half-round profile-wax 3.0 X 1.5mm, Dentaurum,was used), 3)bone perforations were overlied with framework, 4)the framework material volume was kept minimal, 5)abutment necks were polished, 6)the implant frame surface was sand blasted.

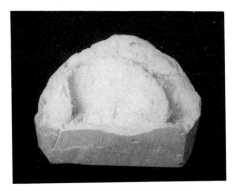
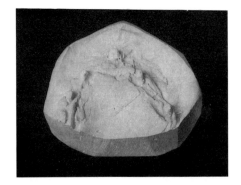

Fig 1:Plaster-model of the free lying maxilla during the first operation.

Fig.2:Five extensions of the implant used as bridge abutments,seen on plaster-model,10 days after first operation.

Five extensions of the implant,situated by teeth 11,14,16,24 and 27 (Fig.2) were used as bridge-abutments.On the bridge-framework (Fig.3),the two anterior crowns were twisted to maintain the proper positioning of the dental-arch,because it was not possible to construct the base of the abutments on the right anatomical locations.This was due to the extensive bone loss and perforations.The cornered palatal surfaces of the crowns were reconstructed into smoother slopes.This reconstructed bridge was incorporated on to the abutments.The bridge-framework in figure 3 was produced as a prototype.

The parts of the implant-framework,lying over perforated bone areas,served as firm bases for the overlying soft tissues.

Second operation and postoperative care

On 14.6.1983 the flaps of the first operation were loosened again.The three perforations were hermetically sutured,after mobilising the inferior nasal and septal mucosae.The implant was inserted between the mucoperiosteal flaps and maxillary-bone . In figure 2 the plaster model of the situation 10 days after insertion is seen.After suturing the flaps,an acrylic palatal plate was hung and fixed firmly with Adams wirings to both zygomatic arches .Its purpose was to hinder dehissences,which could very easily be caused by pneumatic pressure changes,between the oral,nasal and antral cavities.The left sinus was also operated radically.Between the plate and mucoperiostel flap,an antiseptic gauze was placed.The borders of the plate reached the dento-gingival margins and the soft palate.The plate was removed after 10 days (Fig.2).As a precaution the Adams wires

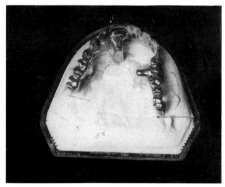

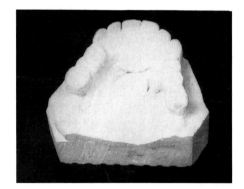

Fig.3: Prototype bridge-framework sitted on the plaster-model,used for construction of the ultimate bridge.

Fig.4:   Plaster-model   with temporary   bridge   fixed   on the implant and the dehissences in the palatal flap.

were left in situ.As we removed the palatal plate,we observed dehissences in the muco-periosteal flap,occuring at the palatal sides of the abutments. Dehissences between the oral, nasal or antral cavities were not observed. We sutured the dehissences in conjunction with flap-mobilisations and fixed the plate once more for a period of 8 days, 3 days after its first removal. In this stage a temporary bridge was fixed on the implant-abutments. Due to dehissences in the palatal flap (Fig.4), one day after its second removal, the plate had to be fixed for the third and last time, for a further 8 days. To close the repeated dehissences -also following definitive plate removal- in conjunction with suturing, Tissucol^R * (a fibrine sticking agent, mixed with calcium-chloride-thrombine solution), Fibrinkleber Human Immuno^R ** (a lyophilised thrombine, mixed with aprotinine-calcium-chloride solution) and Lyodura^R ***(a lyophilised homologe dura), were used.

On the 5th of July 1983 the clinical and x-ray examinations of the patient were almost entirely satisfactory.

In our dental laboratory a complete bridge was constructed. On the 25th of October 1983 it was fixed on the implant-abutments.

RESULTS

During the postoperative five years the patient had no complaints. In this period our clinical and x-ray results were satisfactory as well. There has been no contact with the patient for the past two years.

DISCUSSION

With the exception of sandwich techniques, which are to some extent successful in mandibles, and more recently applied iliac grafts with blood-vessel supplies, iliac or costal grafts used for reconstructing alveolar processes are often resorbed in a short time causing additional bone loss. If the alveolar crest is not high enough, vestibuloplasty is not a solution. Obviously endo-osseous implants are also no means, where bone presence in the anterior maxilla is insufficient. In the present case the only solution to give the patient a complete bridge, was to insert a subperiosteal maxillary implant. In addition, the soft tissues were firmly underlied with the implant parts, which were themselves passed over bone perforations. This enabled

---

* Immuno, Heidelberg
** Immuno, Vienna
*** B. Braun, Melsungen

safer postoperative wound and bone-perforation closures. As a result, we inserted a subperiosteal implant, although these implants have not been favored in recent years.

We believe that, especially in similar frequently seen cases, the future of dental implantology and consequently the success of periodontal health lies in the improvements of operative as well as constructive techniques relating to subperiosteal implants.

REFERENCES

1. Grasser HV (1987) Die Beschichtung von subperiostalen Implanta-ten mit Glaskeramiken. Zahnaerztl Praxis 2:42-45
2. James RA (1983) Subperiosteal implant design based on peri-implant tissue behavior. New York Journal of Dent 53:8
3. Judy KWM, Weiss CM (1976) Totale subperiostale Implantate für unbezahnten Oberkiefer. Entwicklung, Operationstechnik, Prothetik, Gedanken zum Konstruktionsentwurf und klinische Auswertung. Orale Implantologie 4:87-102

© 1991 Elsevier Science Publishers B.V.
Recent advances in periodontology Vol. II,
S.I. Gold, M. Midda and S. Mutlu, eds.

THE ANTIOXIDATIVE EFFECTS OF VARIOUS CHEMOTHERAPEUTIC AGENTS

ERHAN FIRATLI(*),   TAHSİN ÜNAL(**),   NECLA TOKER(**),
PEKER SANDALLI(*),   HASAN MERİÇ(*)
Dept.of Periodontology,Faculty of Dent.(*),& Dept.of Biochemistry,Istanbul
Faculty of Medicine(**),Univ.Istanbul 34390 Çapa,Istanbul,Turkey

INTRODUCTION

Lipid peroxidation in biological membranes is mediated by various bacterial
or host derived oxygen species such as hydroxyl radicals or singlet molecular
oxygen(1).Excessive peroxidation of polyunsaturated fatty acids in biological
membranes is thought to be especially related to inflammation(2,3).

Chemotherapeutic agents are used widely as an adjunct to periodontal therapy
for inhibiting plaque accumulation and reduction of inflammation(4,5).
One can question whether the agents are effective on inhibiting inflammation by
reducing plaque accumulation or have some direct effects by decreasing the
oxidation of tissues during inflammation.

The aim of this study is to determine the antioxidative effects of various
antiplaque agents such as Chlorhexidine (Chx), Sanguinarine (Sn), Listerine
antiseptic (La), and Cetylpridinium Chloride (CPCL).The antioxidative activity
(AOA) of biological fluids is determined by using fresh ox-brain homogenate
according to the method of Stocks et.al.(6).Brain tissue containing large
amounts of polyunsaturated fatty acids provides a suitable medium for lipid
peroxidation.

MATERIALS AND METHODS

Bovine brain was obtained from a recently decapitated ox and brought to the
laboratory packed in ice.The meninges were cleared and coagulated material was
washed off in ice-cold 0.15 mol/L NaCl.Then the cerebrum was chopped into small
pieces and homogenizated for 3 to 4 minutes in a Pott-Elverjem teflon glass
homogenizer in four times its weight of ice-cold phospate saline buffer (40 mmol
/1 KH2PO4/K2HPO4, pH 7.4 in 0.142.mol/L NaCl).The homogenates were centrifugated
for 15 minutes at 1000g.The supernatant was transferred into 10 ml disposable
capped tubes.They were stored at -20°C for 4 weeks.

Stock samples were thawed at room temperature and diluted with three times
their volume with phosphate-saline buffer,without delay.5 ml aliquots of the
diluted homogenate were transferred into 10 ml centrifuge tubes.
Samples of the solutions (Sanguinarine, Listerine Anticeptic, Chlorhexidin and
Cetylpyridinium Chloridine) to be tested were added in different volumes (0.1ml,

0.2ml, 0.3ml,0.4ml) together with the corresponding volumes of phosphate saline (control).

Aliquots for zero-time malonyldialdehyde (MDA) estimates were removed as soon as the mixing was done, by adding 2 ml of Trichloroacetic acid (280 g/l) to 4 ml of homogenate and removing the precipitated protein by centrifugation.For 1 hour MDA estimations, the tubes were transferred to a 37°C shaking water bath and incubation was continued for exactly 1 hour.The reactions were stopped and the protein was removed by Trichloroacetic acid as mentioned above.Approximately 4 ml of supernatant was heated with 1 ml 10 g/L thiobarbituric acid for exactly 15 minutes at 99°C.Absorbances were measured at 532 nm.The ADA of the tested solutions were expressed in terms of percent inhibition of spontaneous oxidation as measured in the control homogenate.The calculation was thus:

$$ADA = (1 - \frac{MDA\ test\ (1hour) - MDA\ test\ (0\ time)}{MDA\ cntr\ (1hour) - MDA\ cntr\ (0\ time)}) \times 100$$

RESULTS

The results were summarized in Table 1 and Graphic 1.

TABLE 1

THE ANTIOXIDATIVE ACTIVITY OF Sn, LA, Chx,CPCL

(The ADA is expressed in terms of % inhibition of spontaneous oxidation as measured in the control homogenate)

Volume	Sn	LA	Chx	CPCL
0.1 ml	72	47	23	12
0.2 ml	93	92	36	15
0.3 ml	99	99	41	19
0.4 ml	99	99	47	23

The ADA of Sn is 72,93,99 and 99 when 0.1 ml, 0.2 ml, 0.3 ml and 0.4 ml volumes were added to the homogenate respectively.The ADA of LA is 47,92,99 and 99 when 0.1 ml, 0.2 ml, 0.3 ml and 0.4 ml volumes were added to the homogenate respectively.The ADA of CPCL is 12,15,19 and 23 when 0.1 ml, 0.2 ml, 0.3 ml and 0.4 ml volumes were added to the homogenate respectively.

DISCUSSION

It has been suggested that lipid peroxidation of biological membranes is related to inflammation(7).The oxidation of gingival tissues during inflammation is enhanced by bacterial or host derived hydroxyl radicals,free oxygen radicals, singlet molecular oxygen and superoxide anions(8).

GRAPHIC 1:The antioxidative activities (%) of Sanguinarine,Listerine Antiseptic, Chlorhexidine and Cetylpyridinium Chloride

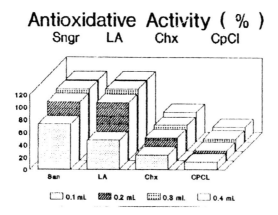

The antioxidative activities (ADA) of various antimicrobial agents which were used in periodontal therapy as an adjunct to control inflammation were studied by using the brain homogenate assay (6) as it was an adequate medium for lipid peroxidation with its high amounts of polyunsaturated fatty acids.

A decrease in the oxidation of host tissues may cause the resolution of inflammatory changes.We therefore tested the antioxidative effects of these agents.

The inhibition of superoxide anion generation of red blood cells(9) and neutrophiles(10,11) by chlorhexidine has been reported recently.But we failed to find a literature on the antioxidative effects of Sanguinarine,Listerine and Cetylpyridinium Chloride.

It has reported that the aromatic compounds were scavengers of hydroxyl radicals,superoxide anions and singlet oxygen(12).A part of the anti-inflammatory action of these agents could therefore be due to the inhibition of free oxygen radical activity.It can be said that these agents have anti-inflammatory property besides their antimicrobial effects.

The mechanism of inhibition of oxidation is still unclear and is under investigation.However,it may be reasonable to assume that the drugs are interacting with the biological membranes and probably with the peroxidative process.

Why Sanguinarine and Listerine have higher ADA than Chx and CPCL is unknown but may be related to their molecular structure and their scavenging capacities.

The results showed that in addition to their antiseptic effects these chemicals have an ADA against spontaneous oxidation.

REFERENCES

1.Toppel Al (1973) Proc Fedn Am Soc Exp Biol 32:1870-1874.

2.Del Maestro RF (1982) Can J Physiol Pharmac 60:1406-1414

3.Del Maestro RF,Bjork J,Arfors KE (1981) Microvascular Res 22:225-270

4.Loe H,Schiott GR,Glavind L,Karring T (1976) J Periodont Res 11:255,270

5.Lamster IB,Alfono MC,Seiger LC,Gordon JM (1983) Clin Prevent Dent 5:12-16

6.Stocks J,Gutteridge JMC,Sharp RJ (1974) Clin Sci Mol Med 47:215-222

7.McCord JM (1974) Science 185:529-531

8.VanDyke TE,Levine MJ,Genco RJ (1985) J Oral Pathol 14:95-120

9.Gabler JMA,Roberts D,Harold W (1987) J Periodont Res 22:150-155

10.Gabler JMA,Bullock WW,Creamer HR (1987) J Periodont Res 22:445-454

11.Goultschein J,Levy H (1986) J Periodont 57:422-424

12.Weiss SJ,King GW,LoBuglio AF (1977) J Clin Invest 60:370-373

© 1991 Elsevier Science Publishers B.V.
Recent advances in periodontology Vol. II,
S.I. Gold, M. Midda and S. Mutlu, eds.

GINGIVAL MANAGEMENT RELATED TO OSSEOINTEGRATED IMPLANTS

ZVI ARTZI, HAIM TAL, OFER MOSES, AVITAL KOZLOVSKY
Department of Periodontology, The Maurice and Gabriela Goldschleger
School of Dental Medicine, Tel Aviv University, Israel

The longevity of osseointegrated implants depends, among other factors, on the health of the surrounding mucosa.

Is a keratinized epithelium less permeable than a non-keratinized one? The current view is that although tissue resistance is determined by the nature of cells and intercellular contacts irrespective of the presence or absence of keratinization (1,2), clinical experience led to the general acceptance that keratinized, masticatory mucosa or skin are more easily maintained or less susceptible to mechanical trauma, such as chewing and tooth brushing, and less vulnerable to inflammation when in contact with dental implants. Furthermore, such an environment according to Schroeder (3), enables the epithelial cells to achieve adhesion easily with the titanium fixtures.

The assumption is that lack of masticatory mucosa and the presence of unwanted marginal soft tissue embracing the implant often causes residual inflammation and can result in peri-implant destruction at a later stage.

Much research was conducted on this topic, from Lang and Loe (4) who declared that inflammation persisted in gingival areas with less than 2 mm of keratinized tissue to the series of studies by Dorfman (5) and Wennstrom (6) with the same conclusion: Facial gingival units with minimal or no attached keratinized gingiva can maintain attachment levels when inflammation is controlled and lack of keratinized gingiva is not necessarily a vulnerable situation. Movable mucosa around the neck of the implant, if maintained, will allow for success.

On the other hand, Langer and Becker (7) found keratinized gingiva a necessity in ceramic restorations in order to maintain peri-implant health; and on examining the distribution of an inflammatory cell infiltrate in wide and narrow zones of keratinized gingiva, Ericsson and Lindhe (8) found that in the wide zone the inflammatory cell infiltrate was confined to the tooth side of the gingiva, whereas in the narrow zone, virtually the entire connective tissue was occupied by inflammatory cells. Kennedy et al. (9)

examined 32 patients with bilateral areas of inadequate attached gingiva and placed a free gingival graft on one side only with the following findings: examination of the patients who did not perform meticulous plaque control and/or discontinued participation in this study for a period of 5 years revealed a re-establishment of gingival inflammation on the control sides associated with additional recession; similar changes were not observed in areas treated by a free graft.

The criteria for the success of implants proposed by Albrektsson et al. (10), do not include a measure of mucosal health. This reflects our lack of knowledge about the physiology of the peri-implant mucosa. We also realize from the above criteria that conventional periodontal indices such as plaque index, gingival index, probing depth, and width of attached gingiva do not appear to be important diagnostic criteria or are not appropriate for assessing the health of the peri-implant tissues and we think it should be re-evaluated.

The first line of defence must be a motivated patient who is effective in accomplishing daily removal of plaque. Soft tissue management is the first step in achieving this target, that is maintaining a clean peri-implant area.

Among mucogingival surgery techniques, the most predicted one is the free gingival graft as has been studied by Rateischak et al. (11), Hangorsky and Bissada (12) and Kennedy et al. (9). Mucogingival surgery in osseointegrated prosthesis can take place prior to the surgical phase, post-surgical phase - prior to the prosthetic phase, and post-prosthetic phase.

Eight patients with lack of attached gingiva, unfavorable vestibulum and/or plaque control alone was unable to maintain a healthy peri-implant environment, went through soft tissue management, i.e., mucogingival surgery, with satisfactory and maintainable follow-up (Figs. 1 and 2).

CONCLUSION

The following parameters are used to monitor the condition of the natural dentition and may perhaps also be used to monitor dental implants: (a) probing depth of 1-3 mm, (b) stable clinical attachment levels, (c) absence of bleeding on probing, (d) low plaque indices, (e) absence of mobility, (f) minimal radiographic crestal

bone overtime, (g) absence of peri-implant radiolucency, (h) absence of discomfort of chewing, (i) absence of discomfort of per-
forming meticulous plaque control, and (j) normal crevicular bacterial flora. When 2 to 3 parameters out of a,b,c,d,h,i deterio-
rate, soft tissue management by the clinician should be considered.
To avoid misinterpretation by our presentation, lack of attached
gingiva per se, when controlled, is <u>not</u> an indication for mucogingival surgery.

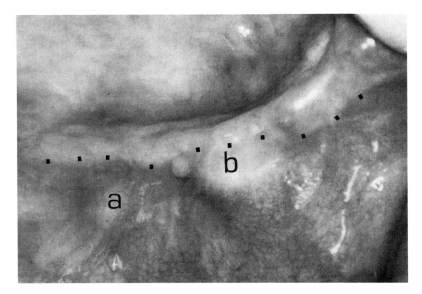

Fig. 1. Pre-exposure: the location of the fixtures are reflected
     through the mucosa (a,b).

To sum up our presentation on the future direction of clinical
practice and research from a periodontal perspective, shown by the
American Academy of Periodontology as a concensus report (13), the
following should be emphasized:

1. Study of gingival parameters as indicators of health, such as
   sulcular fluid flow, bleeding on probing, gingival index,
   plaque index, and microbial index.
2. Pathogenesis of peri-implant disorders and diseases.
3. The importance of the surrounding mucogingival complex and the
   significance of attached keratinized tissue to the long-term
   maintenance of the implant.

4. Number and size of implants necessary to support a prosthesis.
5. The force dynamics of attaching rigid implants to the natural dentition.
6. Post-insertion supportive therapy.

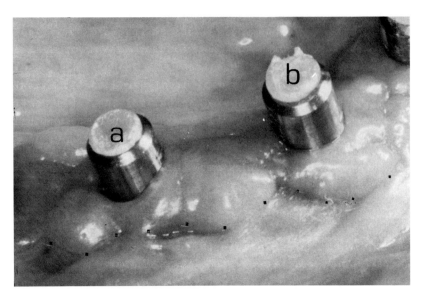

Fig. 2.   Post-exposure: clinical view with a normal keratinized tissue embracing the super structures.

REFERENCES

1. Squier CA (1973) J Ultrastruct Res 43:60
2. Squier CA, Rooney L (1976) J Ultrastruct Res 54:286
3. Schroeder HE (1981) J Oral Maxillofac Surg 9:15
4. Lang NP, Loe H (1972) J Periodontol 43:623-627
5. Dorfman HS et al. (1980) J Clin Periodontol 7:316-324
6. Wennstrom J (1982) Thesis, University of Goteborg, Sweden
7. Langer B, Becker W (1989) In: The Branemark Osseointegrated Implant Chapter 3
8. Ericsson I, Lindhe J (1984) J Clin Periodontol 11:95-103
9. Kennedy JE et al. (1985) J Clin Periodontol 8:667-675
10. Albrektsson T et al. (1986) Int J Oral Maxillofac Implants 1: 11-25
11. Rateischak et al. (1979) J Clin Periodontol 6:158-164
12. Hangorsky V, Bissada N (1980) J Periodontol 51:274-278
13. Proc World Workshop Clin Periodont (1989) Princeton, NJ, USA

© 1991 Elsevier Science Publishers B.V.
Recent advances in periodontology Vol. II,
S.I. Gold, M. Midda and S. Mutlu, eds.

CLINICAL AND HISTOLOGICAL STUDY OF GLASS CERAMICS TOOTH IMPLANTS IN MONKEYS.

HIROSHI KATO, OKITO HONGO, YUTAKA MUKAINAKANO AND MASAMITSU KAWANAMI
Department of Periodontology and Endodontology, Hokkaido University,
School of Dentistry, Kita 13, Nishi 7, Kita-ku Sapporo, Japan.

INTRODUCTION

In recent years many ceramic materials for dental implant have been studied and clinically applied. In these ceramics, bioinert materials such as Zirconia or Alminum Oxide have high mechanical intensity, but they never connect directly with bone tissue. While, bioactive materials such as Hydroxyapatite connect directly with bone, but do not have enough mechanical intensity for tooth implant.

Development of bioactive glass ceramics started by Hench in 1972, and thereafter several glass ceramics with different components were investigated. Recently, a new glass ceramic was developed by Nihon Denki Glass company in Japan. This material has high mechanical intensity and we observed high bio-compatibility of the material with oral tissue in monkeys. It was suggested that this material was useful for the treatment of periodontal bony defect and dental implant.

The purpose of this study was to evaluate bio-compatibility of the newly developed glass ceramic dental implant to oral tissue by using undecalcified histopathological method.

MATERIALS AND METHODS

Implant material.

The glass ceramic tooth implant we investigated had simple form with smooth surface and without retention screws nor grooves. It was composed of CaO 36%, P_2O_5 9%, MgO 11%, SiO_2 43%, CaF_2 very little, and had high mechanical intensity (Table 1).

TABLE 1. Mechanical properties of ceramic materials.

	Hydroxy-apatite	Glass Ceramics	Alminum Oxide(poly)
Bending strength (kg/cm²)	1,000-1,900	2,700	3,000-4,000
Compressive strength (kg/cm²)	5,000-9,000	11,000	25,000-30,000
Modules of elasticity(kg/cm²)	35-120× 10¹	125× 10¹	350-380× 10¹
Hardness (Hv)	700	730	1,800

Experimental animals.
Two adult male Rhesus monkeys were used.
Experimental sites were edenturous areas of upper first molars and
lower first premolars.

Outline of the experiment.
Fig.1 shows outline of the experiment.
At first, 4 upper first molars and 4 lower first premolars were
extracted in order to make edentulous areas. Over 12 weeks after
extraction, glass ceramics were implanted.
At 1 week after implantation, a metal crown was set on each
abutment of 6 implants to get occlusal function, and 2 implants were
remained without metal crown. The periods from implantation to
sacrifice were 5, 9 and 13 weeks. Through the all experimental
period, oral hygiene procedures had been performed by brushing and
scaling 3 times a week.

Fig.1. Outline of the experiment

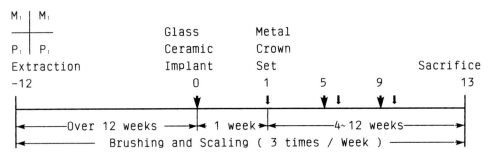

Histological Observation.
Specimens were made with no decalcification. They were embedded in
poliestel resin and cut by hard tissue cutter and stained with
methylene blue and fucusin.

RESULTS and DISCUSSION
Seven of 8 implants were clinically good through the whole experimental period, but only one implant was spontaneously dropped out at
5 weeks after implantation. The reason that one implant was lost was
thought to be that bone might be overheated during drilling or
occlusal force might be too strong after crown was set.
Histological Findings.
In all specimens, new bone formation was observed around implant
teeth. Implants were surrounded with bone tissue and new bone
directly contacted to the implant surface at almost all area (Fig.
2,3,4,5). The surface layer of the implant was faintly stained. This

suggested that implant surface was altered and connected directly with bone (Fig. 6,7).

Connective tissue intervened between implant and bone only in limited area (Fig. 8).

At the bone crest area, new bone formation was observed.

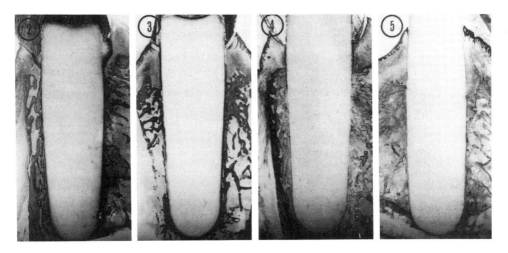

Fig. 2 - Fig. 5.   5,9,13 weeks specimen with occlusion and 13 weeks specimen without occlusion. All specimen is surrounding with newlly formed bone tissue. No marked difference is observed in them.

Connective tissue fibers were running parallel to implant surface above the crest. A small fracture of implant, which was made artifactly during processing specimen, was attaching to the parallel fibers. This suggested that firm connective tissue attachment to the implant were made (Fig. 9). The amount of apical migration of epithelium was within 1 mm from metal crown margin and short junctional epthelium was observed (Fig. 10).

SUMMARY

1. Although the implants had occlusal function at 1 week after implantation, 7 of 8 glass ceramics implant teeth were well maintained clinically, and only one was lost after 5 weeks.

2. In histological observation, most of the implant root surface was connected to compact bone directly. At cervix of the implant, connective tissue attached firmly to implant tooth and short epithelial attachment was also observed.

324

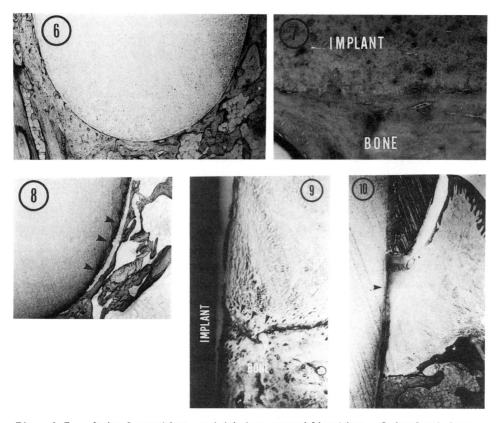

Fig. 6,7.   Apical portion and higher magnification of implant bone
            interface of Fig.4.
Fig. 8.   Connective tissue intervention between implant and bone.
Fig. 9,10. Bone crest and marginal gingiva of 13 weeks specimen.

3. These results suggest that the new glass ceramic implant has
good biocompatibility to alveolar bone and gingiva and is useful as
an implant tooth.

REFERENCES

1. Brånemark PI (1983) J Prosthet Dent 50:399-410

2. Hench LL, Splonter RJ, Allen WC, Greenlee TK (1972) J Biomed
   Mater Res Symp 2:117-141

3. Ericsson RA, Albrektsson T (1984) J Oral Maxillofac Surg 42:705-
   711

© 1991 Elsevier Science Publishers B.V.
Recent advances in periodontology Vol. II,
S.I. Gold, M. Midda and S. Mutlu, eds.

A HISTOLOGICAL STUDY OF THE GLASS CERAMICS IMPLANTS IN FURCATION
BONY DEFECTS IN MONKEYS

MASAMITSU KAWANAMI, YUTAKA MUKAINAKANO, OKITO HONGO and HIROSHI
KATO

Department of Periodontology and Endodontology, Hokkaido University School of Dentistry, Kita 13, Nishi 7, Kita-ku Sapporo,
Japan

INTRODUCTION

In order to regenerate periodontal tissue or fill periodontal
defects, a variety of new technics, such as many kinds of
osseoinductive or osseoconductive materials implant, citric acid
application, guided tissue regeneration technic, have been tried
clinically. Inorganic materials such as hydroxyapatite, beta-TCP,
alminus ceramics, have been comparatively popular, in periodontal
therapy because it is very easy to get commercially.

A new $CaO-P_2O_5-MgO-SiO_2-CaF$ system glass ceramics was developed by Nihon Denki Glass Company in Japan. This is bioactive
cristalized glass material which has better mechanical properties
than hydroxyapatite and better biocompatibility than aluminus
ceramics. Histological investigation of the dental implant of the
glass ceramics was reported in the previous paper. The purpose of
this study was to investigate the effectiveness of the glass
ceramics granules for treatment of furcation bony defects clinically and histologically using undecalcified section method.

MATERIAL AND METHODS

Fourteen furcation regions of premolars and molars in 2 adult
monkeys were used. Before starting the experiment, meticulous
dental brushing and scaling were performed to recover the gingival health for 4 to 8 weeks. After getting gingival health,
baseline examinations was done, which were Plaque Index (1964
Silness and Löe), Gingival Index (Löe and Silness 1963), probing
depth, clinical attachment level and X ray radiography. The same
examinations were performed at 4,6 and 8 weeks later. Surgical
operations were done at baseline, 4 and 6 weeks later in order to
get the 8 week, 4 week and 2 week specimens after glass ceramics
implant, Mucogingival flap was elevated, the buccal interradicular alveolar bone and root cementum at furcation were removed
with low speed rotary round bur and hand chisel to make class II
furcation bony defects and the glass ceramics were implanted at 8
experimental sites (Fig.1). The granules were spherical and the
diameter was 500-840 micrometer. The flap was repositioned and
sutured. At six control sites the flap was also elevated and the
same bony defects were made, but no granules were implanted.
The animals were sacrificed and fixed for light microscopy at 8
weeks later. The specimens were embedded in polyester resin without demineralization, and cut mesio-distally with 200 micrometer
thickness by hard tissue cutter. The section were stained with
methylene blue and Fucsin.

RESULTS

At the results of clinical examination, any clinical problems
or abnormal response at the sites of glass ceramic implantation

were not observed during the experiment. No statistically significant difference in clinical parameters was found between experimental and control sites during the whole experimental periods.
In every radiographs at 2,4 and 8 weeks after the operation,
radiolucency was comparatively lower at furcation region of
experimental sites than at control sites(Fig.2).

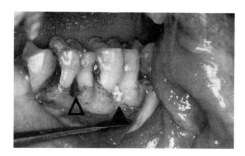 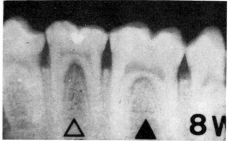

Fig.1. Glass ceramiacs granules were put into a furcation bony
defect of experimental site pointed with a closed triangle.
Fig.2. Radiolucency was comparatively lower at furcation region
of experimental site(closed triangle) than at that of control
site 8 week after the operation.

In histological sections at 2 weeks after the operation. The
granules were observed in interradicular space in experimental
sites(Fig.3). Most of the granules close to the bottom of the
defect, namely close to the remained bone, were directly surrounded by new bone trabecula(Fig.4).

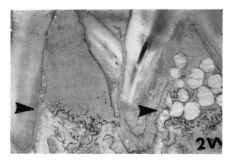 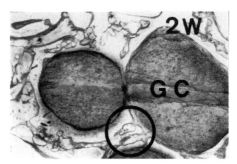

Fig.3. The bottom of the defect was pointed by arrows. The ceramics granules were observed in interradicular space of experimental site.
Fig.4. The granules were directly surrounded by new bone trabecula.

On the some part of surface of the granules, osteoid tissue was also observed. The round nuclear cells were accumulated (Fig.5). New trabecular bone was seen among the granules as well as between the granules and the remaind bone(Fig.6). At the coronal part of the defects new bone was not observed around the granules yet. Methylene blue-stained round nuclear cells were accumulated around on the granules. The top of new bone trabecula was more colonally than in control. But at this point, in both sites, new bone formation was not so much.

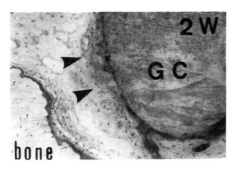 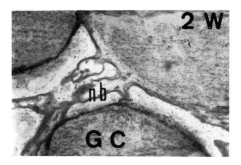

Fig.5. Osteoid tissue was pointed by arrows on the surface of the glass ceramic (GC) granules.
Fig.6. New bone(nb) trabecula was seen between the granules.

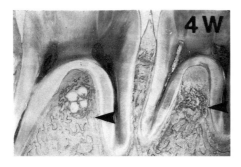 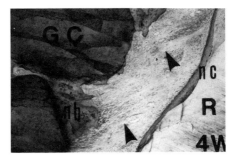

Fig.7. Most of the granules were enveloped with new bone and regenerated trabecula further grew more coronally in experimental site.
Fig.8. New cementum and fibrous structure were regenerated in the space between the granule and root surface.

At the 4 week specimens , little inflammatory infiltration was observed both in experimental and control sites. Most of the granules were enveloped with new bone and regenerated trabecular bone further growed more coronally than at 2 week specimens in the experimental sites(Fig.7). In the limitted area between the glass granules and root surface, new cementum was formed on the root surface which had been surgically denuded and fiberous structure was also regenerated(Fig.8). There was no findings that the granules were directly connected or integrated to the root surface. A few granules at most coronal part of furcation were disappered in most of the specimens. In the control site, new bone trabecula was also regenerated, however, it was not so much as in experimental site.

At 8 week of healing, inflammatory cells were not observed both in experimental and control sites. In experimental sistes, new bone regeneration had reached to the platau and the shape of alveolar crest was rounded to make a space for periodontal ligament(Fig.9,10). In control site new bone was also regenerated little less than that in experimental site(Fig.9).

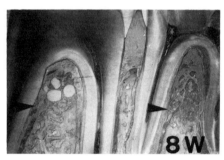
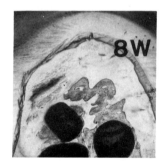

Fig.9. There was not distinct difference of amount of regenerated bone between experimental and control sites at 8 week of healing.
Fig.10. The shape of the bone crest was rounded to make a space for periodontal ligament.

CONCLUSIONS

To determine the efficacy of glass ceramics for treatment of furcation bony defects, the ceramic granules were implanted in class II furcation bony defects made surgically in two monkeys. As controls, non-implanted sites were preserved. Clinical examinations and histopathological observation were performed.

The results obtained were as follows;

1. No clinical problems or abnormal response at the sites of glass ceramic implantation were observed during the experiment.

2. Two and 4 weeks after surgery, remarkable regeneration of bone was shown in the implanted sites. New bone was connected directly to the granules without soft tissues and growed further to the coronal from the granules.

3. Eight weeks after surgery, there was not the distinct difference of amount of regenerated bone between in implanted sites and in control sites.

These results can suppose that the glass ceramic granules has osteoconduction in early stage of surgical bony wound healing.

REFERENCES
1. Hench LL, Splonter RJ, Allen WC, Greenlee TK (1972) J Biomed Mater Res Symp 2:117-141
2. Matsui A (1988) The Quintessence, 7:421-436

© 1991 Elsevier Science Publishers B.V.
Recent advances in periodontology Vol. II,
S.I. Gold, M. Midda and S. Mutlu, eds.

THE PITT-EASY BIO-OSS IMPLANT SYSTEM

DR.J.C.BRINKS
Centre for Oral Implantology,
   Oosterstraat 4   7741 JR   Coevorden (The Netherlands)

INTRODUCTION

In the fast-growing field of oral implantology , the introduction of a new cylindertype of implant ,seems almost too much, but after studying the theory and design of this implant,we decided to place a few . Working with this implant, it proves itself so easy-handling and the results are so good that we are now using this implant as a first choise.

Of course ,we are still using the blades and the subperiosteal implants,but in our office the indication is moving more and more to this excellent implant.

In the last three years we did about 350 cases,and we lost only 12 implants, and what maybe is more important, all the failures happened in the first four weeks after placing the implants and only with four patients. All the loaded implants are still in function and are doing well.

The implant is developped by two famous implantologists of the Pittsburgh university, Prof.Ismail and Prof.Grafelman.

MATERIAL AND METHODS

The Implant. Basicly ,the implant is a selftapping hollow screw were different posts can be screwed in.The apex of the implant is closed and has a small gap ,to prevent rotation after the healingperiod. The material is of course titanium and the screw-thread is coated with titanium-plasma spray (TPS). This screw-thread is so constructed that it, little by little, becomes smaller according as you go from the apex to the neck.Because the the implant is a little smaller at the apex ,you can screw in the implant very easy, till the last two or three rotations. This excellent design provides a very strong initial retention what is important for a good osseo-integration.

The neck is smooth polished and during the healingperiod the implant is covered by a flat coverscrew.In some circumstances is it possible to place a higher coverscrew , to help the gingiva form a collar of healty tissue around the neck of the implant.

The length of the implant is variable from 8mm till 24mm and there are three different diameters, 3,25mm ,3,75mm and 4mm. Till so far there is nothing new ,but what makes this implant so interesting ,is the way the posts are screwed in. Deep in the lower half of the implant is the thread ,this leaves in the upper third of the implant a space ,were the chewingforces will be broken, so that around the neck of the implant less forces will be transferred into the surrounding bone.This could be a way to prevent resorption of bone around the neck of the implant ,as we see often after a few years of been loaded, by other root-formed implants.

There are various types of posts and ,besides of the common posts for crown- and bridgework, we are very pleased with the ball-shaped posts ,whereupon you can build a suprastructure for an overdenture.In our office we like to work with the egg-shaped dolderbar in combination ,with a metal clip in the prosthesis. Because of the ballshape is this suprastructure always fitting !!

The Instruments. The whole system is designed by very experienced implantologists and we found nothing to complain about.From the burs to the setting instruments,and from the coveringscrews to labor-dowelpins, everything is there,nothing to much and nothing to less.The burs have a logical sequence and the marks for the depth of drilling are very obvious.

The Bone. Around the implant there should be 1 till 1,5mm healthy bone. When necessary, you have to shorten the alveolar ridge to create enough width. If it is impossible to create enough width or height ,it could be wise to choose other systems like blades or subperiosteals, or to make artificial elevations with hydroxylappatite and/or bone.

The Surgery. After exposing the bone,is it important to look for undercuttings ,it could be a possible failure in the future when there are to much and to big perforations. Because of the X-ray the surgeon had made his choise ,but every implantologist knows that sometimes you have to change your plans during the operation. It depends what you see after exposing the bone, often needs the bone a cutting to create a better implant-place. Sometimes in the upper-jaw is the bone simply to narrow to place a root-formed implant.

After opening the cortical layer with the highspeed 700 drill, we use a pilotdrill for the first depth-drilling. After this we use a twist drill for the first drilling on the right depth, then we use the spiral precision-drill that suits by the chosen implant. The implant is screwed in and the coverscrew is screwed on. It is better to create a bicortical support for the implant and even when the implant is screwed through the other side of the jaw ,it will heal very well and give a good support for the suprastructure. The incision is sutured and if you wish to do a deepening of the buccal gingiva ,you can do it in the same operation.

 After three months ,the coveringscrews are removed and the impressionposts can be placed. Sometimes you can see these screws already, otherwise you have to expose these coveringscrews what can be done with minor surgery.

The Impression. The impression is made with Xantopren-blue in combination with Silaplast. After screwing on the pitt-dowelpins ,the impressionposts can be exactly replaced in the impression and the technician can make a accurate model,then we follow the normal procedures for crown-and bridge work

The laboratory. The normal procedures for overdentures or crown- and bridgework can be put into practice. You can make every suprastructure removable if you wish, but of course you can cement them too.

The choise depends only from the preference of the implantologist.

RESULTS

Complications. When the surgery is done carefully, with slow speed drilling and much cooling liquid, the complaints will be small. Besides of the normal post-operative pain there is a swelling possible, this depends how far the periosteum has been loosed. The prescription of the right medicaments, to relieve this complaints, should belong to the knowledge of every implantologist. We don't like to prescribe antibiotics because we belief that healthy bone doesn't nead it. When you have bone that needs an antibiotic ,it is better to give up implantology.

Other complications ,like opening the sinus or touching the mandibular nerve belong to the type of complications caused by bad implantology, and how to avoid those failures should be common knowledge of the implantologist.

The Implants. We placed 350 pitt-easy implants and removed 12 implants. The succesrate is 96%. We see the patients every six months and all these patients are also seen by the dental hygienist. All the loaded implants are free of inflammation and very solid. Once in a year we made a X-ray and till now not one of the implants shows loss of bone around the neck.

The 12 implants wich are removed have all shown the same pattern, they were very painfull by touching and the bone around the implant looked like suffering of an ostomyelitis. The implants could be removed very easy , after removal the bone recovered quickly and a few months later we placed implants in the same place again.The implants were lost with only four patients and we never had to remove a loaded implant.

The Suprastructure. 21 implants (6%) are single-tooth replacements, 165 implants (47%) are the base for an overdenture and 152 (43,5%) implants are carrying crown- and bridgework.All those constructions are functionating very well and the patients are enthusiastic.

DISCUSSION

The Pitt-easy Bio-oss implant system has proven to be a valuable contribution in our daily implant practice. The older systems like blades and subperiosteals are not totally out of sight but their indicationrange has become smaller.

Of course three years experience are too short to give a long-term judgement , the Harvard Conference of Implants demands a longer follow up to review this system, and this is right. But the first impressions of this system are very good and a careful follow-up will be needed to see how the long-term results are. Especially the X-ray's will tell us ,in the future, more about the resorpion of bone around the neck of this implant. When it stays the way it looks now ,it is the feeling in our team that we are dealing with an implantsystem what is very suitable for the common dental office and can bring back a healthy mouth to those patients who had gigantic problems with their dentition.

For the younger colleaques this is an ideal system to start with implantology ,it is good for their patients and for themselves.

ACKOWLEDGEMENTS

I like to thank my whole team for their support,enthusiasm and their criticism.

© 1991 Elsevier Science Publishers B.V.
Recent advances in periodontology Vol. II,
S.I. Gold, M. Midda and S. Mutlu, eds.

ADVANTAGES AND LIMITS OF CERAMIC COATINGS
ON TITANE IMPLANTS

ROBERT PIERRE* **& CUISINIER** FREDERIC**

*Dept.of periodont.,Faculté de Garancière, Paris.
**Centre de recherche Odontologique, Faculté de Chir. Dent. de Strasbourg

One objective of today's implantology is to improve the intimate contact between bone and implant. Branemark and his group have largely shown through all their studies the biological benefit of the Titanium (Ti). However Titanium is shown to have a passive action towards biological Tissue.

Hydroxyapatite, then has been used to obtain what GEESINK(6) called a bioactive surface with the bone Tissue. Calcium phosphate ceramics however have only very low biomechanical properties. It is suggested therefore that the benefit of the 2 materials should be combined.

The Ti is used as a substrate and the Ha is projected on the implant's surface. Different techniques for coating Ha on Ti have been reported (1), but only one is commonly used ; the plasma sprayed technique.

Many different results were obtained from numerous studies on the same animal, using pratically the same method (1,3,4,6,10). These studies have compared the healing of the bone around the Ti implant and to its coated alloy using the plasma sprayed technique.The method consists of inserting the test and control implants into the femur of dogs.Three to 52 Weeks later, depending upon the studies, implants are extracted from the femur. The extraction forces are related to the bone implant interface.The results show large variations between studies. This is due to the differencies in the materials and methods involved. The results of all the studies show the biomechanical superiority of coated implant compared with those that are not. The advantage of Ha was apparent from the beginning of the experiment and was evident throughout all the studies.(5)

Whatever the time of analysis, it is possible to show that the coated implant has much more bony interface than Titanium.

A quicker immobilization of the implants is observed. After having reached a peak, the majority of the results show a decrease in value. This is associated with considerable bone remodelling (10).This decreasing period is characterized also by direct mineralization of the bone on the implant with incorporation of Calcium and phosphate from the coating.

Most of the histological analysis have shown the presence of macrophages and giant cells at the bony interface. The disappearance of phagocyte cells is connected with the end of active resorbtion.

This dissolution-degradation phenomena would decrease to a minimum after a few months by absorbtion of biological molecules on the implant surface (4). This development is strongly related to the thichness necessary for the coating.

It was then decided to observe the structural aspect of three coated implants.

MATERIALS AND METHODS

The three implants : IMZ, Biovent, Denar were chosen.

	dense	thickness coating (micronm)	Length	diameter (mm)	Ref.
IMZ	yes	50	13	4	51-1115
BIOVENT	yes	50	13	3,5	
DENAR	yes	50	14	3,8	90089

A sample of each coating material was scraped off with a blade and analysed by electron difraction.

In the second step each implant was observed by scanning electron microscopy.

RESULTS AND DISCUSSION :

The electron difraction pattern, wich is the reciprocal space of the crystal, is an indirect representation of the structure of the coating material.The distances and the angles wich separated the different spots of these patterns are analysed and compared to a simulated reference of Hydroxyapatite.

In the three cases, the coating material observed had a structure related to Ha.

The paralel observation of the surface of each implant using the scanning microscopy shows tree like form of the following sizes.

- 43 microns for IMZ,
- 33 microns for Biovent,
- 14 microns for Denar.

These different measurements seemed to be related to the size of the particles of wich the coating was composed.

In observing the surface perpendicularly, there was evidence of a number of new structures:

- gaps,
- round particles,
- holes,

Their number and distribution were different depending upon the implant.

The surface of the coating seems to be produced by a multiple apposition of layers which make up the whole thichness.

Some time the superimposition of the upper layer is not perfect and deep gaps can be found with different diameter.

- IMZ produced an unequal surface with deep gaps and large openings (of approximately 90*75 micronm).
- In Biovent :The gaps seemed less deep but of the same diameter.
- In Denar the gaps are not well defined due to a better superimposition of each layer.Non-round particles were observed, free of attachment pratically at the surface of the coating.

These different structures will influence the amount and the rate of dissolution and degradation of the coating. The specific surface of the materials is well correlated with the dissolution rate (8).Most of the surface particles or other free structures will be progressively incorporated and degraded by the cellular system (4).These two mechanisms explain the decrease of the Ha layer within a few months.

The size of gaps suggest that bone growth will not be the same in the three cases. The least porous system would allow less uniform tissue calcification within (2).

Past studies have largely shown the importance of coated implant in todays development of implantology. Our observations have indicated that we need more informations on the properties and characteristics of the coated implant materials used in practice.

ACKNOWLEDGEMENTS

The authors thank Dr.TAMSIN S.H. DRYSDALE for the preparation of this manuscript.

REFERENCES

1.   Bloch M.,Kent J.,Kay J.:(1987):Evaluation of hydroxyapatite-coated titanium dental implants in dogs.   J.Oral Maxillo-Surg.:45:601-607

338

2.   Bobyn B., J.,Pilliar R.,Cameron H.,Weatherly G.:(1980):The optimum pore size
      for the fixation of Porous surface metal implants by the Ingrowth of the   Bone.
      Clin.Orth.and Relat.Res.:150:263

3.   Cook S.Thomas K.,KayJ.,Jarcho M.:(1988):Hydroxyapatite-coated Titanium
      for orthopédic Implant applications. Clin.Orthop.and Related Res.:232:225

4.   De Groot K.,Geesink R.,Klein C.,Serekian P.:(1987):Plasma sprayed coatings
      of hydroxyapatite. J.Biomedical Mater.Res.:21:1375-1381

5.   Ducheyne P.,Hench L.,Logan A.,Martens M.,Bursens A.,MulierJ.:(1980):
      Effect of hydroxyapatite impregnation on skeletal bonding of porous
      coated implants.   J.Biomedical Mater.Res.:14:225

6.   Geesink R.,De Groot K.,Klein C.:(1988):Bonding of Bone to apatite-coated
      implants.   J.of Bone and Joint Surgery:70B:1:17

7.   Hayashi K.,Matsugushi N.,Venoyama K.,Kranemaru T.,SugiokaY.(1989):
      Evaluation of metal implants coated with several types of ceramics as
      biomaterials.   J.Biomed.mat.Res.:23:1247

8.   Jarcho M.(1986):Biomaterial aspects of calcium phosphates properties and
      applications .   Dent.Clin of North Am.:30:1:25

9.   Lacefield W.(1988): Hydroxyapatite coatings.   Ann.New York Acad.Sc.10:72

10.   Thomas K.,KayJ.,Cook S.,Jarcho M.,(1987):The effect of surface macrotexture
      and hydroxylapatite coating on the mechanical strengths and histologic
      profiles of titanium implant materials.   J.Biomedical Mater.Res.:21:1395-1414

Reprint requests to:
Dr. PIERRE ROBERT,Unité INSERM U157,4 Rue kirschleger,67000
Strasbourg,FRANCE

© 1991 Elsevier Science Publishers B.V.
Recent advances in periodontology Vol. II,
S.I. Gold, M. Midda and S. Mutlu, eds.

THE COMBINED PERIODONTAL ORTHODONTIC TREATMENT OF SECONDARY MALOCCLUSIONS DUE TO PERIODONTAL DISEASE

SÖNMEZ FIRATLI(*), ERHAN FIRATLI(**), MUSTAFA ÜLGEN(*), PEKER SANDALLI(**), HASAN MERİÇ(**), TÜRKÖZ UĞUR(*)
Dept.Orthodontics(*),& Dept.Periodontology(**),Faculty of Dent.
Univ.Istanbul, 34390, Çapa, Istanbul, Turkey.

INTRODUCTION

Advanced periodontal disease may cause pathological tooth migration,rotation, diastema or increasing of overbite.In such cases orthodontic treatment may be required after periodontal therapy.

In this study,the effect of fixed orthodontic treatment on the continuation of reduced but healthy periodontal tissues is investigated.For this purpose the patients, who have undergone to periodontal-orthodontic treatment, are compared with the periodontally treated patients.

MATERIALS AND METHODS

Patient Selection

12 adults, who were suffering from various periodontal disease and secondary malocclusions, were selected.Patients were chosen according to the following criteria :

1)No history of systemic disease, 2)No antibiotic theraphy in the last 6 months, 3)No periodontal theraphy before. 6 patients, 5 females and 1 male with a mean age of 36.5 (range 21 to 47) were undergone for orthodontic treatment.Other 6 patients, 4 females and 2 males with a mean age of 34.5 (range 25 to 42) were observed as controls.

Periodontal Status

Plaque Index(1), Gingival Index,periodontal pocket depths and clinical attachment levels(2) were carried at baseline, 3 months after periodontal surgery and after orthodontic treatment for the study group and also 15 months after periodontal surgery for the patients comprising control group.PPD and CAL were measured at the line angles of each tooth by a Williams type periodontal probe with an end diameter of 0.5 mm.Serial radiographs were evaluated at every 6 months.

Periodontal Treatment

All patients were treated with scaling, root planing and modified Widman flap surgery.Professional tooth cleaning and scaling were performed to all patients at every 4 weeks during orthodontic treatment or control period.

Orthodontic Treatment

3 months after periodontal surgery,fixed appliance therapy (Edgewise) was evaluated to 6 patients.Hawley appliances were performed for retention.

Statistical Analysis

Anova was performed for all tested variables to evaluate intragroup differences from baseline and intergroup differences at each observation.T-test at paired observations were performed for intragroup differences and student t test for intergroup differences.A p value of less than 0.05 was considered as significant.

RESULTS

Mean orthodontic treatment period was 12.7±5.2 months.The control patients were observed for 15 months after periodontal therapy.No tooth loss was seen during the study period except little root resorption in two orthodontic patients.

PI,GI,PPD (Table 1) were decreased (p<0.001) after periodontal treatment in both groups.The intergroup differences were not significant.Significantly clinical attachment gain was seen in both groups (p<0.001) after periodontal treatment and control group was seen.The final scores of orthodontic treatment group was significantly lower (p<0.001) than the control group (Table 1).

DISCUSSION

The results of this study summarizes that fixed orthodontic treatment in adults with reduced but healty periodontium has not resulted in any further periodontal destruction and tooth loss.The slight increases in each parameter after orthodontic treatment were not statistically significant.In this investigation both groups (study and control) were chosen from adult periodontal patients to evaluate whether orthodontic treatment causes further periodontal tissue damage.

It has spaculated radiographycally that loss of periodontal bone support may occur during orthodontic treatment(3).But the apical root resorptions and the movement of teeth into infrabony defects can mislead to the radiographical view of periodontal destruction.

The need of good oral hygiene,root planing, and surgical elimination of inflammation for a well performed combined periodontal-orthodontic treatment has been reported(4,5).

Our results conclude with the previous studies which has demonstrated that

TABLE 1

THE PI,GI,PPD,CAL VALUES (Mean±SD)

		I	II	III
		Mean±SD	Mean±SD	Mean±SD
PI	Study	2.24±0.54	0.41±0.15	0.44±0.08
	Control	2.01±0.55	0.37±0.11	0.42±0.14
GI	Study	2.38±0.59	0.30±0.09	0.33±0.08
	Control	2.33±0.54	0.31±0.11	0.44±0.19
PPD	Study	4.71±0.86	1.60±0.22	1.80±0.08
	Control	4.53±0.76	1.57±0.18	1.96±0.19
CAL	Study	5.54±0.79	2.28±0.09	2.42±0.13 ⎤ *
	Control	5.67±0.80	2.44±0.22	2.78±0.21 ⎦

I-Baseline, II-After periodontal surgery, III-After orthodontic treatment
for study group and 15 months later after periodontal surgery for control group.
* p<0.001

orthodontic treatment in adults with healthy but reduced periodontal support was
not responsible from marginal bone resorption and clinical attachment loss(6,7).

In this study we also found significantly higher attachment gain in orthodontic
treatment group than the controls.The reason of this may be;

1-The elimination of intrabony defects by the movement of teeth,

2-The stimulation of bone regeneration by moving teeth into infrabony defects(8),

3-The well performed oral hygiene during orthodontic treatment.

Shortly we conclude that fixed orthodontic treatment do not result further
clinical attachment destruction or tooth loss in reduced but healty periodontal
tissues.

REFERENCES

1. Silness J, Löe H (1964) Acta Odontol Scand 22:121-135.
2.Löe H,Silness J (1963) Acta Odontol Scand 21:533-563.
3.Artun J, Urbye KS (1988) Am J Orthod 93:143-148.
4.Ericsson I, Thilander B (1980) Eur J Orthod 2:51-57.
5.Williams S, Melsen B,Agerbaek N, Ashoe V, (1984) Br J Orthod 9:178-184.
6.Melsen B, Agerbaek N, Markenstam G (1989) Am J Orthod 96:232-241.
7.Boyd RL, Leggon PJ, Quinn RS, Eskie WS, Chambers D (1989) Am J Orthod 96:191-196.
8.Gazit E, Lieberman M (1980) Angle Orthod 50:346.

© 1991 Elsevier Science Publishers B.V.
Recent advances in periodontology Vol. II,
S.I. Gold, M. Midda and S. Mutlu, eds.

EXTENSION OF THE GINGIVA PROPRIA AS A PERIODONTAL PROPHYLAXIS
MEASURE

ANTRANIK ESKICI
Dept. of Oral and Maxillofacial Surgery, University Dental Clinic,
A-8036 Graz, Austria

INTRODUCTION
As periodontal diseases augment even in adolescents, periodontal
therapy and periodontal prophylaxis measures are becoming more and
more important also in this group of patients. For this reason periodontal surgery, and in particular the muco-gingival surgery,
has to play a prophylactical role.

MATERIALS AND METHODS
15 patients with gingival recession were treated by extension of
the attached gingiva after initial therapy has turned out ineffectiv
The vestibuloplasty which is used in such cases in Graz will be explained now.

AIMS OF THE MUCO_GINGIVAL SURGERY
1. Maintenance or creation of a gingival border and an adequate
   width of the attached gingiva.
2. Elimination of tension on the free gingiva.
3. In extreme cases creation of an adequate depth in the vestibulum to ensure an optimal oral hygiene (CHARANZA F.A.and CHARRARO
   J.J. 1970, HILEMAN, A.1967, ROSENBERG, M.M. 1960, RAMFJORD, S.P.
   and COSTICH, E.R. 1968).
In the framework of these aims the vestibuloplasty is of a very
great importance.

INDICATION FOR VESTIBULOPLASTY WITH EXTENSION OF THE GINGIVA is
 given when following cases occur:
1. Progressive recession of the gingiva (RATEITSCHAK et al. 1979,
   MARXER et al. 1982, MATTER, J. 1979, 1980, DORFMANN et al. 1982,
   LANG and LOE 1972).
2. Disorders between periodontal membrane and gingiva
3. Extremely coronal displacement of the muco-gingival line.
 We were able to obtain satisfying results by an in principle simple
method in recent years.

TECHNIQUE OF THE OPERATIVE PROCEDURE
 The surgical treatment is mainly effected in the lower front area
under local anesthesia. The vestibular mucosa is mobilized up to the
linea gilandiformis initiating by two vertical mucosal incisions in
each of the areas of the caninus. A horizontal cut across the linea
gilandiformis links the ends of incision - if no attached gingiva is
available, the mucosa is transected 2mm underneath the margo. The
now obtained mucosal flap makes possible to denudate the musculus
mentalis. The muscle is transected at its point of attachment on the
alveolar ridge and pushed down from the periostium as far as an adequate area of the periostium is denudated. The periostium itself remains intact. Subsequently the mucosal flap is fold down by three
sutures in such a way that a mucosal strip of about 5mm lays on the
periostium after sewing up the free border of the mucosal flap with
the periostium (chromic-cut-sutures). The coronapetally remaining
part of the periostium is left to secondary epithlialisation (Fig.1,
2).
 After secondary granulation of the periostium this area is epithe-
lialised from the gingival border so that a new wide attached gingiva can develop (Fig. 3).

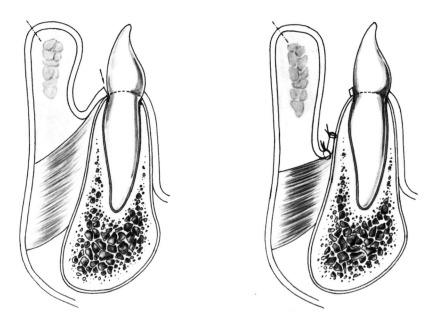

Fig. 1: Mucosa mobile up to the collum dentis
Fig. 2: Vestibuloplasty with fixation of a mucosal strip in the new
        mucosal fold.

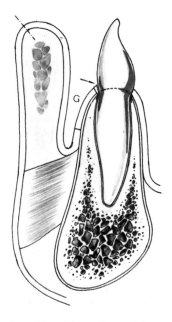

Fig. 3: After formation of the attached gingiva (G).

345

DISCUSSION AND RESULTS
A ten years' observation shows that a obtained by this procedure vestibulum with extended gingiva propria remains in its extension.

Summing up, it may be said that the by the above explained method widening of the gingiva propria seems to represent an improvement in the field of muco-gingival surgery in cases of periodontal diseases. This method is also effectively used within the scope of preprosthetic surgery and in particular in the oral endo-osseous inplantation.

REFERENCES

CARRANZA,F.A. and CARROW,J.J.: Mucogingival techniques in periodontal surgery.
J.Periodont., 41:294, 1970.

DORFMANN,H.S., KENNEDY,J.E., BRID,W.C.: Long itudinal evalnation of free autogenous gingival grafts. A four year report.
J.Periodont. 53:349, 1982.

ESKICI,A.: Spätergebnisse der Mundvorhof- und Mundbodenplastik in 20 Jahren.
Fortschritte der Mund-, Kiefer- und Gesichtschirurgie, Bd.XXI:146, 1976

HILEMAN,A.! Surgical repositioning of vestibule and frenums in periodontal disease.
J.AmDent.Assoc. 55:676, 1976

LANG,N.P., LOE,H.: The relationship between the width of keratinized gingiva and gingival health.
J.periodont. 43:623, 1972

MATTER,J.: Free gingival graft and coronally res'positioned flap. A 2-years follow-up report.
J.Lin.Periodont.

MARXER,M.A., RATEITSCHAK,K.H., HEFTI,A.: Freies Schleimhauttransplantat-Edlan-Mejchar-Operation. Ein Vergleich.
Acta parodont., in: Schweiz.Mschr.Zahnheilk. 92:75/11, 1982

RAMFJORD,S.P. and COSTICH,E.R.! Healing after exposure of periosteum of the alveolar process.
J.Periodont., 39:199, 1968

ROSENBERG,M.M.: Vestibularal alterations in periodontics.
J.Periodont., 31:231, 1960

RATEITSCHAK,K.H., EGLI,U., FRINGELI,G.I.: Recessions: A 4-year longitudinal study after free gingival grafts.
J.Clin.Periodont. 6:158, 179

© 1991 Elsevier Science Publishers B.V.
Recent advances in periodontology Vol. II,
S.I. Gold, M. Midda and S. Mutlu, eds.

THE EFFECT OF FIBRIN ADHESIVE MATERIAL - FAM (TISSUCOL) AND CITRIC ACID ON PERIODONTAL WOUND HEALING

KÖKSAL BALOŞ, İ. LEVENT TANER , ALTAN DOĞAN, TÜLİN OYGÜR Gazi University, Faculty of Dentistry, Department of Periodontology, Emek, Ankara (Türkiye).

INTRODUCTION

Histologic evidence of cementogenesis and new connective tissue attachment to previously diseased root surfaces using citric acid demineralization following root preparation has been reported in animal and human studies [1, 3, 8, 9].

In several studies, tissue adhesive material containing attachment glycoproteins and other plasma factors have been used to aid periodontal regeneration [2,4,5,6,7,10,11].

The purpose of this study was to evaluate the difference in periodontal healing following surgery and citric acid conditioning of root surfaces with or without the application of a fibrin adhesive material (TISSUCOL) in a model closed to bacterial plaque.

MATERIAL AND METHODS

Seven adult experimental dogs with clinically healthy periodontal conditions were used in this study. Experimental procedures were carried out on the mesial and distal roots of the first maxillary molars and canines on both side. Fenestration wounds approximately 8 by 8 mm. were made through the buccal cortical plate to expose part of the roots.

The forty-two fenestration wounds of selected teeth were distributed into four groups. 1) Group C(control), the root surface was planed and irrigated with saline. 2) Group CA (citric acid), the planed root surface was demineralized with citric acid pH.1 for three minutes, 3)Group FAM, fibrin adhesive material was applied to completely cover the planed root surface, 4) Group CA+FAM, fibrin adhesive material was applied to planed and demineralized root surface.

The dogs were sacrificed at the 7, 21 and 42 days. Following routine histological procedures, bucco-lingual sections were cut at a thickness of six micrometers and stained with Hematoxylin and Eosin and Crossmon's Modification of Connective Tissue Stain.

The histological analysis was performed on step serial sections using a calibrated grid mounted in the eyepiece of a microscope

One way ANOVA test was used for statistical analysis.

348

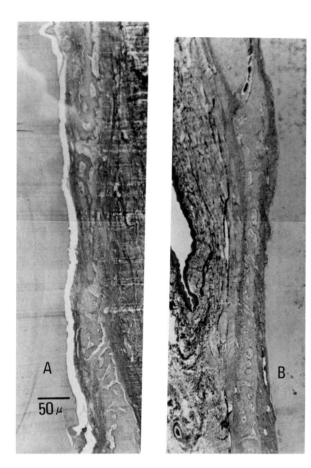

Fig 1. Photomicrograph showing total bone regeneration at forty-two days
A. FAM., B.CA+FAM

RESULTS

Histological Observations

Seven days after surgery. The control and the three different experimental specimens showed clot retention which appeared to be consisting of red blood cells and inflammatory cells enmeshed in a fibrin network. Furthermore, subepithelial tissue was particularly infiltrated by the mononuclear cells and polymorphonuclear leucocytes.

Twenty-one days after surgery Small amount of cementum deposition with connective tissue attachment and bone remodelling was observed in the notch areas. Some specimens showed local root resorption where the exravasated erythrocytes were also found.

TABLE 1 : MEAN PERCENTAGE (X) AND STANDARD DEVIATION (SD) OF NEW
CEMENTUM AND BONE OBSERVED AT 21 DAYS

C E M E N T U M

	FAM X∓SD 64,22∓15,89 (N=5)	CA+FAM X∓SD 46,45∓8,26 (N=4)	CA X∓SD 64,85∓8,26 (N=4)	C X∓SD 15,10∓11,85 (N=4)
FAM X∓SD B 12,91∓8,49 (N=5)		*	NS	**
CA+FAM X∓SD 0 2,2 0∓1, 21 (N=4)	**		*	**
CA X∓SD N 2,72∓1,26 (N=4)	**	NS		**
C X∓SD E 2,45∓2,78 (N=4)	**	NS	NS	

(*) P< 0.05, (**) P<0.01, (NS) NOT SIGNIFICANT

Forty- two days after surgery A new layer of cementum had formed along
the root surfaces thinning through the middle part of the defect in most of the
specimens but some root resorption areas were still observed. All specimens
of group CA+FAM showed new cementum formation and reattachment.

One specimen from both the FAM and the CA+FAM groups showed total
bone regeneration [Fig.1] Some bone and cementum regeneration were also
observed in the CA and control groups.

Results of Histometric Measurements

Results of histometric measurements of new cementum and bone formation
were evaluated as a percentage of the total length of the apico-coronal distance of the defect. The significant probability values are shown in table 1
and 2.

TABLE 2:MEAN PERCENTAGE (X) AND STANDARD DEVIATION (SD) OF
NEW CEMENTUM AND BONE OBSERVED AT 42 DAYS

	C E M E N T U M			
	FAM X∓SD 84,52∓24,1 (N=5)	CA+FAM X∓SD 99,62∓0,52 (N=4)	CA X∓SD 84,52∓14,84 (N=4)	C X∓SD 56,8∓41,1 (N=4)
FAM X∓SD B 75,1∓26,0 (N=5)		NS	NS	*
CA+FAM X∓SD O 68,67∓26,05 (N=4)	NS		NS	**
CA X∓SD N 61,52∓9,69 (N=4)	**	**		*
C X∓SD E 22,50∓20,18 (N=4)	**	**	NS	

(*) $P < 0,05$, (**) $P < 0.01$, (NS) NOT SIGNIFICANT

REFERENCES

1. Albair WB, Cobb CM (1982) J Periodontol 53, 515

2. Caton JG, Polson AM, Pini Prato GP, Bartolucci EG, Clauser C (1986) J Periodontol 57: 385

3. Crigger M, Bolge G, Nilveus R, Egelberg J, Selvig KA (1978) J Peridontal Res 13: 538

4. Nasjleti CE, Caffesse RG, Castelli WA, Lopation DE, Kowalski CJ (1986) J Periodontol 57: 568

5. Nasjleti CE, Caffesse RG, Simith BA, Lopation DE, Kowalski CJ (1987) J Periodontol 58: 770

6. Pini Prato GP, De Paoli S, Clauser C, Bartolucci EG (1983) Int J Periodont Rest Dent 4:49

7. Pini Prato GP, Cortellini P, Clauser C (1988) J Periodontol 59: 679

8. Polson AM, Proye MP (1982) J Clin Periodontol 9: 441

9. Polson AM, Proye MP (1983) J Clin Periodontol 54: 141

10. Ripamonti U, Petit J-C, Lemmer J, Austin JC (1987) J Periodontal Res 22:320

11. Ripamonti U, Petit J-C (1989) J Periodontal Res 24 : 335

© 1991 Elsevier Science Publishers B.V.
Recent advances in periodontology Vol. II,
S.I. Gold, M. Midda and S. Mutlu, eds.

THE EFFECT OF SYSTEMIC TETRACYCLINE AND ORNIDAZOLE ADMINISTRATION ON PATIENTS WITH ADULT PERIODONTITIS

SERDAR ÇINTAN & ÖZEN TUNCER

University of İstanbul,Faculty of Dentistry,Department of Periodontology, Çapa, İstanbul-Turkey

INTRODUCTION

Black pigmented Bacteroides have a significant role in the etiology of periodontal disease.These microorganisms induce tissue destruction by their proteolitic properties which inactivates the complement factors and immunoglobulins (10,11,12).

Recent studies have demonstrated that tetracycline and nitroimidazole derivates could be effective on these microorganisms (4,7).

Improvement on clinical parameters have been demonstrated by Saxer and Guggenheim (1983), Gusperti,Syed and Lang (1986),and Mombelli et al.(1989) when ornidazole was given as adjunct to mechanical debridement.Further more these investigators also showed a significant reduction in the number of black pigmented Bactroides after this treatment.

Several investigators have demonstrated that tetracycline is capable of inhibiting the activity of tissue collagenase (1),

Improvement in clinical parameters and significant reduction of the number of black pigmented Bacteroides have also been demonstrated by Scopp et al. (1980), Kornman and Karl (1982), and Lindhe et al. (1983) when tetracycline were used as adjunct to root planing.

In this study an attempt was made to evaluate the effect of ornidazole and tetracycline HCl compared to control group by clinical histological and microbiological parameters.

MATERIAL & METHOD

The investigation has been realized on 21 patients (14 women and 7 men) with 312 periodontal units and age ranging between 35 to 59. Patients have been designed in three groups namely the tetracycline group,ornidazole group and the controls.An attempt was made to pool the study groups with similar defects and same number of peridontal units from the anterior group of teeth including the first premolars..All subjects received scaling and root planing treatments.Tetracycline administered for two weeks (1 gr/day) for one group;the other group received ornidazole for ten days (1gr/day);and the control group has not medicated with any antibiotics.

Periodontal status of patients have been evaluated before and after therapy with the following parameters: Plaque Index,PI (Silness-Löe,1964), sulcus fluid flow rate,SFFR (mod. Löe&Holm-Pedersen,1965), sulcus bleeding index,SBI (Mühlmann&Son,1971), gingival recession index (Tuncer,1975), pocket probing depths, clinical attachment levels, histological index (Oliver et al. 1969) and microbiological assessments.The results have been compared statistically.

RESULTS

The results indicated that there is a marked improvement in all parameters and assessments of all three groups.

The drugs administered groups showed statistically significant alterations with respect to all parameters.Only the clinical attachment level gains of ornidazole group failed to show statistically significant results compared with the control group. (Figs.1,2,3 and 4)

Results of histological observations revealed significant improvement in index values. Increased activity of collagen was demonstrated at the tetracycline group.

Microbiological samples isolated from the ornidazole and tetracycline groups failed to cultivate black pigmented Bacteroides after treatment.

But these bacteriae which are thought to be strongly related to the periodontal disease are harbored at the cultures of the control group after mechanical treatment.

The findings of this research suggest that the use of tetracycline or ornidazole may be useful as adjuncts to root planing in the treatment of adult periodontitis. It could be emphasized that the use of of microbiological parameters with the clinical ones are useful in evaluating the results of periodontal therapy.

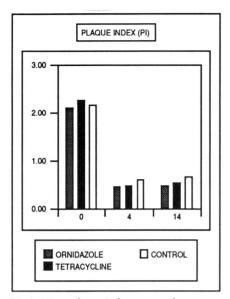

*Fig.1. Mean plaque index scores of
ornidazole, tetracycline and control
groups devided to weeks.*

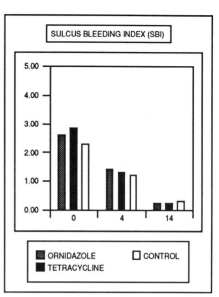

*Fig.2. Mean sulcus bleeding index scores of
ornidazole, tetracycline and control
groups devided to weeks.*

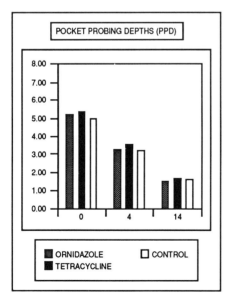

*Fig.3. Mean scores of pocket probing depths
of ornidazole, tetracycline and control
groups devided to weeks.*

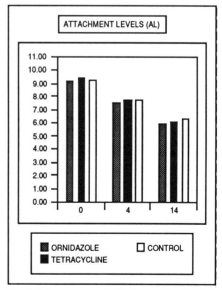

*Fig.4. Mean scores of attachment levels of
ornidazole, tetracycline and control
groups devided to weeks.*

354

REFERENCES

1. Golub,L.M.,Wolff,M.,Lee,H.M., McNamara,T.F., Ramamurthy,N.S., Zambon,J., Ciancio, S.: Further evidence that tetracyclines inhibit collagenase activity in human crevicular fluid and from other mammalian sources.J.Periodont. Res. 20: 12, 1985.

2. Gusperti,F.A., Syed,S.A.,Lang,N.D.: Clinical and microbiological effects of ten days' oral therapy with ornidazole following mechanical treatment of periodontal disease.Acta Parodontologica,96:893,1986.

3. Kornmann,K.S.,Karl,E.H.:The effect of log term low dose tetracycline therapy on the subgingival microflora in refractory adult periodontitis. J.Periodont. 53:604, 1982.

4. Külekçi,G., Güvener,Z., İnanç, D., Balkanlı,O., Küçükkay,S.,Erişen,R.: Endodontik kaynaklı diş apselerinden izole edilen anaerob bakteriler ve ornidazole duyarlıkları.Oral. 2:15,1986.

5. Lindhe,J.Liljenberg,B.Adielson,B.:Effect of long term tetracycline therapy on human periodontal disease.J.Clin.Periodont.10:590,1983.

6. Mombelli,A.,Gusperti,F.A.,Lang,N.P.:Treatment of recurrent periodontal disease by root planing and ornidazole.J.Clin. Periodont. 16: 38, 1989.

7. Saxer,U.P.:Medikamente.Bestandteil der Parodontitistherapie?.Schweiz Monatsschr. Zahnmed.97:87,1987.

8. Saxer,U.P.,Guggenheim,B.:Ornidazole in the treatment of periodontal disease. Acta. Parodontologica.12:137,1983.

9. Scopp,I.W.,Fletcher,P.D.,Wyman,B.S.,Epstein,S.R.,Fine,A.:Tetracycline: A clinical study to determine its effectiveness as long term adjuvant. J.Periodont. 48: 484, 1977.

10. Slots,J.,Listgarten,M.A.:B.gingivalis,B.intermedius and A. actinomycetemcomitans in human periodontal diseases. J. Clin. Periodont. 15:85,1988.

11. Sundquist,G.Carlsson,J.Haenström,L.:Collagenolytic activity of black pigmented Bact. species.J.Periodont.Res.22::300,1984.

12. Van Winkelhoff,A.J.,van Steenbergen,T.J.M., DeGraaf,J.: The role of black pigmented Bacteroides in human oral infections.J.Clin. Periodont. 15: 145, 1988.

© 1991 Elsevier Science Publishers B.V.
Recent advances in periodontology Vol. II,
S.I. Gold, M. Midda and S. Mutlu, eds.

PERIODONTAL HEALTH STATUS AND TREATMENT NEEDS IN THE INDEX AGE
GROUPS IN TURKEY BASED ON CPITN CRITERIA

GÜLÇİN SAYDAM

Associate Professor, Preventive Medicine and Public Health, Dental Faculty of Istanbul
University, Istanbul (Turkey)

İNCİ OKTAY

Professor, Preventive Medicine and Public Health, Dental Faculty of Istanbul University,
Istanbul (Turkey)

An epidemiologic study for assessment of prevalence and severity of oral diseases in Turkey
have been conducted by our research team between June 1987 – June 1988.

This National Oral Health Pathfinder Survey was prepared with the permission and
administrative support of the Ministry of Health and with the financial and technical cooperation
of WHO Regional Office for Europe.

Total sample size of 6290 persons were examined in the survey and periodontal disease
treatment needs were calculated according to the Community Periodontal Index of Treatment Needs
(CPITN) which was developed and agreed for use in field trials by WHO and FDI in 1981 (1).

In this manuscript the CPITN values of some index age groups taken from the global data and
the treatment needs assessed were discussed and evaluated together with periodontal health
targets by 2000.

MATERIAL AND METHOD

The national survey has been conducted in 57 examination sites in 5 cities resembling
different geographic regions of Turkey.

The subjects of this investigation, 1943 people of the index age groups 15–19, 35–44 and
65+ were also examined in the same sites and recorded in oral health assessment form (WHO
1986) (2).

A special probe, 621 WHO periodontal probe was used to collect data utilizing 6 index teeth
16. 11. 26. 36. 31. 46 for subjects under 20 and 17. 16. 11. 26. 27. 36. 37. 31. 46. 47
index teeth   for subjects over 20.

Each tooth was probed gently to determine pocket depth and to detect calculus and bleeding
response in 6 sites; mesiobuccal, midbuccal, distobuccal, mesiolingual, midlingual and
distolingual to resemble 6 sextants of the mouth. Subjects then are classified into the different
treatment needs (2, 3, 4).

Computer analyses were done at WHO Geneva.

RESULTS

The survey results are summarized in 3 tables below.

TABLE 1: PREVALENCE RATES OF CPITN CRITERIA

Age group	Number of ex. per.	Healthy %	Bleeding %	Calculus %	Shallow poc. %	Deep poc. %
15-19	1037	25.75	51.11	21.22	1.83	0.10
35-44	510	3.04	24.49	37.65	28.95	5.87
65 +	387	3.75	21.25	27.50	28.75	18.75

In the index age groups of 15-19, 35-44 and 65+ the percentage of people showing indicators of periodontal disease according to CPITN as bleeding, calculus, shallow and deep pocket is shown in Table 1. The percentage of healthy people who do not exhibit any sign of disease is 25.75% in the age of 15-19 while it is only about 3% in 35-44 and 3.75% in 65 +.

In table 2, the average number of affected sextants per person is shown.

TABLE 2: AVERAGE SEXTANTS OF CPITN CRITERIA PER PERSON

Age group	Num. of ex. per.	Healthy	Bleeding	Calculus	Shallow poc.	Deep poc.
15-19	1037	3.43	2.56	0.44	0.04	0.00
35-44	510	0.86	4.44	2.14	0.85	0.09
65 +	387	0.30	3.09	1.95	0.95	0.40

Mean number of healthy sextants determined is to be 3.43 in 15-19 but it drops to less than 1 sextant in the other two groups. Bleeding and calculus affects the most sextants in 35-44, shallow and deep pockets do not affect more than 1 sextant in any of the age groups.

GRAPH I: AVERAGE SEXTANTS OF CPITN PER PERSON

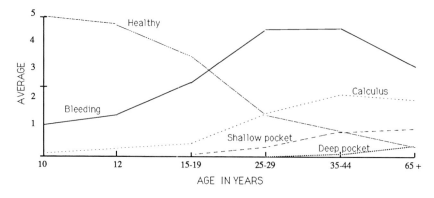

Looking at the graph 1 which was drawn with the values of Table 2,it is observed that bleeding and calculus affects more sextants with the increasing age and bleeding reaches 4.4 sextants maximum in 35-44 while dental calculus too shows high values at the same age declining slowly after, affecting app. 2 sextants in both 35-44 and 65+. Shallow pockets are observed early in 15-19 and deep pockets before 35-44 .

The differences between cities are tested by statistical means and only 15-19 year olds of Gaziantep city was relatively good in respect to Trabzon, Kırşehir and Istanbul and also Muğla was considerably better than Trabzon p< 0.05. Trabzon was the only region where deep pockets were observed.

TABLE 3: TREATMENT NEEDS OF THE INDEX AGE GROUPS

Age group	No. of ex. per.	Treatment I Oral hygiene instruction %	Treatment II Preventive-protective treatment %	ave. sextant	Tretment III Complex treatment %	ave. sextant
15-19	1037	74.25	23.14	0.44	0.10	-
35-44	510	96.96	72.47	2.14	5.87	0.09
65 +	387	96.25	75.00	1.95	18.75	0.40

Required periodontal treatments classified according to CPITN criteria for 3 age groups are found in the Table 4. According to this, oral hygiene instruction, treatment I appears to be needed by 74.25% for 15-19 and almost 100% for the other two groups. Treatment II consists of scaling,professional cleaning and health education must be practiced for 23.14% in 0.44 sextant in 15-19 age group besides treatment I and for 72.47% in 35-44 for app.2.14 sextants. Treatment II is also needed for older group by 75% in app. 1.95 sextants. Complex treatment that includes surgical intervention starts quite early in young age group and needed most in advanced age 65+ by 18.75% in app. 0.4 sextant. Similar to the data given in Table 3, the treatment requirements of Trabzon city in the age group 15-19 is higher than the other cities and Trabzon was the only examination site that needed complex treatment in the age group of 15-19.

DISCUSSION

Our investigation demonstrated that while bleeding is the most frequent observed CPITN indicator in 15-19, it is calculus and shallow pockets for 35-44 and deep pockets for 65+ and pocket formation never reaches 1 sextant in any age group.
Healthy sextants free of bleeding, calculus and pocket formation are estimated to be ave.3.43 in young age group 0.86 in 35-44 and only 0.3 for 65+. In overall country base, the most needed treatment in each group is treatment I, while treatment II is needed exceeding 70% in 35-44 and 65+ besides treatment I. Complex treatment is needed by 5.87% in 35-44 and by 18.75% in advanced age.

According to the provided data, what is mostly needed in terms of periodontal disease in Turkey is mainly the health education to raise the existing health capacity of periodontal tissues and mouth, and other protective and simple preventive methods including professional cleaning and scaling. However it is obvious that these must start to be practiced at early ages covering a wide scale of the population.

The comparision of our data with EEC countries' periodontal health targets of 2000 is as follows (5).

TABLE IV: EEC TARGETS

Age group	Targets of EEC countries for 2000	Survey Results (Turkey, 1988)
18	% 90 with min. 3 sext. (CPITN=0)	% 67.22 for the age group of 15-19
35-44	% 75 with min. 3 sext. (CPITN=0)	% 14.32
65 +	not to exceed 10 % with CPITN=4	% 18.75

As it may be seen above, the values of Turkey by 1988 are quite far from the targets of 2000. However, the situation of many countries in Europe are much the same such as the percentage of 35-44 year olds with CPITN=4 is 30 in Finland, 7.7 in Greece and 3 in the Netherlands, it is 5.87% in Turkey (6).

It is clear that a new service structure and a planning of action to raise oral health capacity which will start early with priority groups then extend to cover the population as much as possible are needed in Turkey for the next 10 years.

REFERENCES
1. Ainamo, J., Barmes, D., Beagrie, G., Cutress, T., Martin, J., Sardo-Infirri, J.: Development of the World Health Organization (WHO) Community Periodontal Index of Treatment Needs (CPITN), Int. Dent. J.: 32(3): 281-291, Sept. 1982
2. WHO: Oral Health Surveys, Basic Methods, Third Ed., Geneva, 1987
3. Wilson, M.A., Clerehugh, V., Lennon, M.A., Worthington, H.V.: An Assesment of the Validity of the WHO Periodontal Probe for Use with the Community Periodontal Index of Treatment Needs, Br. Dent. J., 165: 18-21, 1988
4. Persson R., Svendsen, J., Daubert, K.: A Longitudinal Evaluation of Periodontal Therapy Using the CPITN Index, J. Clin. Periodontal, 16: 569-574, 1989
5. WHO: Prevention Methods and Programmes for Oral Diseases, Tech. Rep. Ser., No. 713, Geneva, 1984
6. WHO: Country Profiles on Oral Health in Europe 1986, ICP/ORH 120, Copenhagen, 1986

© 1991 Elsevier Science Publishers B.V.
Recent advances in periodontology Vol. II,
S.I. Gold, M. Midda and S. Mutlu, eds.

THE METHODS TO APPLY FOR REACHING THE PERIODONTAL HEALTH BY THE YEAR 2000 IN TURKEY

İNCİ OKTAY
Professor, Preventive Medicine and Public Health, Dental Faculty of Istanbul University, Istanbul (Turkey)
GÜLÇİN SAYDAM
Associate Professor, Preventive Medicine and Public Health, Dental Faculty of Istanbul University, Istanbul (Turkey)

INTRODUCTION

In the world, oral health related problems of communities have changed in the late decades and seems will continue to change considerably in the next years too.

Global epidemiological data of many countries show two major trends in the prevalence of oral diseases. The first is the mild to high increment for most of developing countries and the second one is almost sharp decrement of many highly industrialized countries (1, 2, 3, 4).

This success of industrialized countries to lessen the severity and prevalence of oral disease mostly depend upon the application of country wide preventive measures and reorganization of services in regard to the strategy of raising their community's existing oral health situation through preventive and interceptive means.

The planning and implementation of such an oral health programme that intends to diminish oral diseases prevalences involve 5 steps (5).

PROBLEM IDENTIFICATION AND SITUATION ANALYSIS

In this stage, the assesment at prevalence and severity of oral diseases, the kind of services provided by the oral health institutions, the available financial resources and the number of employed dental health personnel are investigated.

The baseline data of periodontal disease have been derived from data of the national oral health pathfinder survey, conducted between June 1987–June 1988 in our country (Reported by Dr. Saydam). Some of the results of the examinations of 6290 people in 5 regions of Turkey are summarized in Table I.

The figures of Table I show that the prevalence rate rises up to 50 % at age 12 whereas it exceeds 90 % after 25–29, exhibiting significantly higher rate in rural areas than the suburban and urban for the age group of 15–19 (p < 0.05).

Considering manpower situation of today, the number of registered dentists in Turkey is approximately 9000 and only 1750 of them are employed in public sector. These dental health services of public sector mainly provide restorative and rehabilitative treatments, and preventive methods are not practiced yet, practically not existing.

TABLE I: PERCENTAGE OF PERSONS WITH PERIODONTAL DISEASE ACCORDING TO CPITN CRITERIA

Age in Years	Number of Subjects Examined	Percentage of Total Persons	Location Type		
			Urban	Periurban	Rural
12	408	50.74	50.77	46.81	55.56
15-19	1037	74.25	71.35	80.75	87.34
20-24	400	87.50	80.33	86.46	93.52
35-44	510	96.96	92.79	98.12	98.28
65 +	387	96.25	94.29	96.15	100.00

SETTING OBJECTIVES

The survey results shown with the comparative periodontal health targets for EEC countries (Table II) demonstrate that the prevalence of periodontal disease in Turkey is quite higher than the expected figures of 2000, and there is an urgent need for planning to improve existing situation.

TABLE II: TARGETS FOR THE YEAR 2000 CONCERNING PERIODONTAL DISEASES AND THE RESULTS OF THE ORAL PATHFINDER SURVEY

Targets for the Year 2000	Survey Results	Requirements for Achieving the Targets	Index Ages of 2000	Requirements for the next 10 Years
90 % of the age group of 18 with min. 3 healthy sextants (CPITN=0)	67.22 % for the age group of 15-19	Increase the rate by 22.78 %	8 year olds of 1990	To conserve the existing rate of 90.27 % for the next 10 years
75 % of the age group of 35-44 with min. 3 healthy sextants (CPITN=0)	14.32 %	Increase the rate by 60.68 %	25-34 year olds of 1990	Planning to increase the existing rate of 25.40 %
Deep pockets not to exceed 10 % in 65 + (CPITN=4)	18.75 %	Decrease the rate by 8.75 %	55 + year olds of 1990	Planning to decrease the of 14.81 % to 10 %

However, many factors, primarily the insufficiency in number of dentists of public sector in respect to the high population of the country (app. 55,000,000) besides lack of resources does not allow for covering of all age groups under a comprehensive preventive oral health care programme.

Selecting priority groups are among the most common approaches in such communities with moderate resources and unable to mount personnel in intensive preventive programmes, and it is the young adults for Turkey to improve periodontal health for the next 10 years. The achievement of this target is closely related to the implementation of preventive methods in the age group of 12-14 which is about 3,600,000 by 1985 census.

In addition to this, the fact that periodontal diseases do not require complex treatments in this age group is another reason to consider 12-14 year olds as a priority group (Table III, IV). 50 % of them can be reached in secondary schools.

TABLE III: PERCENTAGE OF PERSONS WITH PERIODONTAL DISEASE IN THE AGE OF 12-14

Number of Subject	Prevalance Rate (Total)	Location Type		
		Urban	Periurban	Rural
1106	57.83	56.70	61.47	69.82

TABLE IV: PERCENTAGE OF PERSONS WITH CPITN INDICATORS IN THE AGE OF 12-14

Healthy	Bleeding	Calculus	Shallow Pockets	Deep Pockets
40.06	43.97	13.31	0.56	0.00

TABLE V: TREATMENT NEEDS ACCORDING TO CPITN CRITERIA IN THE AGE OF 12-14

OHI	Prophylaxis		Complex Treatment	
%	%	mean number of sextants	%	mean number of sextants
57.83	13.86	0.31	0.00	0.00

SELECTING PREVENTIVE MEASURES-PLANNING OF PROGRAMME IMPLEMENTATION

The prevalance of periodontal disease, the types of treatments needed, financial resources and the number of dental personnel in Turkey are important factors in selecting the necessary preventive measures.

Naturally, the initial preventive measure is dental health education that involves teaching correct tooth brushing and dental flossing which can solve most of the problems.

40 % of the age group of 12-14 are healthy and 43.97 % of those with periodontal disease indicators according to CPITN (mostly bleeding) can be healed by individual oral hygiene instruction only.

13.86 % of people that have periodontal disease need scaling and cleaning, called prophylactic treatment or professional cleaning, and these are the second group of instructions that must be included in a preventive programme (Table V) (5).

So called preventive measures that will be implemented in the age group of 12-14 now in Turkey will provide some reductions in periodontal disease prevalance rate of 15-19 year olds and elder groups of tomorrow.

At this stage, the cities that have relatively high number of dentist employed in public institutions can be chosen as pilot regions and immediate preventive programmes can start in priority groups.

A cooperation and coordination between various ministries as the Ministry of Health, National Education and Labour may enable dentists employed in these institutions to take part in community based preventive programmes.

Also a protocol can be designed with above mentioned ministries and dental boards to facilitate the contribution from dentists employed in the private sector for such programmes, and this can be coordinated through local dental boards.

"Community Oral Health Clinics" that will carry out primary health care including care of urgent needs too may be established in far future.

In long term, the designation for employment of more dentists in public institutions regarding dentist/population ratios of country's different regions seems to be very important in planning. As a 5th step, the parameters are used to evaluate the implemented programmes.

REFERENCES

1. WHO: More Tooth Decay in Third World than in Industrialized Countries, WHO Press 36th World Health Assembly Press Release, WHA/5-9 May 1983

2. Waldman, H.B.: Dental Services in England, Wales and the United States: A Comparison of National Survey Data, JADA, Vol. 106: 167-170, 1983

3. WHO: Prevention Methods and Programmes for Oral Diseases, Teeh. Rep. Ser. No. 713, Geneva, 1984

4. Sheiham, A.: Future Patterns of Dental Care-Manpower Implications for Industrialized Countries, Br: Dent. J., Vol. 166/7: 240-242, 1989

5. WHO: Prevention of Oral Disease, WHO Offset Publication, No. 103, Geneva, 1987

6. Sağlık Bakanlığı: Özet İstatistiki Bilgiler, Nisan 1989

© 1991 Elsevier Science Publishers B.V.
Recent advances in periodontology Vol. II,
S.I. Gold, M. Midda and S. Mutlu, eds.

PROSTAGLANDIN E_2 LEVELS IN ODONTOGENIC CYST FLUID

MUKADDES CANBAZ,TÜLİN ÖZBAYRAK,AYŞEGÜL TELCİ,A.RIZA ADHAMİ,ÖZEN DOĞAN,
HİKMET ÖZ

Department of Biochemistry,Istanbul Faculty of Medicine,University of
Istanbul,Çapa-Istanbul,(Turkey)
Department of Oral Surgery,Faculty of Dentistry,University of Istanbul
Çapa-Istanbul (Turkey)

Pain during operation, in spite of local anesthesia, is one of the phenomena to be clarified in odontogenic cysts. Recent studies have shown that agents responsible for pain are prostaglandins which increase in inflammatory processes (3).

In our study we determined the PGE_2 concentrations in odontogenic cyst material of 29 patients (20 male, 9 female), according to the investigations concerning prostaglandins and the hypothesis mentioned above. Odontogen cyst types were not taken into consideration. I^{125} labeled PGE_2 RIA kit (NEN-Dupont) was used. Values obtained from the cyst material were compared to the blood and urine PGE_2 levels of the control group consisting of 21 healthy subjects (8 male, 13 female).

INTRODUCTION

Two phenomena associated with jaw cysts require extensive clarification osteolysis, which is characteristic of and often pathognomomic for different types of cysts and pain sensation, which can not be eliminated even with exact anesthesia. Recent studies have shown that agents responsible for pain are prostaglandins which increase in inflammatory responses (3,4).

Odontogenic cysts originate from the embryonic oral cavity epithelium. Studies concerning various odontogenic cysts have not been able to clarify the reasons for their development. However it has been shown that they cause bone lysis. Pain during odontogenic cyst operation does not disappear completely in spite of local anesthesia. The most important reason of this phenomenon is prostaglandin and leukotriene synthesis. Experiments have shown that prostaglandins act as mediators and modulators in osteolysis and cyst expansion. For this reason, we wanted to determine PGE_2 levels in odontogenic cyst fluid and compare the results to the PGE_2 levels in blood and urine of the control group made up of healthy subjects.

364

TABLE I

PGE$_2$ LEVELS IN ODONTOGENIC CYST FLUIDS IN 29 PATIENTS

Patients No.	PGE$_2$ ng/g
1	25.17
2	23.00
3	19.76
4	18.87
5	25.17
6	23.00
7	29.00
8	28.50
9	27.50
10	21.25
11	26.70
12	19.20
13	20.80
14	25.00
15	8.70
16	12.00
17	10.56
18	18.40
19	19.80
20	27.63
21	23.00
22	-
23	28.90
24	25.30
25	28.50
26	27.90
27	24.80
28	39.00
29	30.29

TABLE 2

BLOOD AND URINE PGE$_2$ CONTENTS IN CONTROL GROUP(21 HEALTHY SUBJECTS)

	Blood	Urine
PGE$_2$(average values)	6.78±1.50 pcg/g	2.50±0.21 ng/ml

MATERIAL AND METHODS

Uninfected odontogenic cyst fluids were obtained from 29 patients (20 male and 9 female) at the Department of Oral Surgery, Faculty of Dentistry, University of Istanbul. Blood and urine samples were taken from 21 healty subjects (control group). PGE_2 I^{125}-RIA kit (NEN-Dupont) was used. Odontogenic cyst, blood and urine contents of PGE_2 was determined by radioimmunoassay according to the methods of Hauenstein, et al.; Dray et al; Frölich et al. (3,1,2) respectively. Findings were analyzed Student's-t test.

RESULTS

As shown in table 1, the average level of PGE_2 contents in odontogenic cyst fluids obtained from 29 patients is 22,68 ng/g. The lowest level is 8,70 ng/g and the highest level is 39,00 ng/g. According to the literature, PGE_2 level in blood is appoximately 3-5 pg/ml (4). But the average of our PGE_2 findings in blood is 6,78 ng/g in control group. This value is very close to the value mentioned above. The levels of PGE_2 in odontogenic cyst fluid is significantly higher than blood PGE_2 levels in control group ($p < 0.001$). There is also statistically significant changes between urine PGE_2 levels in control group and in odontogenic cyst fluids, which were obtained from 29 patients.

DISCUSSION

Recent studies have shown that agents responsible for pain during operation of jaw cysts are prostaglandins which increase inflammatory processes. In our study we determined the PGE_2 levels in odontogenic cyst material of 29 patients, according to the investigations concerning prostaglandins and the hypothesis mentioned above.

The increase in prostaglandin E_2 values in odontogenic cyst fluid were found to be statistically significant ($p < 0.001$) compared to the control group. This finding shows that prostaglandins have definite bioactivity in the formation of inflammation and pain, and it also shows the relation between pain sensation and subsequent in prostaglandin synthesis.

SUMMARY

Pain during operation, in spite of potent local anesthesia, is one of the phenomena to be clarified in odontogenic cysts. Recent studies have shown that agents responsible for pain are prostaglandins which increase in inflammatory processes.

In our study we determined the PGE_2 quantities in odontogenic cyst material of 29 patients, according to the investigations concerning prostaglandins and the hypotheses mentioned above. Odontogenic cyst types were not taken into consideration, I^{125} labeled PGE_2 RIA Kit (NEN-Dupont) was used. Values obtained were compared to the blood and urine PGE_2 values of the control group made up of healthy subjects.

The increase in prostaglandin E_2 values in odontogenic cyst fluid were found to be statistically significant ($p < 0.001$) compared to the control group. This finding shows that prostaglandins have definite bioactivity in the formation of inflammation and pain, and it also shows the relation between pain sensation and subsequent increase in prostaglandin synthesis.

REFERENCES

1. Dray F, Charbonnel B (1975) Radioimmuno assay of PGF_2 , E_1 and E_2 in human plasma. Eur J Clin Invest, 5:311

2. Flolich JC, Wilson TW, Sweetman BJ, Simigel M, Nies AJ, Carr K, Watson TJ, Oates A (1975) Urinary prostaglandins identification and origin. J Clin Invest 55:763

3. Haunstein H und Schettlev D (1985) Untersuchungen uber Prostaglandine bei kieferzysten. Dtsch Zahnargil 40:595

4. Schroer K (1984) Prostaglandine und verwendete verbindungen. Thieme, Stuttgart

© 1991 Elsevier Science Publishers B.V.
Recent advances in periodontology Vol. II,
S.I. Gold, M. Midda and S. Mutlu, eds.

DIAGNOSIS OF PERIODONTAL DISEASE ACTIVITY BY SCINTIGRAPHY

ISIK ADALET(x), ERHAN FIRATLI(xx), SEMA CANTEZ(x), PEKER SANDALLI(xx),
HASAN MERIÇ(xx), ALI GORPE(x)
(x) Istanbul Faculty of Medicine, Dep. of Nuclear Medicine
(xx) Univ. Istanbul, Faculty of Dent., Dept. Periodontology, 34390 Capa,
Istanbul.

INTRODUCTION

Periodontal disease destruction is currently thought to occur with bursts
of activity and remission periods (1). Nuclear medicine techniques identify
the alveolar bone loss before the radiographs. The use of bone seeking
radiopharmacological uptake (BSRU) as an indicator of periodontal disease
activity has been reported.

In this study the usefulness of scintigraphic techniques were studied to
predict the periodontal disease activity and current attachment loss.

MATERIAL AND METHODS

Ten patients who are suffering from adult periodontitis (2) and 6
periodontally healthy volunteers were selected for this study.
Selection Criteria:
1- The patients and the volunteers were systematically healthy,
2- They did not use any antibiotics or metabolic drugs on the last 6 months,
3- No periodontal therapy was evaluated before,
4- They did not carry any endodondic lesion or fracture of jawbones and no
orthodontic treatment was performed during the last 1 year.
Periodontal Implications:
Plaque Index (PI) (4), Gingival Index (GI) (5), Periodontal Pocket Depths
(PPD) and Clinical Attachment Levels (CAL, the distance between cemento-
enamel junction and pocket depth) were measured at baseline and after 6th
month. Serial periapical radiograms were taken at these times. The negative
difference of CAL between baseline and 6th month interval accepted as clinical
attachment loss or in other words, active diseased sites.
Method of Scintigraphy:
Two hours after 20 mCi Tc 99m MDP (Technetium 99m methylene diphosphonate)
injection, anterior images of cranium were taken. By using Siemens Orbiter
Gamma Camera and Micro Delta computer 800.000 counts were obtained. The
uptake of each area was calculated visually and by computer.
Computer Analysis:
To determine the maxillary and mandibular activity of each person right

and left premolar and molar regions were blocked. The orbit bases were also blocked as controls. The following formula was used to calculate each areas activity.

$$\left| \frac{\text{Total counts of a region} - X1}{\text{Total counts of orbit} - X2} \right|$$

X1: Mean total maxillary (or mandibular) counts of controls
X2: Mean total orbital counts of controls

These scintigraphy results compared respectively the areas that accepted as clinically active sites. True positive, true negative, false positive, and false negative values were calculated. The significance of PI, GI, PPD, and CAL in both groups interpreted by using t-test at paired observations.

RESULTS

Patient group was consisted of 5 females and 5 males, total 10 patients. Control group was consisted of 6 persons (5 females and 1 male). PI, GI, PPD, and CAL mean values of patient group were summarized in Table 1 and controls in Table 2.

In this study, 40 sites were evaluated and regional activity values greater than 1 were accepted as scintigraphically active. We found 28 active sites according to scintigraphy in which 25 sites showed clinical attachment loss in 6 months period (real positive). 3 sites which showed activity but not clinical attachment loss were accepted as false negative. Moreover 9 stable sites appeared with clinical attacment loss (false negative) and 3 stable sites appeared with no clinical attachment loss (true negative).

Table 1. Mean values of PI, GI, PPD, and CAL of patient group.

	Baseline	6 months later	Significance
PI	1.43±0.45	1.35±1.67	$p > 0.05$
GI	1.33±0.47	1.27±0.46	$p > 0.05$
PPD	3.25±0.58mm	3.70±0.69	$p < 0.001$
CAL	4.37±0.6mm	4.93±0.66	$p < 0.001$

Table 2. Mean values of PI, GI, PPD, and CAL of control group.

	Baseline	6 months later	Significance
PI	0.36±0.12	0.39±0.15	p>0.05
GI	0.29±0.14	0.32±0.13	p>0.05
PPD	1.53±0.45mm	1.56±0.47	p>0.05
CAL	1.62±0.47mm	1.59±0.38	p>0.05

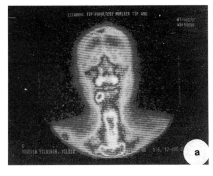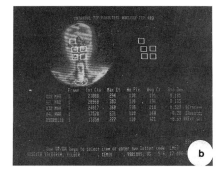

Figure 1. The scintigraphic image of a patient with disease activity (a), and values (b).

DISCUSSION

Clinical, radiological, immunological, and microbiological methods are available to diagnose periodontal disease activity. In recent years the usefulness of nuclear medicine techniques to diagnose the periodontal disease activity has become available.

Disease activity can be diagnosed by radiographs which were performed at 6th months intervals. But these results demonstrate the previous activity instead of present situation. Immunological tests indicate the immunity of the host to the microorganisms associated with disease activity. The microbiological tests give information related to the microbial flora of the site, not of the host.

However bone scintigraphy shows the metabolic changes associated with bone resorption at the time being. The radiopharmaceutical agent Tc 99m MDP accumulates on the surfaces hydroxylappatite crystal. The precipitation of the MDP on hydroxylappatite surfaces was related with, 1. osteogenesis, 2. turnover rate of bone, 3. local blood flow. The uptake of MDP increases with these factors. In periodontal diseases these three factors were increasing (3). In this study we have been able to show the uptake increases in the sites with clinical attachment loss. Scintigraphy indicated a 89.3% diagnostic accuracy. Jeffcoat et al. mentioned 83% (6) and 83.3% (7) diagnostic accuracy in dogs. Reddy et al. (8) and Reddy (9) have mentioned 88% diagnostic accuracy in humans. Our results are very similar to these findings.

As a result, we can conclude that scintigraphy is a useful, quick and easily performed method to diagnose periodontal disease activity.

REFERENCES

1. Haffajee AD, Socransky SS, Goodson JM (1983) J Clin Periodontol 10:257-265

2. Goodson JM, Haffajee AD, Socransky SS (1984) J Clin Periodontol 11:348-359

3. Page RC, Schroeder HE (1982) Periodontitis in man and other animals. A comprehensive review Karger GmbH Zurich pp:222-239

4. Silness J, Loe H (1964) Acta Odont Scand 22:121-135

5. Loe H, Silness J (1963) Acta Odont Scand 21:533-563

6 Jeffcoat MK, Williams RC, Kaplan ML, Goldhaber P (1985) J Periodont Res 20:301-306

7. Jeffcoat MK, Williams RC, Kaplan ML, Goldhaber P (1985) J Periodont 56: Special Issue:8-12

8. Reddy MS, English RJ, Jeffcoat MK, Williams RC, Tumeh SS (1989) J Periodont 60:730

9. Reddy MS (1990) J Periodont 61:309

© 1991 Elsevier Science Publishers B.V.
Recent advances in periodontology Vol. II,
S.I. Gold, M. Midda and S. Mutlu, eds.

371

THE USE OF HYDROXYLAPATITE IN PERIAPICAL-PERIODONTAL DEFECTS-CASE REPORT

PEKER SANDALLI,BARIŞ TUNALI
Department of Periodontology,Faculty of Dentistry,University of
Istanbul (Turkey)

INTRODUCTION

Hydroxylapatite,which is an alloplastic implant material,has
recently found wide application possibilities in dental surgery.In
this study,emphasis is given to the fact that usage of hydroxylapatite has also yielded successful results in periapical-periodontal
defects.We may classify the implant materials developed recently as
follows:

   1 - Calcium phosphate

      -Hydroxylapatite (HA,non resorbable)

     Periograf,Calcitite,Durapatite

      -Tricalcium phosphate(TSP,resorbable)

   2 - Bioglass

   3 - Calcium sulfate (1).

As hydroxylapatite has such characteristics as to activate the
new bone formation,to support bone cavities and to possess biocompatible features,it has the widest field of application among others
in periodontal surgery.When the investigations carried out are examined,it is stated that there is a large number of researches related with this subject,and that hydroxylapatite has yielded considerably promising results at clinical,histological and immunologic
levels in these studies (2,3,4,5,6,7,8).

CASE REPORT

In our case,a 23 year old a male patient applied at our clinic
with complaints of loose incisers.Clinical examination revealed a
pocket depth of 10 mm in this region,whereas the dental mobility
was 2-2,5 degrees.Besides the vestibul was observed to be deficient
in this region.Hower, in the radiograms obtained ,the presence of a
periapical-periodontal defect was detected.In the vitality test
carried out,these 3-1 and 3-2 teeth were detected to be non-vital.

In our treatment,scaling was first applied on the patient,after
which canal treatment was performed on teeth no 3-1 and 3-2.Moreover
root planing was made in this region under anesthesia.At 5 days,

flap operation was performed in this region.During operation,the canals of these teeth were filled with zinc-phosphate cement.Periapical-periodontal lesion,however,was curretted thoroughly to identify clearly the mandibular hard facets.No usual reaction procedure was performed in the roots of both teeth in the defect but Durapatite crystals were implanted instead.The flap was closed with interdental sutures and the region covered with Co-pac.The patient was given antibiotics and radiographs of the region requested. A week later the sutures were removed,followed by the coverage of the region for the second time by paste for a week.

The second stage of our treatment consisted of Edlan-Merjhar operation which was applied 2,5 months after the first surgery to deepen the shallow vestibule in this region.At 5-month results of these procedures,it was observed that the pocket depths,which were originally 10 mm,and dental mobility which was initially 2-2,5 degrees, were all reduced to 2-3 mm and 0-1 degrees,respectively,with the establishment of sufficient vestibular depth.

After wards,the patient was taken under periodic control.But one year after regular control for five months,the patient was lost to follow-up for 1,5 years,only to show up 3 years after his first operation,during which time his oral hygiene had considerably disproved clinically.THe pocket-depths were clinically observed to increase,and the mobility to reach 1,5-2 degrees.Radiographically,resorption could be traced in the supporting tissue surrounding the tooth.A year later,i.e.,4 years after the first operation,the patient referred to as again for a control,where it was observed that pocket-depths reached 7mm,and the mobility 2-2,5 degrees but the tooth had no vertical mobility.Radiographically,a marked resorption was traced around the tooth.THe paitent reported that he sometimes had complaints of tooth ache in that dental region.Presently,it is intemded to retain the same tooth in the mouth for some moretime, and to extract it to replace with a bicortical implant.

DISCUSSION

Clinical results abtained by the application of hydroxylapatite in intraosseous periodontal lessions,correlate well with the results obtained by the other investigation in this subject.The application of a graft material to periapical lesions without the performance of a resection procedure in the anatomic root of the tooth, however,constitutes another aspect of our study,which introduces

a new approach to such cases.The reason why Edlan-Merjhar operation
technique was selected in deepening the vestibule is that no graft
bed was prepared in this technique as,for example,in free dental
graft,and therefore it had no dircet relation with the connective
tisue which covered the hydroxylapatite crystalls and that vestibular deepening could be aachieved at a larger filld.

   In conclusion,we may say that,hydroxylapatite is an alloplastic
material employed not only in filling the cavities of the extracted cysts or in the elevation of shallow alveolar crest,but also in
periodontal defects.

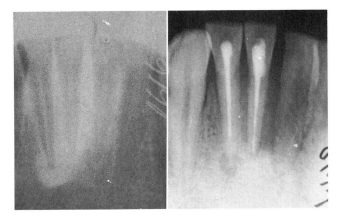

The radiographical image of the patients first and four years
after the flap surgery.

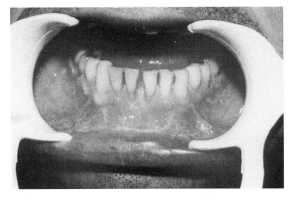

The clinical appearance
of the case's four years
after the flap surgery.

REFERENCES

1. Rateitschak KH,Rateitschak EM,Wolf HF,Hassel TM (1985) Color Atlas of Periodontology 215

2. Benque EP,Gineste M,Heughebaret M(1985) J Biologie Buccale 13:271-282

3. Ganeles J,Listgarten MA,Evian CI(1986) J Periodontology 75:133-140

4. Grigolato P,Parabita GF,Troletti GD,Zanetti U,Beremzi A,Marocolo D (1984) Estr da Minerva Stomatologica 33

5. Hartmann HJ (1986) TD Quintessenz 4:303-314

6. Kenney EB,Lekovic V,Sa Ferreina JC,Han T,Dimitrijevic B,Carranza FA (1986) J Periodontology 75:76-83

7. Meffert RM,Thomas JR,Hamilton KM,Brownstein CN (1985) Periodontology 46:63-73

8. Sapkos SW (1986) J Periodontology 57:7-12

© 1991 Elsevier Science Publishers B.V.
Recent advances in periodontology Vol. II,
S.I. Gold, M. Midda and S. Mutlu, eds.

GINGIVAL FIBROMATOSIS: A CLINICAL, GENETIC AND DERMATOGLYPHIC STUDY

BAHAR KURU, SELCUK YILMAZ, METIN ATASU, MUSTAFA CARPAR

M.Ü. Dental Faculty, Periodontology Dept., Istanbul, Turkey

INTRODUCTION

One of the problems concerning dentistry is the fibrous lesions seen in oral cavity originated from different etiological factors. Being an undetermined etiological case Gingival Fibromatosis (GF) presents some problems in identification and treatment. As it stresses both the hereditary and histopathological characteristics, the term Hereditary Gingival Fibromatosis is used (3), (4), (6). When there is no evidence of genetic transmission the condition is called idiopathic (1), (5). Besides its manifestation as an isolated feature it may also occur with some other abnormalities or diseases or as a constituent of certain syndromes (8). In some syndromes, the abnormalities of extremities particularly of fingers or toes can be observed in addition to GF.

This study is designed to present three patients with GF and their family members and to report on the findings obtained by dermatoglyphics in order to find out whether there is a relation between the highly genetically controlled palmar and plantar pattern types and ridge counts and gingival embryology and whether they show the same characteristics seen in isolated GF (8). In the treatment a different operation technique was performed.

MATERIAL AND METHODS

Three families comprising 8 members in total, 3 of which manifesting GF were analysed. Pedigrees were drawn up and the mode of genetic transmission was analysed. The digitopalmar and plantar dematoglyphics were taken in 3 patients and their family members. The results of dermatoglyphics taken from the Turkish population served as the control data (2).

Family Reports:

Case I : Analysing the family history GF was found. The idiopathic enlargement was present from birth. Class II/I malocclusion and openbite was detected. The patient was 16 years old and GF was accompanied by hearing loss, ear deformity, mental retardation, and hypoplasia of fingers and nails.

Case II : In this 18 year old patient GF was found isolated and idiopathic. The onset had occurred with the eruption of permanent teeth. Openbite and Class III malocclusion was detected.

Case III : In this family GF was recognized as isolated and genetic Class II/I malocclusion was detected.

RESULTS

The minor abnormalities of the fingers and palms were detected in autosomal dominant inherited isolated cases. Dermatoglyphics are recently being used in diagnosis in the field of medicine and dentistry. Distorted dermatoglyphics may suggest the disharmony in the development. In the fingertip patterns the whorls were the most frequent form followed by ulnar loops. An increase in total finger ridge counts the presence of border tri in the IV interdigital region, the axial triradius (t) position being moderately distal (t`) and the presence of border triradii (t^b) and the plantar loop in I-III-IV region were also very frequent (8).

Our results are shown in Tables I, II, III, IV.

As a result the dermatoglyphic findings differ according to the type of GF. It is for this reason that we attach significance to the use of dermatoglyphics in diagnoses. By means of dermatoglyphics, the relation between the embryonic development and GF could be established and GF may be considered as the result of abnormal cell division at the 14th and 21st weeks of embryonic development of mesodermal structures.

In treatment ledge and wedge, gingivectomy, internal bevel gingivectomy or their modifications can be used for GF in a case which shows enlargement on the whole attached gingiva and for sometimes it appears as palatally hanging tissues, standard gingivectomy is uncomfortable and unappropriate because of exposing a very large raw gingival surface (7). Instead the modified split thickness flap is used. In this technique,

a) the marginal outline of the palatal mucosa is scribed by an incision at a 90° angle leaving a blunt margin,

b) the remaining tissue is thinned by an internal bevel incision, and

c) the flap is reflected and snipped and the wound is left to primary healing.

The problems in GF can be solved with this technique which is somewhat more difficult because of the necessity to project precisely the margin of the incised bevels, particularly on the crestal aspect where it will coincide with the crestal margin of bone and dermatoglyphics being a step forward to the future studies needs to be enriched with data taken from various GF cases.

TABLE I: Finger-tip patterns of the cases of
GF and their family members

	LEFT					RIGHT				
	V	IV	III	II	I	V	IV	III	II	I
FAMILY I										
CASE	U	U	U	R	U	U	U	U	W	U
BROTHER	U	U	U	W	U	U	U	U	R	W
MOTHER	U	W	W	R	W	U	W	W	W	W
FATHER	U	U	U	U	U	U	U	U	U	U
FAMILY II										
CASE	W	W	W	W	W	U	U	U	W	U
MOTHER	U	W	U	R	U	U	U	U	U	U
FAMILY III										
CASE	U	W	W	W	U	U	W	W	W	U
SISTER	U	W	W	W	U	U	W	U	U	U

U: Ulnar loop; R: Radial loop; W: Whorl

TABLE II: Finger-tip ridge-counts and total finger ridge-counts

	LEFT											RIGHT											
	V		IV		III		II		I		TOTAL	V		IV		III		II		I		TOTAL	TRC
	r	u	r	u	r	u	r	u	r	u		r	u	r	u	r	u	r	u	r	u		
FAMILY I																							
CASE	10	–	12	–	11	–	–	4	18	–	55	5	–	9	–	12	–	–	4	8	–	38	93
BROTHER	7	–	14	–	12	–	12	8	21	–	66	14	–	14	–	12	–	–	10	20	14	70	136
MOTHER	15	–	19	4	13	19	–	19	21	17	93	11	–	21	–	4	16	13	19	15	18	85	178
FATHER	10	–	13	–	12	–	7	–	17	–	59	6	–	5	–	9	–	6	–	19	–	45	104
FAMILY II																							
CASE	14	15	19	15	13	10	9	20	19	–	80	14	–	19	–	13	–	14	20	14	–	86	166
MOTHER	14	–	16	19	9	–	–	4	21	–	67	10	–	16	–	17	–	16	–	22	–	81	148
FAMILY III																							
CASE	14	–	12	7	14	7	16	9	18	–	70	14	–	12	8	15	5	15	11	18	–	74	148
SISTER	11	–	12	16	11	4	11	14	18	–	74	14	–	9	15	11	–	14	–	20	–	74	144

TABLE III: Palmar configuations and palmar a-b ridge counts

FAMILY I	LEFT HAND									RIGHT HAND									Palmar a. bridge count
CASE	IV	t	4	(3)						IV	t	4	(3)						104
BROTHER	III	t	4	(3)						III	t	4	(3)						80
MOTHER	III	IV	t	5	(3)					III	t	4	(3)						76
FATHER	III	H	t	t^b	4	(3)				III	H	t	t^b	4	(3)				84
FAMILY II																			
CASE	IV	H	t"	t	4	(1)				IV	H	t"	t	4	(3)				104
MOTHER	IV	H	H	t"	t	t^b	4	(3)		III	H	H	t"	t	t^b	4	(3)		82
FAMILY III																			
CASE	IV	H	t	t^b	4	(3)				III	H	t	t	4	(5')				86
SISTER	IV	H	H	H	t"	t	t^b	4	(1)	III	H	H	H	t"	t	t^b	4	(5') 84

TABLE IV: PLANTAR CONFIGURATIONS

	LEFT FEET								RIGHT FEET							
FAMILY I																
CASE	I	I	III	e	f	p'	4		I	II	III	f	p	p'	4	
BROTHER	I	I	III	e	f	p'	4		I	II	III	f	p	5		
FATHER	I	e	4						I	I	III	e	f	p	4	
FAMILY II																
CASE	I	I^f	Y	f	h	4			I	I	I^f	Y	e	f	p'	h 4
MOTHER	I	III	Y	f	p'	h	4		I	III	f	p'	4			
FAMILY III																
CASE	I	II	III	f	p"	z	4		I	I	II	III	f	p'	z	4
SISTER	I	I	III	e	f	p'	z	3	I	I	III	e	f	p'	z	3

REFERENCES

1. Aksoy Y,Parlar A,Demir O (1987) Northeast Soc Perio 10:14-1

2. Atasu M (1979) J Ment Defic Res 23:111-121

3. Carranza FA (1984) Glickman's Clinical Periodontology.W.B. Saunders,Philadelphia

4. Çağlayan F,Şengün D (1987) HÜ Dişhek Derg 11:57-60

5. Lindhe J (1982) Textbook of Clinical Periodontology. W.B. Saunders, Philadelphia

6. Lucas RB(1972) Pathology of Tumours of the Oral Tissues.Churchill Livingstone,Edinburgh,London

7. Schluger S,Yuodelis RA,Page RC (1978) Periodontal Disease. Lea Febiger,Philadelphia

8. Skrinjaric I,Bacic M (1989) J Perio Res 24:303-309

© 1991 Elsevier Science Publishers B.V.
Recent advances in periodontology Vol. II,
S.I. Gold, M. Midda and S. Mutlu, eds.

THE PERIODONTAL EVALUATION OF CROWNS PREPARED BY DENTAL STUDENTS

YASEMİN FOROOZESH(*), UTKU ONAN(**), NURTEN TURAN(***), GÜLDEN IŞIK(**)

(*)Dept. Prostodontics, Faculty of Dentistry, Univ. ISTANBUL
(**)Dept. Periodontology, Faculty of Dentistry, Univ. ISTANBUL
(***)Dept. National Health, Cerrahpaşa Faculty of Medicine, Univ. ISTANBUL

INSTRUCTION

There are some main factors affecting the success of fixed prosthodontic treatments. As we may breifly define this factors as anatomic, esthetic, static, physiologic andhygenic which all these must be considered completely and carefully
during the maintenance of these prosthesis. Both clinical and laboratory studies
must be based on these main factors.

By the way we desided to examine the single crowns which are prepared in our
clinics by the students from the periodontal health point and we aimed to investigate PI and SBI values of the gingiva before and after these applications.

MATERIALS AND METHODS

44 patients who are in need of crown restorations were investigated before and
three weeks after the applications,PI and modified SBI measurement were evaluated
on interprominal areas and buccolingually following parameters of Silness-Löe plaque index and modified sulcus bleeding index(6).

FINDING

In 88 test region a total of 44 crown restorations mesial+distal and vertibul+
oral plaque index scors were calculated before and three weeks after treatment and
printed on table 1.

TABLE 1

PI VALUES

Total PI values found before and three weeks after treatment

n=88	Before Treatment		After Treatment	
PI Scores	Approximal region	Vestibul+Oral region	Approximal region	Vestibul+Oral region
0	10	18	17	39
1	37	48	59	47
2	25	17	11	1
3	16	4	1	1

STATISTICAL ANALYSIS OF PI

x^2 analysis were applied and differences between the investigated regions were calculated(reduced, not changed, increased PI scores) on table 2.

TABLE 2

REGION INVESTIGATION

x^2 analysis and the calculations of the investigated regions

Regions	PI ratio(reduced)	PI ratio(no change)	PI ratio(increased)	Total
Vestibul+Oral	44(50%)	35(40%)	9(10%)	88
Mesial+Distal	44(50%)	31(35%)	13(15%)	88
Total	88	66	22	176

$x^2=0.96$

SBI VALUE CORELATIONS

TABLE 3

MESIAL+DISTAL SBI VALUES COMPARISON

Mc Nemar test calculation of SPI values of Mesial+Distal region before and three weeks after treatment.

	Before treatment		
	+	−	Total
+	34	17	51
−	26	11	37
Total	60	28	88

After treatment

z=1.37

TABLE 4

VESTIBUL+ORAL SBI VALUES COMPARISON

Mc Nemar test calculation of SPI values of Vestibul+ Oral region before and three weeks after treatment.

		Before treatment		
		+	−	Total
After treatment	+	15	11	26
	−	21	41	62
	Total	36	52	88

z=1.76

STATISTICAL ANALYSIS OF SBI

The bleeding index difference between before and three weeks after the treatment and the ratio between the investigated regions were determined(table 3,4).

The critical value of Mc Nemar test was z=1.96 and since our calculations were below this level we can say that there was no significant difference between the ratios. On tho calculated regions the difference of SBI values on Mesial+Distal was found 58% on Vestibul+Oral region 30% and the difference(ξ=3.87, P<0.001) was accepted significant.

RESULTS

In the recent years the relationship between the crowns and the gingiva have been researched by several researchers and some obtained the same results, on the other hand, some obtained different. We also made an analysis of the crowns done by the students to the patients who came to our clinics from a periodontal aspect by making the SBI and PI'es and then compared the results with the literature.

As a result, the crowns prepared by dental students made no harms from the periodontal aspect.

DISCUSSION

Looking at the publications roughness of the surface appears to be very important. Belger, Waerhaug and Volcansky, stated that such retantive surfaces tend to plaque formation and this irritates the epithelial tissue of the gingiva(1,7,8). Larato, mentioned that the crown margin below the gingival level causes the plaque formation and forming the deep gingival sulcuses. In some cases they stated that the inflammatory cells also verify the matter(3).

Our results are in accordance with the above statements. The calculation in this research(table 2) shows that:-

-In 50% of the total 88 test regions, PI scores were reduced in both Vestibul+Oral and Mesial+Distal.

-In 40% of the total 66 test regions, PI scores in Vestibul+Oral and 35% in Mesial +Distal were unchanged.

-In 10% of the total 22 test regions, PI scores in Vestibul+Oral and 15% in Mesial +Distal were increased.

We may consider that the above PI rate increase is because of 13.6% of the patients had a previous treatment of periodontal therapy and application of partial veneer on 37.9% of the patients, finally the surface of the crown restorations not being properly polished(7).

SBI statistical calculationns showed no meaningful values, however after the treatment SBI on Vestibul+Oral and Masial+Distal shows a difference of P<0.001. This indicates that physiological and mechanic cleaning difference of these regions, which is though to be hard to clean the interproximal areas(2,4,5).

REFERENCES

1. Belger L. : Kuron-Köprü Protezleri,Prof.DR.Nazim Terzioğlu Matb.İstanbul 1986.

2. Berran Ö., Özpınar B., Akgünlü A. : Margin lokalizasyonları farklı uygulanan dişlerin Buccal-Lingual ve Mezial -Distal yüzlerindeki Gİ ve PLİ değerlerinin karşılaştırılması, D.D.D.,1, (2);93-106,1980.

3. Larato, D.C. : Effects of artificial crown on gingival pocket depth, J. Prost. Dent., 34 (6); 640-643, 1975.

4. Sıgurd, P.R. : Periodontal aspects of restorative dentistry. J.Oral. Rehabilitation. 1; 107-126, 1974.

5. Sıgurd, P.R. : Aesthetics, periodontology, and restorative dentistry, Quintess Inter. 9; 581-588, 1985.

6. Tuncer, Ö. : Periodontoloji propedötik; Bozok Matbaası, İstanbul 1984.

7. Volchansky, A., Cleaton, Jones, P.and Retief, D.H. : Study of surface characteristics of natural teeth and restorations adjacent gingiva, J. Prost. Dent. 31(4); 411-421, 1974.

8. Waerhaug, J. : Histologic consideration which govern where the margins of restorations should be located in relation to the gingiva. The Dent. Clin of north. Am. 4;161-176, 1960.

© 1991 Elsevier Science Publishers B.V.
Recent advances in periodontology Vol. II,
S.I. Gold, M. Midda and S. Mutlu, eds.

RESEARCH OF THE EFFECT OF DIFFERENT TREATMENT PLANS ON THE PATIENTS WITH JUVENILE PERIODONTITIS

ASLAN Y.GÖKBUGET & ÖZEN TUNCER

University of Istanbul, Faculty of Dentistry, Dept. of Periodontology, Çapa Istanbul-Turkey

INTRODUCTION

Periodontosis (Orban & Weinmann, 1942) or Juvenile Periodontitis (Manson & Lehner 1974) is a disease of the periodontium occuring in an otherwise healthy young individual. Other terms that have been used to describe this or smilar disorders are e.g. "Diffuse Bone Atrophy", "Deep Cementopathia" (Gottlieb 1923, 1928) or "Precocious Periodontitis" (Sugarman & Sugarman, 1977).

Juvenile Periodontitis is characterized by rapid loss of connective tissue attachment and alveolar bone at more then one tooth in the parmanent dentition. According to current concepts two basic forms of Juvenile periodontitis may exist. In one form, localized Juvenile periodontitis, only the first molars and the incisors are involved in the disease process. In the second form, generalized Juvenile periodontitis, most teeth in the dentition are affected (Lindhe, 1984)

MATERIAL AND METHOD

Patients selection has been based on Bear's criteria (1971) for Juvenile periodontitis. The study has been conducted on 109 periodontiums of 12 young girls aged between 17-23 years, having no systemic disorders. In grouping of the patients, age and deffects have been taken into consideration. The patients have been devided into two groups. The first group has been treated with the classical oral hygiene programme, scaling, modified Widman flap. To the other group besides this classical treatment plan, systemic tetracycline of 250 mgx4/day and chlorhexidine mouth wash 0.2% has been prescribed for two weeks.

In the research plaque index (PI) (Silness-Löe, 1964), sulcus bleeding index (SBI) (Mühlemann-Son 1971), sulcus fluid flow rate (SFFR)

(Mod. Löe & Holm-Pedersen 1965), gingival recession index (Tuncer 1975), pocket probing depth (oclusal stand), attachment level (oclusal stand), bacteriological and histological evaluation (Oliver et al. 1969) has been determined. The patients were followed over a period of three months.

RESULTS

As a result, significant decrease in measurements and indexes were obtained in patients with juvenile periodontitis (Fig.1,2,3 &4). The antibiotic administered should be effective for the patogenes.

The tetracycline used in the research fulfills this. Although some researchers favor it, the use of antibiotics is under discussion. The results of our study show that, as in all periodontal therapies, the important aspects in the treatment of juvenile periodontitis are a good diagnosis, patient/dentist cooperation, optimal plaque control and maintenance care. The treatment plan can be supported with tetracycline.

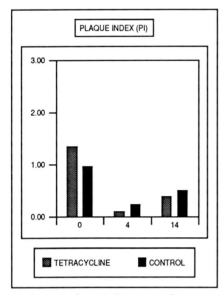

Fig.1. Mean plaque index scores of tetracycline and control groups devided to weeks.

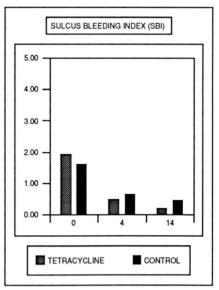

Fig.2. Mean sulcus bleeding index scores of tetracycline and control groups devided to weeks.

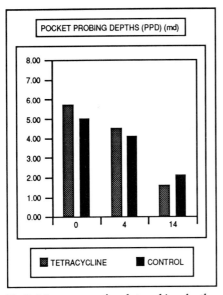

Fig.3. Mean scores of pocket probing depths
of tetracycline and control groups
devided to weeks.

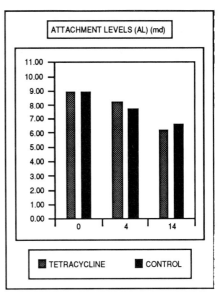

Fig.4. Mean scores of attachment levels of
tetracycline and control groups
devided to weeks.

REFERENCES

1. Baer, P.N.: The Case for Periodontosis as a Clinical Entity.
    J.Periodontol. 42:516, 1971

2. Ciancio, S.G., Genco, R.J.: Periodontal, Tedavide Antibiyotik
    Kullanımı Üzerine. TD Quintessence, 9:755-758, 1986.

3. Christersson, L.A., Slots,J., Rosling, B.G., Genco, R.J.: Microbio-
    logical and Clinical Effects of Surgical Treatment of Localized
    Juvenile Periodontitis. J. Clin. Periodontol. 12:465-476, 1985.

4. Genco, R.J., Christersson, L.A., Zembon, J.J.: Juvenile Period-
    ontitis. Inter. Dent.J. 36:168-176, 1986.

5. Lindhe,J., Liljenberg,B.: Treatment of Localized Juvenile Peri-
    odontitis, Results After 5 Years. J. Clin. Periodontol. 11:399-
    410, 1984.

6. Listgarten, M.A.: Nature of Periodontal Diseases: Pathogenic
    Mechanisms. J. Periodontal Res. 22:172-178, 1987.

7. Mandell, R.L., Socransky, S.S.: Microbiological and Clinical Ef-

fects of Surgery Plus Doxycycline on Juvenile Periodontitis. J. Periodontol. 59(6): 373-379, 1988.

8. Slots, J., Rosling, B.G.:Suppression of Periodontopathic Micro-flora in Localized Juvenile Periodontitis by Systemic Tetracy-cline, J. Periodontol. 10: 465-486, 1983.

9. Tuncer, Ö.: Periodontoloji. Propedötik, Bozak, İstanbul, 1984.

10. Zambon, J.J., Christersson, L.A., Genco, R.J.: Diagnosis and Treatment of Localized Juvenile Periodontitis, JADA 113(2): 295-299, 1986.

© 1991 Elsevier Science Publishers B.V.
Recent advances in periodontology Vol. II,
S.I. Gold, M. Midda and S. Mutlu, eds.

ESTHETICS IN PERIODONTAL TREATMENT

AKIRA HASEGAWA and ITARU MIKAMI
Department of Periodontics, The Nippon Dental University, School of
Dentistry at Niigata, 1-8 Hamaura-cho, Niigata-shi, Japan.

INTRODUCTION

The needs of dental patients are changing. At earlier stages, patients only needed to control pain and at latter stages to recover normal function. Now prevention and esthetics are considered routine. Our concern as a profession is for the health of the mouth and associated functions. Contemporary oral health means not only freedom from pathological conditions but also concern for esthetic dentistry.

Significant progress in dental esthetics is occurring in every dental field. Periodontics also offers many possibilities that will result in esthetic improvement.

The esthetic problems most frequently encountered by periodontisits are:
1. Gingival inflammation
2. Gingival hyperplasia
3. Gingival recession
4. Blunted papilla
5. Deformed anterior alveolar ridge
6. Gingival pigmentation

The treatment procedure for gingival inflammation, hyperplasia and recession have been established as routine.

For blunted papilla, we have just started to improve the necessary technique. This procedure has to be evaluated, after longterm follow-up. The purpose of this report is to present the treatment procedure of deformed anterior alveolar ridge and gingival pigmentation.

DEFORMED ANTERIOR ALVEOLAR RIDGE

For deformed anterior alveolar ridge(Fig. 1), we have been using hydroxylapatite block to augment a ridge depression(Fig. 2). The surgical procedure of my department is as follows.

1. Surgical approach is made from the labial side. The first parallel vertical incisions are made from the gingival margin of the adjacent teeth up to about 5mm beyond the mucogingival junction, and are shallow enough not to reach the periosteum.
2. The second incision, which constitutes a horizontal incision, is performed shallowly just in the mucosa of the lip.

3. A partial thickness flap is reflected. By this reflection, the submucosal connective tissue is exposed in the mucosa of the lip and the periosteum is exposed from the mucogingival junction. Once the periosteum is exposed, a horizontal incision is made therein, then the full thickness reflection is completed(Fig.3).

4. Hydroxylapatite block is contoured using an air turbine fitted with a fine diamond point.

5. Properly arranged hydroxylapatite block is put on the alveolar ridge (Fig.4).

6. The flap is replaced and sutured. The exposed periosteum area is protected with collagen membrane.

Compared with onlay graft or subgingival connective tissue graft, this surgical procedure needs no donor site. Compared with hydroxylapatite granule, this surgical technique is effective for apico-cornal loss, leaving less postoperative shrinkage(Fig.5,6).

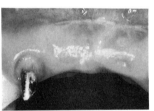

Fig. 1.   Fig. 2.

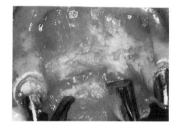
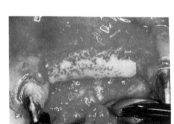

Fig. 3.   Fig. 4.

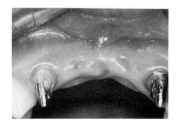

Fig. 5.

Fig.1. Deformed alveolar ridge.
   2. Hydroxylaptite block.
   3. Flap is reflected by partial and full thickness.
   4. Hydroxylapatite is put on the alveolar ridge.
   5. Postoperative view.

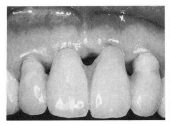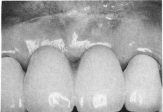

Fig.6. Pre and postoperative restoration

To prevent jaw defects caused by bone cysts, we use beta tricalcium phosphate block(Fig.7). Beta tricalcium phosphate is resorbed and replaced by bone when implanted in bony environments. Numerous methods have been proposed for filling bone cavities after the extirpation of cysts. The aim is to fill the empty space left by the extirpation of diseased tissue. In this regard, it is well known that bone grafts produce the most favorable result. But bone is difficult to obtain, especially in Japan. For this reason, we use beta tricalcium phosphate. The surgical procedure is as follows:

1. The incision is made through the mucosa in the labial vestibule.
2. Following extirpation of the cyst(Fig.8), beta tricalcium phosphate block is inserted and packed(Fig.9). By pressing with an instrument, the block is easy to break and fill every space of the cyst.
3. After ensuring correct density in filling, the mucosal flap is sutured and the closure is completed(Fig.10). Beta tricalcium phosphate block is easily obtainable and easy to work with.

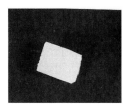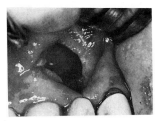

Fig.7. Beta tricalcium phosphate block.

Fig.8. Empty space left by the extirpation of cyst.

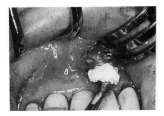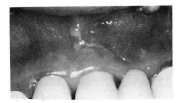

Fig.9. Beta tricalcium phosphate is inserted.

Fig.10. Postoperative view. The depression is minimum.

GINGIVAL PIGMENTATION

Oral pigmentation occurs in all races. Melanin pigmentation is the most common and the patient requests depigmentation for cosmetic reasons(Fig. 11). There are several methods for removing melanin pigmentation. The surgical procedure is the most popular. Laser and cryosurgery have also been reported. Hirshfeld's method which use phenol and alcohol is simple and painless. The method is as follows:

1. The area is isolated with cotton rolls and dried with air.
2. A very small pledget of cotton is dipped into 90 percent phenol, lightly blotted to remove excess phenol and applied carefully to the pigmented area. The surface turns white almost immediately (Fig. 12).
3. Twenty seconds after the application, the phenol is neutralized with 95 percent alcohol and the patient then rinses with water.
4. The area is dried again and the procedure is repeated once.

Within twenty-four hours, the cauterized tissue sloughs off, usually leaving a painless bright red area which heals completely within a week or ten days. By the end of that time, the mucous membrane appears perfectly normal in color and texture with no evidence of the former pigmented condition(Fig. 13). If the pigmentation returns, it is probably because insufficient depth was reached, allowing some melanoblasts to remain. In this case, the process is then repeated. This method was reported by Hirshfeld in 1951 and is simple and painless. So if recurrence occurs, it is easy for patients to undergo the therapy again.

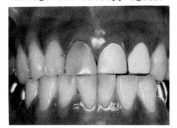

Fig. 11.   Fig. 12.

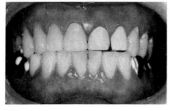

Fig. 11. Melanin pigmentation.
   12. 90 percent phenol is applied to
      the pigmented area.
   13. View after treatment.

Fig. 13.

The gingival frame and color around the teeth form an essential component to a beautiful smile. The periodontist can offer a significant contribution to the successful, corrective cosmetic treatment plan.

© 1991 Elsevier Science Publishers B.V.
Recent advances in periodontology Vol. II,
S.I. Gold, M. Midda and S. Mutlu, eds.

PERIODONTOLOGY — ORTHODONTICS INTERRELATIONSHIP AND ADHESIVE SPLINTS IN RETENTION THERAPY

ORHUN BENGİSU, SERVET DOĞAN, EVREN EVERENOSOĞLU

Department of Periodontology and Orthodontics, Faculty of Dentistry,
Ege University, Bornova, 35100 İzmir (Turkey)

INTRODUCTION

Malocclusion and malalignment of teeth do not directly lead to periodontal destruction. For this reason they do not cause a serious threat for periodontal health
in well motivated patients and orthodontic alignment/realignment of those teeth is
not a routine procedure in their periodontal treatment course. On the other hand,
malocclusion and malalignment of teeth change the oral enviroment of an avarage
patient in such a way that plaque accumulation and growth is favored, while its
elimination becomes harder. Thus, it can easily be said that there are many occasions when changing the position of one or several teeth is an essential part of
periodontal treatment.[1] They can be divided into two main groups:

1. Factors **predisposing** the initiation or progression of periodontal disease
1.1. Tooth crowding makes daily plaque removal difficult or sometimes impossible.
1.2. Root approximation leads to insufficient interseptal bone which may later
     contribute to deep interproximal crater formation.
1.3. Open contacts cause food impaction which can produce rapid distruction of the
     interproximal periodontal structures.
1.4. Increased overbite and other deformities such as rotation, inclination, etc.
2. Pathologic migrations which are the **results** of advanced periodontal disease.
2.1. Medial diastema or general spacing of teeth in the anterior segments.
2.2. Spacing of teeth combined with proclination of upper incisors.
2.3. Rotated and tipped bicuspids and molars with collapse of the posterior occlus-
     ion and reduced height of bite.

Thus, the overall treatment plan for a patient with advanced periodontal disease
often involves minor tooth movement to (1) eliminate predisposing factors which
may impede the overall success of periodontal treatment,(2) reestablish a satisfactory occlusion,(3)have a better esthetics,(4) make chewing comfortable,(5)produce
a favorable response in intrabony pockets,(6) assist in improving gingival and
bony deformities,(7) reorient abutment teeth into better axial inclinations to
allow parallel preparations for bridges,(8) correct phonetic problems.

FACTORS TO BE CONSIDERED IN ORTHODONTIC THERAPY OF PATIENTS WITH ADVANCED PERIODONTAL DISEASE

Periodontium. Since the periodontium around the teeth, which will be moved, is not
healthy, thorough debridement of root surfaces must be done to resolve the existing inflammation before the orthodontic force is applied.[2]During the course of

orthodontic therapy, special care should be taken to maintain a very high standard of plaque control in order to prevent a lateral periodontal abcess formation.

Periodontal surgery. Excision of the fibrotic gingiva, which may prevent the movement of teeth should be done before the initiation of the orthodontic treatment. Apart from this, any periodontal surgery contemplated should preferably be delayed until after the completion of active orthodontic therapy,[3] because, (1) gingival contours may be improved or even the intrabony pockets may be eliminated after the completion of orthodontic therapy and therefore surgery should no more be necessary, (2) although the intra-alveolar fibers of the periodontal ligament are replaced during tooth movement, supra-alveolar fibers are not (but may be merely stretched) and cause relapse. During the surgery, those elastic fibers are cut and after healing, they are attached to a different part of root surface and provide a biologic retention by minimizing the risk for and degree of relapse.

Reduced height of the attachment apparatus is not a contraindication to orthodontic therapy, provided that it is non-inflammatory, because teeth with reduced but healthy periodontium respond to orthodontic forces just like teeth with normal support.Furthermore, those teeth can move back to alignment remarkably quickly and the orthodontic phase of treatment is usually not prolonged.

Age is not a contraindication to orthodontic treatment, but in the elderly, the tissue response to orthodontic forces is slower and this means that hyalin zones, which may prevent tooth movement temporarily, may form more easily in adults. In order to prevent this and to allow time for tissue reorganisation, the orthodontic forces applied in adults should preferably be **light** and **interrupted.**

Patient problems. It is far more difficult for an adult individual to adapt to an orthodontic appliance than for a child. Phonetic adjustment to a removable appliance generally requires more time in adults. Furthermore, there is always a risk of using it sporadically. However, a **fixed appliance** is usually better tolarated by adult patients, although in the beginning, it may be difficult to accept it for esthetic reasons.[4] The selection of proper anchorage may also present a major problem if the patient is partially edentulous or has reduced amounts of alveolar bone.

Retention. The retention period is generally long in adults, owing to the decreased ability of the periodontal tissue to react to mechanical stimuli. Thus, **permanent retainers** must be applied to adults to prevent risk for relapse. When removable retainers are used, the dentist is too dependent on the cooperation of the patient. Therefore, **fixed** retainers must be preferred in adults. A proper retainer should keep each orthodontically treated tooth in the acquired position. It should be designed to be as inconspicuous as possible, yet strong enough to achieve its objective. It should also allow the patient to achieve proper plaque control and and should not be deleterious to the periodontal tissues or cause speech problems. Adhesive splints have all these properties and moreover they are pretty esthetic **and** do not require irreversible tooth preparation.

CASE PRESENTATIONS

We treated several cases according to principles described above. Only two selected cases are presented here, one as the **cause** (Fig.1-4) and the other as the
result of periodontal disease (Fig.5-8). In all cases, adhesive splints were appli-
cated as permanant-fixed retainers and removal of orthodontic appliances delayed
after their bonding on to the teeth.

Case No.1 : A 35 year old woman had to be treated orthodontically, because tooth
crowding on mandibular anterior incisors had made plaque control impossible and
fibrous hyperplasia and pseudo-pockets had aroused (Fig.1). Tooth 41 was extracted
during the gingivectomy operation to create space for the proper alignment of the
remaining incisors by means of a sectional light arch wire (Fig.2). Six months
later, an adhesive splint was fabricated (Fig. 3) and bonded for permanent retention (Fig.4).

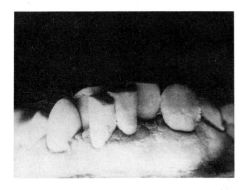

Fig. 1

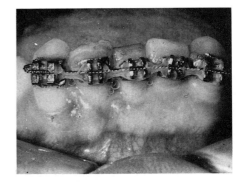

Fig. 2

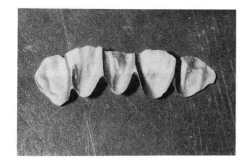

Fig. 3

CASE NO. 1

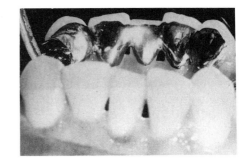

Fig. 4

394

Case No.2 : A 25 year old woman had to be treated orthodontically because of pathological tooth migration (Fig.5, Fig.6). After a meticulous debridement and achievement of plaque control, the spaces were closed by means of a sectional arch wire
and an Alastic chain (Fig.7). In the meantime, root surfaces were debrided at regular intervals to prevent an abcess formation and a further attachment loss. After completion of orthodontic therapy, additional surgical pocket elimination was
carried out and retention was performed by means of an adhesive splint (Fig.8).

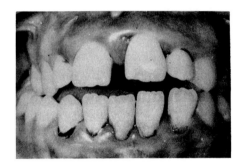 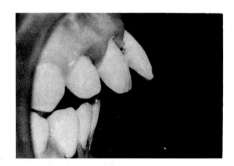

Fig. 5   Fig. 6

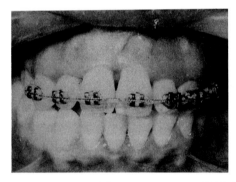

Fig. 7   CASE NO. 2   Fig. 8

REFERENCES

1. Hirschfeld L (1978) In: Schluger S, Yuodelis RA, Page RC (eds) Periodontal
   Disease. Lea and Febiger, Philadelphia, pp 422-435
2. Jenkins WMM, Allan CJ, Collins WJN (1986) Guide to Periodontics, William
   Heinemann Medical Book Ltd. London, pp 52-53, 143
3. Thilander B (1985) In: Lindhe J (ed) Textbook of Periodontal Therapy. Munsgaard
   Copenhagen, pp 480-499
4. Tayer BH, Burek MJ (1981) A survey of adult's attitudes toward orthodontic
   therapy. Am J Orthod 79(3):305-315

POSTER PRESENTATIONS

© 1991 Elsevier Science Publishers B.V.
Recent advances in periodontology Vol. II,
S.I. Gold, M. Midda and S. Mutlu, eds.

GINGIVAL HYPERPLASIA ASSOCIATED WITH CALCIUM ANTAGONISTS

MASAHARU SHIRAKAWA, KEIICHIRO KAWAMURA AND HIROSHI OKAMOTO
Dept. of Endodontol. and Periodontol., Hiroshima Univ. School of Dent.,
1-2-3, Kasumi, Minami-ku, Hiroshima, (Japan)

INTRODUCTION

In recent years, calcium antagonists have been widely used for circulatory diseases such as essential hypertension and angina pectoris in Japan. As their side effects, gingival hyperplasia due to the continued use of nifedipine has been observed and it has been pointed out that both the clinical and histopathological patterns closely resemble that of hyperplasia due to diphenylhydantoin (1-4). We have observed gingival hyperplasia in three patients who were administered nifedipine and other calcium antagonists for an extended period. This report persents the clinical findings and therapeutic course of these cases.

CASE REPORT 1

The patient is a 49-year-old male who visited our hospital with a chief complaint of severe halitosis. Two years previously he had an attack of angina pectoris and thereafter he has received oral administration of nifedipine at 40 mg/day and diltiazem at 120mg/day. Oral examination revealed marked hyperplasia of the papillary gingiva of the lower and upper anterior teeth particularly of the lower anterior teeth with the involved gingiva being firm and elastic(Fig. 1). Redness and swelling of the gingiva were remarkable in whole mouth, but bleeding and plus discharge were observed only in a few teeth. Mobility of 1-2 degree was confined to some molars. Probing pocket depth was more than 6 mm at the molars and more than 4 mm at the anterior teeth. Much deposition of dental calculus was observed. His oral hygiene was poor with O'Leary's PCR being 100 %.

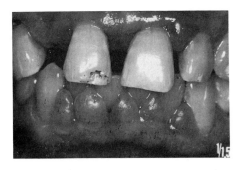

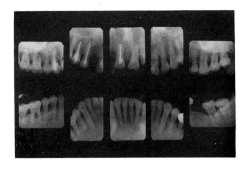

Fig. 1. Clinical feature at initial visit (Case 1). Nodular type hyperplasia of lower anterior gingiva.

Fig. 2. Radiograph at initial visit (Case 1).

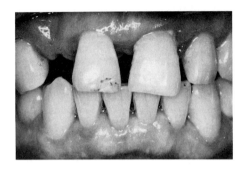

Fig. 3. One year and nine months following gingivectomy (Case 1).
No recurrence of hyperplasia.

Radiologically, deep vertical bone resorption observed in the molar region
with only slight horizontal resorption in
the lower anterior tooth region (Fig. 2).

As for the course of therapy, following
initial therapy in which adequate plaque
control was made, gingivectomy was performed of the lower anterior tooth region.
Nifedipine and diltiazem have been continued to administer to the patient. To
date no tendency of hyperplasia has been
observed during the postoperative course
of one year and nine months (Fig. 3).

CASE REPORT 2

The patient is a 50-year-old male who visited our hospital with a chief complaint of gingival enlargement. Seven years prior to the first examination he
suffered cerebral hemorrhage and thereafter oral administration of nicardipine
has been continued at 60 mg/day. Three years ago he had an attack of angina
pectoris and thereafter oral administration of diltiazem at 90 mg/day has been
added. Oral examination revealed remarkable gingival hyperplasia in both the
upper and lower jaws with the surface being irregular, solid, elastic and firm,
and nodular in part (Fig. 4). Remarkable redness, bleeding, pus discharge were
observed in almost all the teeth. A large number of teeth showed mobility exceeding degree 2. Probing pocket depth of more than 6 mm was seen in all the
teeth. PCR was poor with the value being 100%. Radiologically, in both the
upper and lower jaws, vertical and/or horizontal resorption involving more than
2/3 of the alveolar bone were observed (Fig. 5).

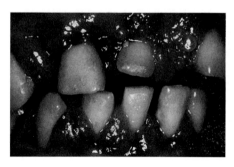

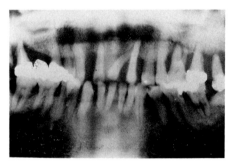

Fig. 4. Clinical feature at initial visit
(Case 2). Remarkable gingival hyperplasia of upper and lower gingiva.

Fig. 5. Radiograph at initial visit
(Case 2).

As for the course of therapy, following consultation with his physician, administration of nicardipine and diltiazem was suspended and initial therapy was commenced. Hyperplasia decreased following suspension of drug therapy and almost disappeared four months later. At present subsequent one year course, no evidence of recurrence of hyperplasia has been observed(Fig. 6).

Histopathologically, marked epithelial hyperplasia and acanthosis with irregular elongation of rate peg, and proliferation of the connective tissue of the lamina propria of the gingiva were observed. In addition, there were sites disappearance of collagen fibers due to infiltration of inflammatory cells from the inner margin of the gingiva(Fig. 7).

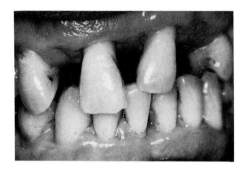

Fig. 6. One year and four months following the suspension of drugs. Hyperplasia disappeared.

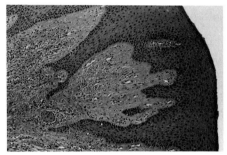

Fig. 7. Marked epithelial hyperplasia and acanthosis with irregular elongation of rate peg.   H. E.

CASE REPORT 3

The patient is a 47-year-old male who visited our hospital with a chief complaint of masticatory disturbance.   From two years ago oral administration of

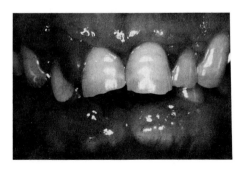

Fig. 8. Clinical feature at initial visit (Case 3). Marked hyperplasia right upper cuspid region.

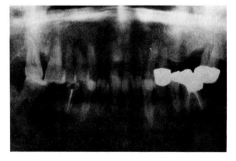

Fig. 9. Radiograph at initial visit (Case 3).

nifedipine at 30 mg/day has been made for hypertension. Oral examination revealed remarkable gingival hyperplasia particularly at the upper right cuspid region
and redness, bleeding of the gingiva of the upper and lower jaw(Fig.8). Mobility
of degree 1-2 was observed in a few teeth and probing pocket depth was more than
6 mm. His oral hygiene showed O'Leary's PCR of 50%. Radiologically, in both the
lower and upper jaws, vertical and/or horizontal resorption involving more than
2/3 were observed(Fig.9).

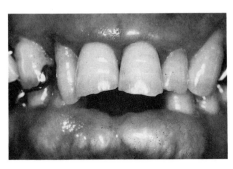

Fig.10. Ten months following the suspension of drug. No signs of
repeated hyperplasia with drug
restoration.

As for the course of therapy, following
consultation with his physician, oral administration of nifedipine was suspended
and initial therapy was commenced and PCR
improved to 16%. Following suspension of
drug therapy, hyperplasia gradually decreased and three months thereafter it
almost completely disappeared. As elevation of blood pressure was observed, drug
therapy was restored again, but at present subsequent six months after disappearance there has been no evidence of
recurrence of hyperplasia(Fig.10).

CONCLUSION

Three cases of gingival hyperplasia associated with the administration of nifedipine and other calcium antagonists were reported. In Case 1 initial periodontal therapy and gingivectomy were performed while continuing the oral administration of nifedipine and diltiazem; in Case 2 initial periodontal therapy was performed after suspending the oral administration of nicardipine and diltiazem; and
in Case 3 initial periodontal therapy was performed after suspending the oral ad-
ministraton of nifedipine and drug administration was restored again. In all the
cases, disappearance of gingival hyperplasia was observed.

There are many unknown points in the developmental mechanism and in the incidence rate of this entity. Local factors such as inadequate plaque control might
have played an important role, but it is suggested that the appearance of the
gingival hyperplasia is related to the administration of calcium antagonists.

REFERRENCE

1. Ramon Y, Behar S, Kishon Y and Engelberg IS (1984) Int J Cardiol 5:195-204
2. Lederman D, Lumerman H, Reuben S and Freedman PD (1984) Oral Surg 57:620-622
3. Lucas RM, Howell LP and Wall BA (1985) J Periodontol 56:211-215
4. Barak S, Engelberg IS and Hiss J (1987) J Periodontol 58:639-642

© 1991 Elsevier Science Publishers B.V.
Recent advances in periodontology Vol. II,
S.I. Gold, M. Midda and S. Mutlu, eds.

COLLAGENASE AND COLLAGENASE INHIBITORS FROM HUMAN PERIODONTAL LIGAMENT CELLS

KICHIBEE OTSUKA, MITSUHIRO OHSHIMA, FUMIYUKI KUWATA, YOSHINORI SASAI, and KANTARO SUZUKI

Department of Biochemistry, Nihon University School of Dentistry, 1-8-13 Kanda Surugadai, Chiyoda-ku, Tokyo 101 (Japan)

INTRODUCTION

The attachment loss and bone matrix resorption of the periodontium are major problems in periodontitis. Much of the connective tissue degradation in periodontal diseases is mediated by proteolytic enzymes. Previous studies on the enzymatic tissue degradations have focused on the action of proteinases, mainly collagenase, released by invading polymorphonuclear neutrophils, macrophages and bacteriae. However, metalloproteinases released by interstitial cells of the periodontium not only control the turnover of the matrix, but also are involved in attachment loss and bone matrix resorption.

SOMERMAN et al. (1) have suggested that collagen secretion of periodontal ligament cells (PDL cells) in comparison with that of gingival fibroblasts were significantly high, whereas, the collagenase activity of the PDL cells, which is necessary to the turnover of the tissue collagen, was hardly detectable according to RICHARDS and RUTHERFORD (2).

To clarify the action of collagenase on the mechanism of collagen turnover and/or extensive degradation of collagen in periodontitis, we attempted to quantify the collagenase and collagenase inhibitors secreted by cultured human PDL cells. We found collagenase activity in the conditioned medium of the PDL cells cultured could be detected after 10mM dithiothreitol (DTT) treatment of the medium. Therefore, DTT treatment was necessary to inactivate the collagenase inhibitor for quantification of collagenase.

In this presentation, we have quantitated of collagenase secreted by the PDL cells and compared the collagenase inhibitors with those of gingival fibroblasts as a control.

MATERIAL AND METHODS
Cell culture

A pair of human periodontal ligament and adjacent gingiva were kindly provided by a volunteer, who was undergoing dental treatment at Nihon University Dental Hospital. The sample of periodontal ligament attached to the middle one-third of the root surface was collected by careful scrape with a scalpel, avoiding contamination of neighbor tissues. The gingival connective tissue specimen was taken from free gingiva adjacent to the extracted tooth using a surgical knife and cut into small pieces on a glass plate. Several fragments of each explant were placed on the bottom of 60-mm Petri dishes and covered with 24x32-mm Thermanox coverslips, and incubated with culture medium: α-MEM supplemented with 10% (v/v) heat-inactivated fetal bovine serum and antibiotics. Both cell populations were grown to confluence for two to three weeks and then subcultured by trypsinization. For gel filtration chromatography, confluent cells of PDL cells and GF were cultured for 1-4 days in serum-free culture medium, respectively. Harvested media from two cell populations, collected daily, were pooled and concentrated by precipitation with 90% saturated ammonium sulfate. The precipitates were dialyzed against the collagenase assay buffer (50 mM Tris-HCl/100 mM NaCl/5 mM $CaCl_2$/0.05%(w/v) Brij 35/ 0.02%(w/v) NaN_3, pH 7.4). Subsequently, media concentrates were prepared for gel filtration chromatography.

Gel Filtration Chromatography

Two samples concentrated were chromatographed on an Ultrogel AcA 54 gel filtration column (1.6x90-cm), equilibrated with collagenase assay buffer at 4 °C, respectively. The sample was fractionated at 10 ml/h with 2.05 ml fractions collected. Each fraction was assayed for collagenase and collagenase inhibitor.

Enzyme and Inhibitor Assays

For routine collagenase and collagenase inhibitor activities, radiolabelled type I collagen (specific radioactivity: 1.2×10^8 dpm/mg) as substrate was prepared by metabolic labeling of PDL cells according to the method of OVERALL et al. (3) using $[^{14}C]$proline. Prior to collagenase assay, each fraction from AcA 54 gel was treated with DTT to inactivate the collagenase inhibitor and dialyzed. Collagenase and collagenase inhibitor activities were assayed as described by TERATO (4) with slight modification. Latent collagenase was routinely activated by 1 mM APMA. Following a 30-min preincubation at 35 °C, the assay was continued with 2 h incubation at 35 °C. For inhibitor assay, aliquots of sample were preincubated with active human gingival collagenase for 30 min at R.T. before adding the substrate. The assay mixtures were followed to proceed at 35 °C for 2 h. For all assays, the reactions were terminated by adding of o-phenanthroline and dioxane. Each aliquot of the supernatant was counted in a Liquid Scintillation Spectrometer.

One unit (U) of collagenase was defined as the amount of protein which hydrolyzed 1 µg of native soluble collagen per minute. One unit (U) of collagenase inhibitor was defined as the amount of protein required for 50 % inhibition of 2 U of collagenase.

Fluorography

The reaction mixtures for collagenase activities, containing [^{14}C]proline-labeled collagen were terminated by addition of electrophoresis sample buffer to a final concentration of 2 M urea, 2 % (w/v) SDS and 2% (v/v) mercaptoethanol in LAEMMLI stacking gel buffer (5). The reaction products by collagenase were separated by SDS-polyacrylamide gel electrophoresis (SDS-PAGE) on discontinuous 7.5% cross-linked polyacrylamide gels (7x8-cm) with a 4% cross-linked polyacrylamide stacking gel in the buffer system of LAEMMLI (5). The gels were subsequently processed for fluorography and exposed to KODAK SB-5 x-ray film at -80 °C for three or four days.

RESULTS

The ammonium-sulfate-precipitated enzymes and inhibitors from PDL cells and GF cultures were fractionated by gel filtration on an AcA 54 resin (Figs. 1 and 2). The latent collagenase was found to elute as a single peak (Mr 30000) whereas the inhibitor activity was resolved into two peaks (Mrs 32000 and 70000).

Figure 3 shows the SDS-PAGE fluorographs for collagenase activity of PDL cells and GF.

DISCUSSION AND CONCLUSION

The collagenase activity can be regulated by specific inhibitors such as tissue inhibitor of matrix metalloproteinases, which is synthesized by mesenchymal, epithelial and inflammatory cells. The gingival fibroblasts produced much collagenolytic enzymes when cultured in the presence of some cytokines, whereas little activity for PDL cells (2). WANG et al. (6) has reported on ConA stimulation of collagenase synthesis by human gingival fibroblasts. PETTIGREW et al. (7) detected collagenase inhibitors in cultured media derived from PDL cells, and demonstrated these inhibitors were different from

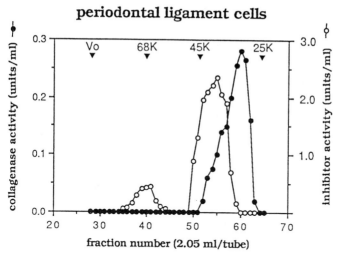

Fig. 1 Elution profile of collagenase and collagenase inhibitors

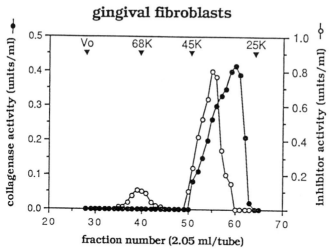

Fig. 2 Elution profile of collagenase and collagenase inhibitors

periodontal ligament cells

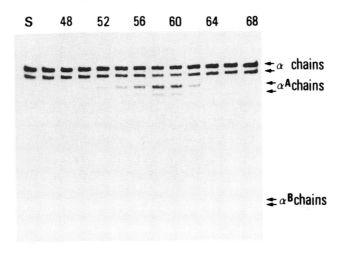

gingival fibroblasts

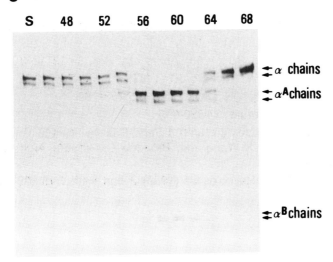

Fig. 3 SDS-PAGE fluorographs showing cleavages in collagen substrates by fractionated samples.

those of gingival fibroblasts. MEIKLE et al. (8) reported on the characteristic difference between latent collagenase and inhibitor-bound collagenase. Therefore, we proposed a hypothesis. If it is possible to inactivate the collagenase inhibitor, we would be able to quantitate the collagenase activity of PDL cells.

The collagenase inhibitor in cultured media derived from PDL cells was inactivated by pretreatment with dithiothreitol (DTT). Therefore, we could detect the latent collagenase secreted by PDL cells, and developed a method for the quantitative assay of collagenase activity.

From the behavior on gel filtration chromatography, the molecular weights of collagenases from both PDL cells and GF were estimated to be 30K. And two collagenase inhibitors were contained both in PDL cells and GF: approximate Mrs of 32K and 70K. Two collagenase inhibitors of PDL cells and gingival fibroblasts were resistant to APMA, and a marked difference on the amounts of collagenase inhibitors between PDL cells and GF was apparent.

These results indicated that the regulation of collagen metabolism in PDL cells was different from that of GF, in respect of producing amounts of collagenase inhibitors.

REFERENCES
1. Somerman MJ, Archer SY, Imm GR, Foster RA (1988) J Dent Res 67: 66-70
2. Richards D, Rutherford RB (1988) Archs oral Biol 33:237-243
3. Overall CM, Wiebkin OW, Thonard JC (1987) J Perio Res 22:81-88
4. Terato K (1976) Biochim Biophys Acta 445:753-762
5. Laemmli UK (1970) Nature 27:680-685
6. Wang HM, Hurum S, Sodek J (1983) J Perio Res 18:149-155
7. Pettigrew DW, Sodek J, Wang HM, Brunette DM (1980) Archs oral Bio 25:269-274
8. Meikle MC, Heath JK, Reynolds JJ (1986) J oral Pathol 15:239-250

© 1991 Elsevier Science Publishers B.V.
Recent advances in periodontology Vol. II,
S.I. Gold, M. Midda and S. Mutlu, eds.

THE EFFECTS OF CONCANAVALIN A ON COLLAGENASE SECRETION BY CULTURED HUMAN PERIODONTAL LIGAMENT CELLS

MITSUHIRO OHSHIMA, FUMIYUKI KUWATA, KICHIBEE OTSUKA, YOSHINORI SASAI, and KANTARO SUZUKI

Department of Biochemistry, Nihon University School of Dentistry, 1-8-13 Kanda Surugadai, Chiyoda-ku, Tokyo 101 (Japan)

INTRODUCTION

A number of studies have shown that metalloproteinases produced by interstitial cells of the periodontium mainly cause the loss of connective tissue attachment (1). Particularly, collagenases are suspected to play an essential role in the collagen degradation of periodontium during the course of periodontitis. To examine the effects of concanavalin A (Con A) on collagenase secretion of human fibroblasts, we developed a simple and inexpensive enzyme assay method after inactivation of the inhibitors in cultured media. Con A is known to exert various stimulatory effect on cells in culture depending on the cell type studied. For example, Con A stimulates the biosynthesis and secretion of plasminogen activator by macrophages and enhances production of a lymphocyte factor which in turn stimulates collagenase production by macrophages (2). Furthermore, WANG et al. (3) reported that the collagenase synthesis of human gingival fibroblasts was stimulated by Con A. However, the mechanism by which Con A induces the increase in collagenase synthesis is not clear.

In this investigation, we examined whether Con A stimulate the collagenase production of human periodontal ligament cells.

MATERIAL AND METHODS

Cell culture

Four pairs of human periodontal ligaments and adjacent gingivae were kindly provided by four different volunteers, who were undergoing dental treatment at Nihon University Dental Hospital. Samples of periodontal ligament attached to the middle one-third of each root surface were collected by careful scrape with a scalpel, avoiding contamination of neighbor tissues. The gingival connective tissue specimens were taken from free gingivae adjacent to the extracted teeth using a surgical knife and cut into small pieces on a glass plate.   Several fragments of each explant were placed on the bottom of 60-mm Petri dishes and covered with 24x32-mm Thermanox coverslips, and incubated with culture medium: α-MEM supplemented with 10% (v/v) heat-inactivated fetal bovine serum and antibiotics. Both cell populations were grown to confluence for two to three weeks and then subcultured by trypsinization as described by OHSHIMA et al. (3).   At the 6th or 7th passage, each cell population was seeded into 6-well plates (Falcon) with approximately $6x10^4$ cells/well and incubated for two weeks in culture medium.   The cells were washed twice with α-MEM and then incubated in serum-free α-MEM with various concentration of Con A (0, 0.04, 0.2, 1.0, 5.0, 25 μg/ml) for three days.   The media were collected and stored at 4 °C until dithiothreitol (DTT) treatment.

Enzyme Assays

For routine collagenase activity, radiolabelled type I collagen (specific radioactivity: $1.2x10^8$ dpm/mg) as substrate was prepared by metabolic labeling of PDL cells according to the method of OVERALL et al. (5) using [^{14}C]proline. Prior to collagenase assay, each medium was treated with 10 mM DTT to inactivate the collagenase inhibitor and dialyzed against collagenase assay buffer.   Collagenase activity was assayed as described by TERATO (6) with slight modification.   Latent collagenase   was routinely activated by 1 mM APMA.   Following a 30-min preincubation at 35 °C, the assay was continued with 1 h incubation at 35 °C, but in the presence of 1 mM APMA.   For all assays, the reactions were terminated by adding of o-phenanthroline and dioxane.   An aliquot of the supernatant was counted in a liquid scintillation spectrometer.

One unit (U) of collagenase was defined as the amount of protein which hydrolyzed 1 μg of native soluble collagen per minute.

DNA content

The determination of DNA content of cells was carried out using Hoechist 33258 described by LABARCA and PAIGEN (7).   The fluorescence was measured with a fluorescence spectrophotometer at an excitation wavelength of 356 nm and an emission wavelength of 492 nm using calf thymus DNA as a standard.

The results in the figures were expressed as the mean and standard deviation of 3 wells or 4 cases by mU/μg DNA.

RESULTS

The effect of Con A on collagenase secretion by 4 pairs of PDL cells and GF are shown in Fig. 1.   Except one case of GF, the collagenolytic responce of Con A-treated PDL cells and GF were not dose-dependent and both cell populations were observed a similar collagenolysis in the absence of Con A.   The mean and stndard deviation of 4 cases are shown in Fig. 2.   The GF have approximately 2-fold higher collagenase activity than PDL cells.   However, Con A failed to stimulate collagenase production by PDL cells and GF.

DISCUSSION
        Several reports have described the relationship between the periodontal tissue degradation and gingival collagenase (8).   However, the collagen degradation in periodontal ligament tissue causes the loss of connective tissue attachment during the course of periodontitis.   Therefore, we attempted to investigate the regulation of collagen metabolism by the collagenase derived from PDL cells.
The collagenase activity can be also regulated by specific inhibitors such as tissue inhibitor of matrix metalloproteinases, which is synthesized by mesenchymal, epithelial and inflammatory cells.   The gingival fibroblasts produced much collagenolytic enzymes when cultured in the presence of some cytokines, whereas little activity for PDL cells (9).   PETTIGREW et al. (10) detected collagenase inhibitors in cultured media derived from PDL cells, and demonstrated these inhibitors were different from those of gingival fibroblasts. MEIKLE et al. (1) reported on the characteristic difference between latent collagenase and inhibitor-bound collagenase.   In view of these papers, PDL cells can be produced collagenase inhibitors which are different from those of gingival fibroblasts.   Therefore, we proposed a hypothesis.   If it is possible to inactivate the collagenase inhibitor, we would be able to quantitate the collagenase activity of PDL cells.
        The collagenase inhibitor in cultured media derived from PDL cells was inactivated by pretreatment with DTT.   But DTT also inhibits active collagenase.   To solve this problem, after treatment with DTT, crude solution containing inactivated inhibitor and latent forms of collagenase was dialyzed against assay buffer, and DTT was removed before collagenase assays.   As a result, collagenase inhibitors secreted from PDL cells and GF were inactivated by DTT treatment.   So, we found a method for quantitation of collagenase derived from PDL cells.   Previously, WANG et al. (3) has demonstrated Con A stimulated the collagenase synthesis by human gingival fibroblasts.   And they detected small amounts of collagenase

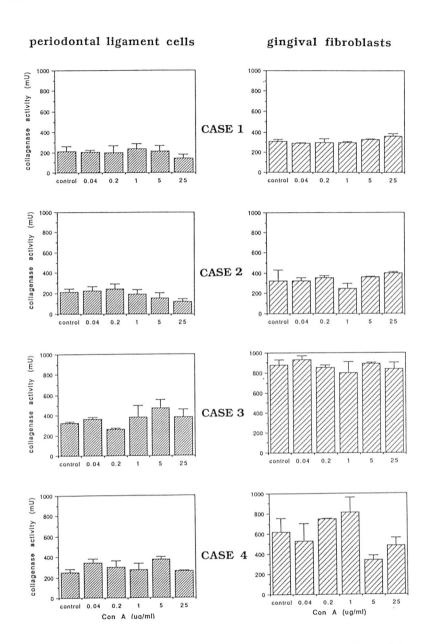

Fig. 1. The effect of ConA on collagenase activity of PDL cells and GF. PDL cells and GF were treated with increasing amounts of ConA and conditioned media were harvested after 3 days. The media were treated with DTT and dialized against collagenase assay buffer and assayed for collagenase after APMA activation. Monolayers were assayed for DNA content and the collagenase activity are expressed per µg DNA. Results are means and standard deviations of triplicate wells.

periodontal ligament cells   **gingival fibroblasts**

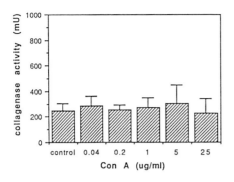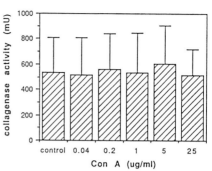

Fig. 2. The effect of ConA on collagenase activity of PDL cells and GF. Results are means and standard standard deviation of 4 cases shown in Fig.1.

activity when cultured in the absence of Con A whereas we were able to detect the collagenase activity because samples were treated with DTT to inactivate the collagenase inhibitors.

These results might suggest Con A reduce the production of collagenase inhibitor rather than stimulate the collagenase production.

REFERENCE
1. Meikle MC, Heath JK, Reynolds JJ (1986) Archs oral Biol 15:239-250
2. Wahl LM, Wahl SM, Mergenhagen SE, Martin GR (1975) Science 187:261-263
3. Wang HM, Hurum S, Sodek J (1983) J Perio Res 18:149-155
4. Ohshima M, Kuwata F, Otsuka K, Saito R, Sato K, Shioji S, Suzuki K (1988) J Nihon Univ Sch Dent 30:208-217
5. Overall CM, Wiebkin OW, Thonard JC (1987) J Perio Res 22:81-88
6. Terato K (1976) Biochim Biophys Acta 445:753-762
7. Labarca C, Paigen K (1980) Anal Biochem 102:344-352
8. Kowashi Y, Jaccard F, Cimasoni G. (1979) Archs oral Biol 24:643-650
9. Richards D, Rutherford RB (1988) Archs oral Biol 33:237-243
10. Pettigrew DW, Sodek J, Wang HM, Brunette DM (1980) Archs oral Biol 25:269-274

© 1991 Elsevier Science Publishers B.V.
Recent advances in periodontology Vol. II,
S.I. Gold, M. Midda and S. Mutlu, eds.

CHARACTERISTICS OF HUMAN ALVEOLAR BONE DERIVED CELLS OBTAINED FROM DIFFERENT AGE GROUPS

KENJI FUJIKAWA, KUNIHARU SUZUKI, KOJI TANAKA, SHINICHI EBASHI MASAO MAENO[*], KICHIBEE OTSUKA[*] and SEIDAI MURAI

Depts. of Periodontology and Biochemistry[*], Nihon University School of Dentistry, 1-8-13, Kanda Surugadai, Chiyoda-ku, Tokyo, 101 (JAPAN)

INTRODUCTION

It is generally known that the degree of periodontal breakdown increases with aging, but physiological changes in osteoblast's characteristics are not clearly identified. Recently, we have developed a cell culture system of human alveolar bone derived cells (HAB cells), and identified that HAB cells have osteoblast-like characteristics[1]. Then, we attempted to determine alteration of the cell specificities in relation to aging.

MATERIALS and METHODS

Isolation and culture of human alveolar bone derived cells[2]

Human alveolar bone blocks were obtained from 13 patients in the range of 22 to 59 years old (6 males and 7 females), who were undergoing ostectomy or osteoplasty. After removing adjacent soft tissues, the bone blocks were fragmented to small pieces and treated with sequential digestion of bacterial collagenase. After the enzyme digestion, these fragments from individuals were separately placed into 60mm dishes and maintained at 37°C in a humidified atmosphere (95% air and 5% CO_2) with α-minimum essential medium (α-MEM) containing 15% fetal bovine serum and antibiotics (penicillin G, gentamicin and fungizone). HAB cells were subcultured until third passages for this experiment. Cells migrated from individual bone were classified into two different groups; one named HAB-Y included from 22 to 49 years old, the other named HAB-O was over 50. Average ages of HAB-Y and HAB-O were 36 ± 8.9 and 55 ± 2.9 years, respectively.

Human gingival fragments were voluntarily provided from 7 out of 13 patients. Small pieces of human gingival connective tissues were placed into 60mm dishes and cultured under the same condition of HAB cells. Human gingival fibroblasts (HGF) were also used utilize as a control.

<u>Determination of mineralized nodule formation[3)]</u>
The cells from each tissue were seeded at a density of 1.4 x 10^5 cells/35mm-dish and cultured for 42 days; the culture medium was changed every 3rd day.   At day 42, cell layer on the bottom of the dish was directly fixed with neutral buffered formalin solution, and stained with alizarin red S or von Kossa technique to detect calcium mineral deposits.

<u>Assays of enzyme activities</u>
Alkaline phosphatase (ALPase), acid phosphatase (ACPase) and tartrate resistant acid phosphatase (TRAP) activities were directly measured in 96-well tissue culture plates.   HAB cells and HGF were seeded at a density of 5 x 10^3 cells/well and cultured for 35 days. ALPase activity was determined using 8mM p-nitrophenylphosphate (p-NPP) and metal ions (Mg^{2+}, Zn^{2+}) in 50mM glycine-NaOH buffer at pH 10.5. ACPase activity was determined using 8mM p-NPP and 50mM acetate buffer at pH 4.0. TRAP activity was determined using 8mM p-NPP, 10mM sodium tartrate and 50 mM acetate buffer at pH 4.0.   Each enzyme reaction was performed at 37°C for 30min and terminated by the addition of 1N NaOH.   After the termination, the absorbance of released p-nitrophenol (p-NP) was measured at 405nm using Titertek Multiscan (Flow Laboratories. Inc.).   One unit (U) of each enzyme activity was calculated as micromoles of p-NP liberated per minute, and specific activity was shown as mU per 10^4 cells.   The results of HAB-Y, HAB-O and HGF were analyzed with Mann-Whitney's U-test.

<u>Analysis of protein synthesis</u>
The harvested cells from each tissue were seeded at a density of 1.4 x 10^5 cells/35mm-dish and cultured for 14 days.   To analyze the protein synthesis, each cell population was exposed to 2 μCi of ^{14}C-proline in 1.0 ml of α-MEM containing 1% FBS and 50μg of ascorbic acid for 24 h on day 14 to 16.

<u>Quantitation of collagenous proteins to total protein synthesis</u>
Radiolabeled proteins were treated with bacterial collagenase in the presence of 25mM $CaCl_2$ and 62.5mM N-ethylmaleimide at 37°C for 90min.   Undigested non-collagenous proteins were precipitated by the addition of 5% tannic acid and 10% trichloroacetic acid (TCA).   After the suspension was centrifuged at 5000 rpm for 5 min, the super-natant was collected (S-1).   The precipitate was resuspended, and again centrifuged with the same condition to obtain the second supernatant (S-2).   Both S-1 and S-2 were combined, and this

solution was dealt with collagenous protein (COL). The precipitates were dissolved in 5mM DDT and 0.5% SDS, and heated at 100°C for 30 min to obtain the non-collagenous protein (NCP). Radioactivities were determined by scintillation counting, and ratio of collagenous protein to total protein synthesis was calculated by following formula described by Wong and Cohn[4].

Proportion of collagenous proteins for total protein = (COL / (COL + 5.4 x NCP)) x 100

RESULTS and DISCCUSION

The appearance of HAB cells in spite of ages showed more polygonal shape than that of HGF, which had typical spindle shape. HAB cells formed mineralized nodules, which were stained with alizarin red S and von Kossa technique. Different sizes of mineral deposits were seen in both HAB groups without any difference in numbers, intensity and size between HAB groups. ACPase and TRAP activities showed the same level (approximately 0.3 mU/10^4 cells)(Figs.2,3), However, HAB-Y showed the high ALPase activity (0.87~1.25 mU/10^4 cells) compared with HAB-O (0.29~0.56 mU/10^4 cells) during day 14 to 21(Fig.1). Ratio of collagenous proteins to total protein synthesis was examined by calculating the amount of ^{14}C-proline incorporation described by Wong and Chon[4]. Total protein synthesis of HAB-Y and HAB-O was 2.6 and 2.1-fold higher than HGF's; respectively, based on ^{14}C-proline incorporation. HAB-Y produced 18.8% of collagenous proteins of total proteins, while HAB-O produced 16.9%. Slight difference was recognized in the collagenous protein synthesis between each group. Compared with collagenous protein synthesis of HGF, both HAB cells showed greater collagenous protein production. According to some properties of HAB cells in terms of polygonal appearance, mineralized nodule formation, high ALPase activity and high collagenous protein synthesis, HAB cells are osteoblast-like cells. Futher, the characteristics of HAB-Y showed the superior to the HAB-O in respect of ALPase activities and collagenous protein synthesis. Although HAB cells from older ages somehow lost osteoblastic characteristics, further research is needed to evaluate whether sex hormones and/or the physiological condition[5] (postmenopause, osteoporosis et. al.) effect to alter HAB cells' characteristics.

416

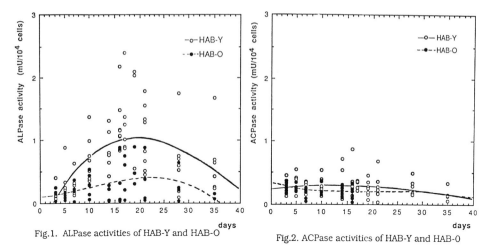

Fig.1. ALPase activities of HAB-Y and HAB-O

Fig.2. ACPase activities of HAB-Y and HAB-O

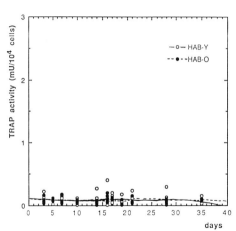

Fig.3. TRAP activities of HAB-Y and HAB-O

REFERENCES

1.Suzuki K., Fujikawa K., Tanaka K.,Ito K.and Murai S. (1990) JDR 69: special issue, 432.

2.Suzuki N.,Isokawa K.,Maeno M.,Otsuka K.,Toda Y.and Suzuki K. (1989) Jap. J. Oral Bio. 31:622-625.

3.Bellows C.G., Aubin J.E.,Heersche J.N.M. and Antosz M.E.(1986) Calcif. Tissue Int. 38: 143-154.

4.Wong G.L.and Cohn D.V. (1977) in Mecanism of localized bone loss: Horton J.E.,Tarpley T.M. and Davis W.F. 47-59.

5.Koshihara Y.(1989)The Tissue Culture.15:58-61.

© 1991 Elsevier Science Publishers B.V.
Recent advances in periodontology Vol. II,
S.I. Gold, M. Midda and S. Mutlu, eds.

A CROSS SECTIONAL STUDY OF CYCLOSPORINE INDUCED GINGIVAL
OVERGROWTH IN LIVER AND HEART TRANSPLANT PATIENTS.

SOMACARRERA, ML ; HERNANDEZ, G ; MOSKOW, B.S.

Complutense University , Madrid (Spain) & Columbia University
, New York, N.Y. (USA).

INTRODUCTION

Cyclosporine A (CsA) is indicated as an immunosuppressive
agent for the prevention of organ rejection in transplant
patients, as well as for other
applications, as illustrated in
Figure 1.

The mechanism by which
cyclosporine inhibits the
rejection response is highly
specific. The drug inhibits the
interleukin-2 production by T-
helper lymphocytes and
suppresses proliferation and
generation of T-cytotoxic
lymphocytes (2,3).

However, CsA has various
side effects (4,5) - Figs. 2,3.
We will now discuss the CsA-
induced gingival hyperplasia in
transplant patients.

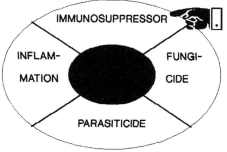

Figure 1
CsA APPLICATIONS

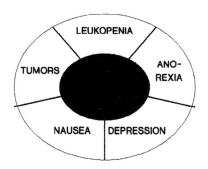

Figure 2
CsA SIDE EFFECTS - 1

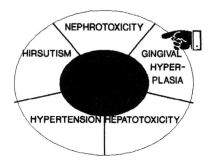

Figure 3
CsA SIDE EFFECTS - 2

418

MATERIAL AND METHODS

The 61 patients reported here were studied in the Puerta de Hierro Hospital and in the Faculty of Dentistry (Complutense University, Madrid) following heart or liver transplant. The 46 patients undergoing CsA treatment (Fig.4) made up the study group, while as the 15 patients being treated with Azathioprine served as control group (Fig.5).

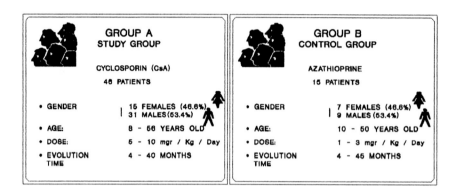

Figure 4
CsA-TREATED STUDY GROUP

Figure 5
AZAT.-TREATED CONTROL GROUP

Time elapsed since transplant took place ranged from 4 to 14 months (recent transplant patients, 3 months or less, were excluded, as well as edentulous patients)

Measured parameters were:

1.- Plaque Index (O'Leary System - Indiana University)

2.- Gingival Condition (idem)

3.- Hyperplasia Index (Harris-Ewalt,modified)

4.- CsA Daily Dose (mg/Kg/day)

5.- CsA Plasma Concentration (Radio Immunoassay, Sandoz method)

These observations were statistically analyzed to test the significance of the impact of the CsA treatment (vs. the control group), as well as to test the significance of the association of the various parameters with the Hyperplasia Index.

RESULTS

The CsA treated study group showed an 80 % Hyperplasia incidence, as opposed to a 0% incidence among the Azathioprine treated control group. (Fig.6)

Within the CsA treated study group, the Hyperplasia Index ranged from 0 to 3 (Fig.7); no patient showed a level 4 Hyperplasia.

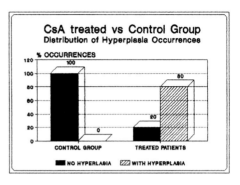

Figure 6
HYPERPLASIA INCIDENCE
CsA TREATED VS. CONTROL

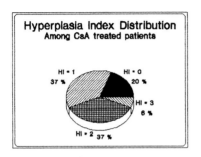

Figure 7
HYPERPLASIA DISTRIBUTION

Those patients with low Hyperplasia levels had a generalized hyperplasia distribution, while as those with high Hyperplasia levels showed a predominantly anterior location.

The association between these parameters and the Hyperplasia Index was then tested. Fig.8 shows the three parameters whose association was above that required for a p<0.001 significance level (CsA Plasma Concentration, Plaque Index and Gingivitis Index. The association with CsA daily dose and with age did not reach this significance level, while as the time elapsed since the transplant date did not show any association.

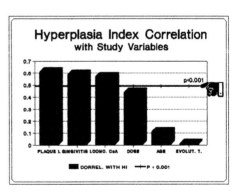

Figure 8
ASSOCIATION WITH
HYPERPLASIA INDEX

As for the Plaque and Gingivitis Indexes, they were also very highly associated among themselves.

CONCLUSIONS

Based on the fact that none of the 15 Azathioprine treated control patients showed Hyperplasia, as opposed to the 80% incidence among CsA treated patients, we concluded that Cyclosporine A treatment was the essential (sine qua non) factor for Gingival Hyperplasia in this population.

The CsA plasma concentration was found to be a highly significant factor ($p < 0.001$), much more significant than the oral dose.

The Plaque level was also identified as a highly significant factor ($p < 0.001$). Gingivitis also presented a high association with Hyperplasia; however, due to its very high cross-association with the Plaque Index , it is likely that the Plaque level induces both Gingivitis and Hyperplasia.

REFERENCES

1.   Sandoz (1989) Sandimmun Practical Guide. Basle,Switzerland

2.   Wish JB (1986) Immunologic Effects of Cyclosporine. Transplant Proc. 18,3:15-18.

3.   American Medical Association (Council on Scientific Affairs) (1987) Introduction to the Management of Immunosuppression. JAMA 257:1781-1785.

4.   Rostock MH, Fry HR, Turner JE (1986) Severe Gingival Overgrowth Associated with Cyclosporine Therapy. J.Periodontology, 57,5:294-299.

5.   Daley TD, Wysocki GP, Day HB (1986) Clinical and Pharmacologic Correlations in Cyclosporine-induced Gingival Hyperplasia. Oral Surg. Oral Med. Oral Pathol., 62:417-421.

© 1991 Elsevier Science Publishers B.V.
Recent advances in periodontology Vol. II,
S.I. Gold, M. Midda and S. Mutlu, eds.

AN ULTRASTRUCTURAL STUDY OF LANGERHANS CELLS IN NORMAL AND INFLAMMED GINGIVA

HERNANDEZ, G.; SANCHEZ, G.; MOSCOW, B.S.
Faculty of Odontology, Complutense University, Madrid (Spain). Columbia Univ.,
New York, N.Y. (U.S.A.)

INTRODUCTION

Langerhans cells (LC) are clear dendritic cells which are sometimes seen in
the suprabasal layers of skin and oral epithelium. They are concerned with the
processing and presentation of antigens to T-lymphocytes and, therefore, are
considered to be protective to the epithelium (1). LC have been previously
studied in normal and inflammed gingiva and while some investigators have
described their presence in the sulcular and oral epithelium, others have failed
to find these cells in junctional and pocket lining epithelium (2) (using
monoclonal antibodies -OKT6- as a marker). This absence has been interpreted as
a factor promoting a state of immune tolerance in the epithelium, since
diffusion of plaque antigens through Langerhans cell deficient junctional
epithelium or pocket lining epithelium may lead to an inappropiate immune
response in gingiva (3). In this sense it has been suggested that variations in
the number of LC may either result from different bacteria elucidating different
responses or merely reflect different responses to similar plaque antigens (4)
penetrating the surface of oral epithelium.

The aim of this paper is to describe the presence and ultrastructural
characteristics of LC in sulcular and periodontal pocket epithelium both in
normal and diseased gingiva.

MATERIAL AND METHODS

Healthy gingiva group

Biopsies were obtained from five children (9-13 yr) undergoing orthodontic
treatment, and with gingival index (Löe and Silness) near to 0. Extraction of
the tooth with adherent gingival tissue including sulcular and junctional
epithelium was performed. Once fixed, the soft tissue was dissected from the
tooth using scalpels and two samples corresponding to sulcular and junctional
epithelium were removed and processed for Electron Transmission Microscopic
examination.

Diseased gingiva group

Ten patients diagnosed as having a severe periodontitis (Type IV) were
selected. None of them had any history of systemic disease. All of them had
indication for periodontal surgery. The region where the biopsy was going to be
taken was left unscaled until periodontal surgery was performed.

The biopsy specimen was collected at the time of surgery from the area showing more than 6 mm of periodontal pocket depth during the initial examination. The sample included the whole periodontal pocket wall, gingival margin and the connective tissue underlying the pocket lining epithelium. Once washed, the tissue was dissected using scalpels and pieces of 1 cubic mm were selected from five different areas corresponding to: marginal gingiva, sulcular epithelium and upper, medium and lower thirds of the periodontal pocket. A sample of the connective tissue corresponding to the middle area beneath the periodontal pocket was also obtained.

Transmission Electron Microscopy proccedure

Inmediately after removal, the biopsies were placed in a fixative containing Karnowsky solution (2% paraformaldehyde and 2.5% glutaraldehyde buffered in sodium cacodylate) for four hours and postfixed in 1% osmium tetroxide for 1.5 h., dehydrated in alcohol and embedded in Epon.

Slides were obtained and stained with toluidine blue for observation under light microscopy in order to identify clear cells. The fields containing clear cells were selected and ultrathin sections were prepared and contrasted with uranyl acetate and lead citrate for observation with E.M.

RESULTS

Langerhans cells were observed in sulcular epithelium of healthy gingiva, most of them in the suprabasal and spinous cell layers (Fig. 1a). They were characterized by presenting clear cytoplasm with a moderate number of mitochondrias, Golgi Apparatus, a few lysosomes and rough endoplasmic reticulum. Dendritic projections were seen in most of the specimens examined (Fig. 1b). Nuclei were usually round or ovoid and few characteristic Birbeck granules were observed in the citoplasm (Type II cells) (Fig. 1a). Ocassionally indeterminate clear cells (with no specific granules) were seen in the lower areas of the sulcular epithelium.

LC in the epithelium of the pocket wall showed several changes in comparison to normal biopsies. Most of the nuclei were indented or irregular with sparce heterochromatin (Fig. 2a). Mitochondria with dense matrix were numerous in the cytoplasm. Profiles of rough endoplasmic reticulum and Golgi Cisternas were not prominent, and Centrioles were observed in the cytoplasm of some LC (Fig. 2b). Although charateristic and numerous Birbeck granules with raquet shape (terminal vesicles) were frecuently observed (Type I cells), typical rod-shaped granules with a central bar were the most numerous (Fig. 2a). Some LC were noted which displayed intracytoplasmic polimorphic granules similar to those seen in proliferative cells of Histiocytosis X (Fig. 2c).

LC in the lining pocket epithelium were commonplace in the upper areas.

However, LC could be observed (except for 4 biopsies) in the middle region of pocket wall. Only one LC appeared in the lower region of pocket epithelium. Direct interactions between LC and keratinocytes and extracellular material were also observed. Cell membrane invaginations and vermipodia-like cytoplasmic processes ocurred frequently.

In the connective tissue one cell with ultrastructural characteristics corresponding to a Langerhans cell precursor (clear indeterminate cell) was

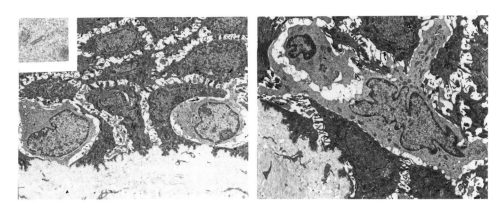

Fig. 1. LC in basal and suprabasal layers of the sulcular epithelium of healthy gingiva (1a) showing specific granules in the cytoplasm (1a -top left-) and dendritic projections (1b).

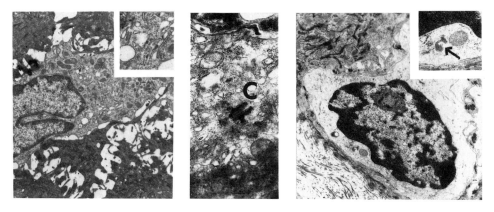

Fig. 2. LC in the upper and middle areas of pocket epithelium. Note the presence of numerous organelles, indented nucleous and Birbeck granules (arrows -top right-) (2a). Centrioles are occasionally present in the cytoplasm (2b) and cytoplasmic structures resembling Histiocytosis X granules can be observed (arrow -top right-) (2c).

observed crossing the high endothelium of a postcapilar venule and included inside the cytoplasm of an edothelial cell (peripolesis mechanism) (Fig. 3).

Our results suggest that LC may be present in the pocket epithelium, and can play a role in the defense mechanisms at this level since they present characteristics of activated cells. To our knowledge, this is the first description of the possible mechanism used by LC to migrate from the blood vessels.

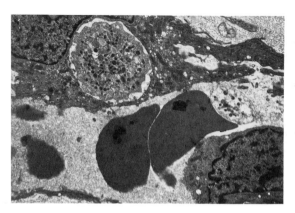 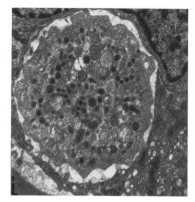

Fig. 3. LC precursor with clear cytoplasm and numerous organelles inside the cytoplasm of an endothelial cell.

REFERENCES
1. Stingl G, Katz SI, Clement L, Green I, Shevach EM (1978) Immunologic func-
    tion of Ia-bearing epidermal Langerhans cells. J Immunol 121:2005-2013.

2. Newcomb GM, Powell RN (1986) Human gingival Langerhans cells in health and
    disease. J Periodont Res 21:640:652.

3. Newcomb GM, Powell RN (1986) The ultrastructure of human gingival Langerhans
    cells in health and disease. Arch Oral Biol 51:727-734.

4. Baelum V, Fejerskov O, Dabelsteen E (1989) Langerhans cells in oral epithe-
    lium of chronically inflamed human gingival. J Periodont Res 24:127-136.

© 1991 Elsevier Science Publishers B.V.
Recent advances in periodontology Vol. II,
S.I. Gold, M. Midda and S. Mutlu, eds.

ULTRASTRUCTURAL STUDY OF BONE CELLS AND MATRIX INCIDENT IN EXPERIMENTAL
PERIODONTITIS

HIROAKI KOKATSU,KOHJI HASEGAWA,REIJI TAKIGUTI*

Department of Periodontics,The first Department of Oral Anatomy*,Showa
University Dental School,2-1-1 Kitasenzoku,Ohta-ku Tokyo,JAPAN

INTRODUCTION

Periodontitis results in both acute and chronic episodes of osseous resorption and one cell intimately involved in this process is the osteoclast.
But a large number of mononuclear cells,notably fibroblasts and macrophages,
have often been observed in close contact with osteoclasts and resorbed bone
surface.The purpose of this study was to examine the process of bone destruction and the ultrastructural features of the cells and the bone matrix in
resorbing site induced by experimental periodontitis.

MATERIAL AND METHODS

65 male Wistar rats ,weighing an average of 200g at the beginning of the
experiment,were utilized in this study.

To induce periodontitis and the following
bone resorption,a defect was prepared with
an endodontic reamer in the proximal
surfaces of the right upper 1st and 2nd
molars of the rats.The left molars remained
as a control.(fig 1)

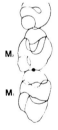
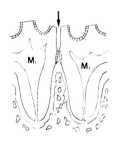

After the experimental period (7,14,and
21days),the animals were fixed with 2.5%
glutaraldehyde-1% paraformaldehyde in 0.1M
sodium cacodylate buffer(PH7.4).

fig 1

①The process of the bone resorption

To observe the process of the bone destruction process,the gingiva and the periosteum and cellular ingredients were disolved with 4% sodium hypo-chlorite .The tissues were rinsed in 0.1M sodium cacodylate buffer(PH7.4) and dehydrated through a graded ethanol series ,critical point dried ,and coated up to 6nm thick.They were observed with a field emission type scanning electron microscope(SEM,Hitachi,S-700) at 25KV.

②SEM observation of the resorbing bone matrix

After fixation,to reveal three-dimensional ultrastructure of bone matrix , both the gingiva and the periosteum were peeled off,and cellular ingredients and amorphous matrix of bone were digested with 1% tripsin(Type1,Sigma) for 5 days.The specimens were conductluely stained with 1% osmium tetroxide and 2% tannic acid and followed in turn by dehydration through a graded ethanol series,placement in isoamyl acetate,critical point dried,and coated up to 6nm thick.They observed with a field emission type SEM at 25KV.

③The ultrastructural features of the cells on the resorbing site

After fixation,the speciments were decalcified with 10% EDTA.

1)Routin sectioning

They were post fixed with 1% osmium tetroxide .They were blockstained with 1% uranyl acetate,dehydrated through a graded ethanol series,and embedded in Epon 812.Ultrathin sections were cut with a diamond knife on a microtome, stained with uranyl acetate and lead citrate,examined with a transmission electron microscopy(TEM,Hitachi,HU-12A) at 75KV.

2)Acid phoshatase(ACP) cytochemistry

The speciments were cutted with a microslicer less than 50μm and incubated in the following media for 30 min at room temperature.The medium for in-oganic trimetaphosphatase according to Doty and Schofield(1) consisted of 0.6mM sodium trimetaphosphate(Sigma) as a substrate,4.5mM acetate buffer,and 4mM lead acetate as the capture reagent,its final PH was adjusted to 4.0 using 0.1M nitric acid. After incubation,the sections were postfixed with 1% osmium tetroxide for 3h at 4℃ and block stained with an ethanolated uranyl acetate for 2h at room temperature.All the specimens were subsequently processed for embedding and TEM observation as described above.

RESULTS

①The process of the bone resorption
The alveolar bone resorption took
place in alveolar crest of interdental areas in 14 days after the
preparetion, and followed by longitudinal. On the day 21th, the
concave bone loss appeared in the
buccal area. (fig 2, 3, 4, 5)

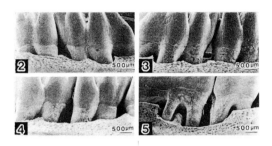

②SEM observation of the resorbing bone matrix
SEM showed many resorbed lacunae in
the alveolar bone in interdental
areas. Ultrastructural differences
in each resorption lacuna were
distinctive. (fig6, 7)

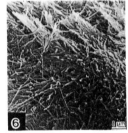
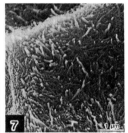

③The ultrastructural features of the cells
　on the resorbing site
On the resorbed bone surface revealed
by TEM many typical osteoclasts,
macrophages, and mononuclear cells resorbing collagen fibrils were observed.
ACP activity of these osteoclasts were
detected as electron-dense precipi-
tations of lead phosphates in vacuoles,
rough endoplasmic reticulum (rER) and
among the ruffled border and in bone
matrix abutted on the osteoclast. (fig8)
The mononuclear cells resorbing

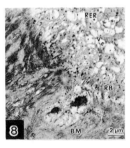
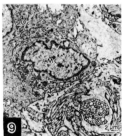

428

collagen fibrils were observed adjacent to the osteoclasts. (fig 9)
These collagen fibrils within the tubular membranous organelles of the mononuclear cells had a periodic striated structures. (fig10)
The macrophages adjacent to the bone resorbed surfaces had many
mitochondrias and cytoplasmic processes towards the bone matrix.ACP activity
of these macrophages was demonstrated in whole cytoplasm and adjoining bone
matrix. (fig11) Many osteoblasts,which remained the resorbed area, seemed to
be inactive and unproductive on account of their undeveloped organells.
(fig12)

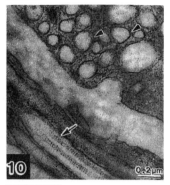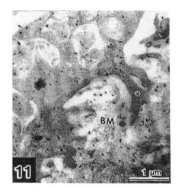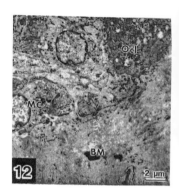

DISCUSSION

Our findings indicated that,in the experimental periodontitis osteoclasts
and other cells were associated with destruction of both organic and inorganic matrix of bone,while osteoblasts were in″ resting ″ stage because of
only a little cytoplasm.The bone resorption due to the experimental periodontitis might be massive and rapid different from the resorption process
of remodelling.The loss of collagens and bone minerals might occur either by
a decrease in the formative elements or an increse in the destructive ele-
ments.The changes in ultrastructures of resorption lacuna matrix result from
the resorption phage,that is coincident with the resorbing activity of the
cells described above.

REFERENCES

1. Doty,S.B and Schofield,B.H.(1972) Electron microscopic localization of
   hydrolytic enzymes in osteoclasts. Histochem.J.,4,245-258.

© 1991 Elsevier Science Publishers B.V.
Recent advances in periodontology Vol. II,
S.I. Gold, M. Midda and S. Mutlu, eds.

TWO-COLOR FLOW CYTOMETRY ANALYSIS OF PERIPHERAL BLOOD LYMPHOCYTE SUBSETS IN ADULT PERIODONTITIS PATIENTS

TAKESHI YAMANAKA , [1]TOSHIAKI SHIBUTANI, [1]YUKIO IWAYAMA, [2]MASATOSHI UEDA, JYUNYA KANEHISA AND HIROSHI TAKEUCHI

Dep. of Oral Pathol., [1]Dep. of Periodontol., School of Dent., Asahi Univ., 1851-1, Hozumi, Hozumi-cho, Motosu-gun, Gifu, Japan and [2]Dep. of Periodontol., Osaka Dent. Univ., 1-5-31, Ootemae, Chuo-ku, Osaka, Japan.

INTRODUCTION

It is widely accepted that host immune responses are involved in the pathogenesis of periodontal disease. Also, the question of whether excessive immune responses, especially B cell activity, play a destructive role in periodontitis has been discussed[1, 2] because of the coincidence of a dense B cell infiltration with advanced periodontitis lesion[3, 4]. Considering the immune system, we have noticed the possibility that excessive B cell proliferation is induced not only by the periodontopathic plaque bacteria but also by the T cell regulation dysfunction. In order to better understand such a possibility, the lymphocyte subsets in the peripheral blood of adult periodontitis(AP) patients and the healthy age-matched control group were analyzed by using two-color flow cytometry analysis and compared. Furthermore, the fluctuations of the lymphocyte subsets of the patients were also analyzed after three months of initial treatment.

MATERIAL AND METHODS

Patients. Thirty patients with moderate to severe generalized AP between the ages of 27 and 57 years were selected for this study. They were compared with healthy, age-matched control group(forty individuals, ranging from 29 to 51 years) with no radiographic or clinical evidence of periodontitis. Both the patients and healthy individuals had no general dysfunction.

Cell separation. Peripheral blood lymphocytes(PBL) were separated by centrifugation on Leukoprep(Becton Dickinson Inc., Mountain View, CA, U.S.A.) at 900 g 10 min. The isolated cells were washed three times with phosphate buffered saline(PBS, 0.01M, pH 7.2) and were resuspended at 1×10^7 cells/ml in PBS for immunofluorescent staining.

Reagents. All monoclonal antibodies were obtained from the Becton Dickinson Inc., Mountain View, CA, U.S.A. Anti-Leu-2a(CD8), anti-Leu-3a(CD4) and anti-Leu-4(CD3) antibodies were conjugated with fluorescein isothiocyanate(FITC) and anti-Leu-8, anti-Leu-15(CD11b), anti-HLA-DR and anti-Leu-16(CD20) antibodies with phycoerythlin(PE).

Two-color immunofluorescence staining. The distributions of PBL subsets were detected by using the combinatios of CD3+HLA-DR, CD4+Leu8, CD8+CD11b and CD20. PBL were stained with FITC and PE conjugated monoclonal antibodies simultane- ously and the cells were incubated for 30 min at 4℃, washed three times with PBS, and resuspended with PBS. Flow cytometry analysis was performed with a model FCS-1(Japan Spectroscopic, Hachioji, Japan).

Cell counting. The forward angle light scatter(0° scatter), which is indica- tive of the size of the cells and the 90° scatter, which provides a measure of the complexity of the internal structure of the cells were used for establish- ing a gate for the lymphocyte region. In determining the percentage of positive cells, a marker was set on the negative control cytogram so that 3% or less of the cells were in other areas. By using this marker, the percentage of fluo- rescent lymphocytes in the specific antibody-stained sample cytogram was calcu- lated.

Follow-up. 9 of those patients were re-examined 3 months after the initial treatment to observe the fluctuations of PBL subsets.

Statistical method. Welch's t-test was used to determine statistical signifi- cance.

RESULTS AND DISCUSSION

The results of flow cytometry analysis from 30 patients and 40 healthy indi- viduals are shown in table-1. There were no significant differences in the per- centage of $CD3^+$ T cells and $CD4^+$ helper/inducer T cells in AP PBL and normal PBL. However, the percentage of $CD8^+$ suppressor/cytotoxic T cells was signifi- cantly lower than that of control(Fig.1), while the percentage of B cells($CD20^+$) in AP PBL was greater than that of control. The results of two-color analysis are also shown in table-1. The percentage of $CD8^+CD11b^+$ suppressor T cell subset was significantly lower than the control(Fig.2). In the $CD4^+$ population, $CD4^+$ Leu8$^-$ helper T cell showed decreased value, while the suppressor inducer T cells were greater than the control group.

Re-examinations were performed in 9 of those patients to observe the fluctu- ations of PBL subsets. In the present study, single-color analysis showed no significant fluctuations in both of the CD4 and CD8 subsets, so that the CD4/CD8 ratios in the patients with AP kept almost the same as the ratios found in the initial examination. However, two-color analysis demonstrated that CD4$^+$Leu8$^-$ helper T cell subsets were increased and CD4$^+$Leu8$^+$ suppressor inducer T cell subsets were decreased in most of the patients. In the CD8 population,   the CD8$^+$ CD11b$^+$suppressor T cell subset showed a slight decrease in most of the patients. Significant increase of CD4$^+$Leu8$^-$/CD8$^+$CD11b$^+$ ratio was found in four cases(Fig.

TABLE-1

Flow cytometry analysis of PBL subsets

Monoclonal antibodies	Patients (n=30)	Control (n=40)
CD3	63.98 ±10.76	61.26 ±10.55
CD4	37.50 ±10.93	36.50 ± 7.73
CD8	24.01 ± 8.54*	28.87 ± 7.15
CD20	9.06 ± 4.52**	5.86 ± 2.92
CD4⁺Leu 8⁻	7.59 ± 3.81**	11.68 ± 3.52
CD4⁺Leu 8⁺	30.52 ±10.37*	25.51 ± 7.53
CD8⁺CD11b⁻	17.99 ± 7.23	19.95 ± 7.07
CD8⁺CD11b⁺	5.37 ± 4.35**	9.34 ± 3.11
CD3⁺HLA-DR⁺	5.16 ± 2.14 (%)	4.16 ± 1.76# (%)
CD4/CD8	1.82 ± 0.92	1.43 ± 0.78
CD4⁺Leu8⁻/CD8⁺CD11b⁺	1.74 ± 1.55	1.41 ± 0.70

* P<0.05, ** P<0.01, # n=7

CD 8

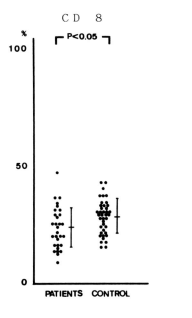

CD8⁺ CD11b⁺

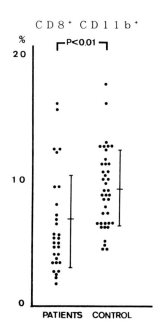

Fig.1. Single-color analysis showed a significant decrease in the percentage of suppressor/cytotoxic T cells in patients with AP as compared to the controls.

Fig.2. Two-color analysis showed a significant decrease in the percentage of CD8⁺CD11b⁺ suppressor T cells in patients with AP as compared to the controls.

3, Fig. 4). CD20⁺ B cells were decreased remarkably except for two increased cases.

Recently, Katz et al.[5] have shown a marked increase of CD4/CD8 ratio in some of the patients with rapidly progresseive periodontitis and indicated the possibility of pathogenesis of this lesion by cellular immune response. We have also demonstrated a high ratio of CD4/CD8 in patients with AP and pointed out

432

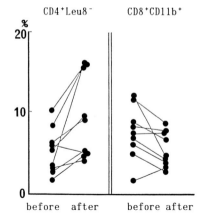

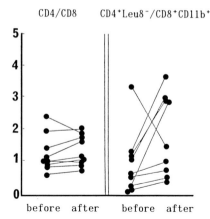

Fig. 3. CD4⁺Leu8⁻ helper T cells increased and CD8⁺CD11b⁺ suppressor T cell subsets showed a slight decrease in most of the patients.

Fig. 4. The CD4/CD8 ratios were stable in most of the patients with AP; however, the CD4⁺Leu8⁻/CD8⁺CD11b⁺ ratios increased in four cases.

enhanced helper T cell activity and/or impaired suppressor T cell activity which seem to underlie the development of an advanced B cell lesion[6]. Although the role of B cells infiltrated in the periodontitis lesion is still unclear, our data suggests that a decrease of suppressor T cells might have an important role to establish the B cell predominant lesion considering the enhancement of B cell activity by T cell regulation.

ACKNOWLEDGMENTS

This work was supported by Grants-in-Aid(62570820) from the Ministry of science, Education and Culture of Japan and a Miyata Research Aid.

REFERENCES

1) Davenport, R.H. et al.: Histometric comparison of active and inactive lesions of advanced periodontitis. J.Periodontol. 53: 285-295,1982.

2) Garant,P.R. et al.: The distribution of plasma cells in naturally occurring periodontitis lesions in rats. J. Periodontol. 54: 227-235, 1983.

3) Seymour, G.J. and Greenspan J.S.: The phenotypic characterization of lymphocyte subpopulations in established human periodontal disease. J. Periodont. Res. 14: 39-46,1979.

4) Reinhardt, R.A. et al.: In situ lymphocyte subpopulations from active versus stable periodontal sites. J. Periodontol. 59: 656-670, 1988.

5) Katz, J. et al.: Peripheral T lymphocyte subsets in rapidly progressive periodontitis. J. Clin. Periodontol. 15: 266-268, 1988.

6) Takeuchi, H. et al.: Helper-to-suppressor T-cell ratios in adult and juvenile periodontitis by single- and two-color flow cytometry analysis. Dentistry in Japan. 26: 123-131, 1989.

© 1991 Elsevier Science Publishers B.V.
Recent advances in periodontology Vol. II,
S.I. Gold, M. Midda and S. Mutlu, eds.

COMPARATIVE STUDY OF THREE DIFFERENT PERIODONTAL PROBES

ITIR GRUBER, YUNG HAN, EBERHARD SONNABEND

Clinic of preventive dentistry and periodontology, University of Munich,

Goethestr. 70, 8000 München 2 (West Germany)

INTRODUCTION

Epidemiological studies confirm that periodontal diseases occur in nearly all human beings and that they constitute one of the main causes of premature loss of teeth(1). Nevertheless they are often detected only in an advanced and severe stage. The increase in the number of periodontally injured patients and the demand for early therapy induced clinicians to record periodontal changes at an initial stage and to register them completely.

Currently, the periodontal probe is one of the most important diagnostic appliances in the hand of the periodontologist. Apart from clinical inspection, periodontal indices and x-ray findings there are practically no other means of assessing periodontal symptoms (2). Clinical probing with adequate instruments is a basic necessity in determining depth, topography and type of the periodontal pocket (3).

It was found that probing force and form of the probe have decisive influence on the result of probing. Consequently, new types of probes with defined pressure were developed(4). Up to this day this probes were hardly ever used by clinicians. Reduced tactile sensation led to additional errors in attachment loss measurement (5). On the other hand, a probe with a spherical tip developed by the WHO seemed to gain popularity (6).

It was the aim of our study to examine the probing depth differences and measuring errors related to the use of three different periodontal probes. We intended to determine differences in measuring results and tried to find a relation between probing depth and clinical status of the pocket.

MATERIAL AND METHODS

100 patients of both genders (Age: 46.8±14.2 years) complaining about gum problems were examined in our department. Examination was done systematically beginning from the distalmost right upper molar and continuing clockwise till reaching the distalmost lower right molar.

The degree of gingival inflammation was assessed using the Sulcus Bleeding Index (SBI, 7) and the level of oral hygiene was gauged by determining the Approximal Plaque Index (API, 8). Pocket depth measurements were limited to the Ramfjord teeth (9), i.e. 16, 21, 24, 36, 41, 44, and were done by only one examiner. Any missing Ramfjord tooth was substituted by the distalnext tooth (10). On every tooth, 6 sites were measured (mesiobuccal, buccal, distobuccal, mesiolingual, lingual, distolingual).

The succession of the different probes was randomly switched from tooth to tooth to make up for a possible influence of the anterior probing on the measured pocket depth. Measurements were recorded in 0.5 mm steps. The following probes were used:

1. **PCP-11:** The tip has a diameter of 0.45 mm. The sections between 3 and 6 and between 8 and 11 mm are coded in black color.

2. **P-WHO:** For examination and recording of treatment needs (Community Periodontal Index of Treatmant Needs: CPITN) we used a probe that was developed by the WHO " Oral Health Unit" in 1978 (6, 11). Its tip ends in a spherical structure of 0.5 mm of diameter. It is supposed to help in the detection of subgingival calculus and to avoid excessive probing of gingival pockets. the section between 3.5 and 5.5 mm is color coded.

3. **Borodontic®:** This probe was developed with the aim of improving reproducibility of pocket depth measurements in clinical studies. It is provided with a joint and a spring that usually limits probing force to 0.25 N. The tip of this probe has a diameter of 0.64 mm. The sections between 2 and 4 mm, 6 and 8 mm and 10 and 12 mm are coded in black color.

 All measurements were statistically evaluated. The means of each couple of probing depth measurements groups were examined using the t-test for independent samples in order to find significant differences depending on the type of probe used. The limit for a significant relation was set at a probability of error of $p \leq 0.05$.

RESULTS

 The group of 100 patients examined in our study showed an Approximal Plaque Index of 61%($\pm$31.4) and a Sulcus Bleeding Index of 43.5%($\pm$32.5).

3534 pocket depth measurements were grouped according to tho following criteria:

 At first, mean values for each type of probe were calculated. They showed a maximum for P-WHO and a minimum for Borodontic. The mean values for PCP-11 and P-WHO had a slight difference of 0.04 mm whereas PCP-11 and Borodontic differed by 0.33 mm. Both differences were significant at the p≤0.001 level. After that, only the 956 "deep pocket" measuremants were evaluated which showed a probing depth higher than 3 mm when gauged with the Borodontic probe.

In accordance with the results mentioned above, the highest mean value was found for P-WHO and the lowest for the Borodontic probe. PCP-11 and Borodontic showed a difference of only 0.04 mm which was not significant (p≤0.427).

Differences between PCP-11 and P-WHO were not significant, either (p≤0.149), whereas a significant difference between P-WHO and Borodontic could be proved (p≤0.0029).

At last, patients were divided into two groups according to the degree of gingival inflammation as gauged by the Sulcus Bleeding Index. Group 1 contained 55 patients with a SBI> 30% and group 2 45 patients with a SBI≤30%. The SBI mean values were 66.9%±25.1 for group 1 and 15%±9.1 for group 2.

In group 1 no significant differences between PCP-11 and P-WHO(p≤0.724) and between PCP-11 and Borodontic(p≤0.092) could be found (**Fig.1**). However, differences between P-WHO and Borodontic were significant (p≤0.045).

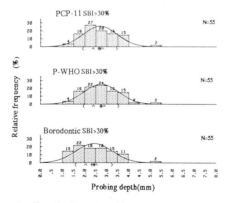

Figure.1: Shows the distrubution of probing depths with each of the periodontal probes for group 1.

In group 2 no differences between PCP-11 and P-WHO could be proved (p≤0.744). On the other hand, significant differences were present between PCP-11 and Borodontic (p≤0.013) and between P-WHO and Borodontic (p≤0.006, **Fig.2**).

436

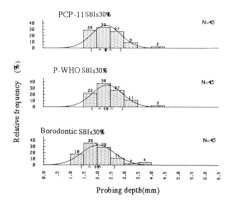

Figure.2: Shows the distrubution of probing depths with each of the periodontal probes for group 2.

CONCLUSIONS

No significant differences could be found between pocket depth measurements with the PCP-11 and P-WHO probe. There was always a significant difference between measurements with P-WHO and Borodontic. Differences decreased with increasing probing depths.

Differences between PCP-11 and Borodontic were not significant in pockets with probing depths of at least 3 mm and belonging to the patients with a high degree of gingival inflammation.

These findings could be explained by the fact that the examiner can apply a higher force with the immobile types of periodontal probe like P-WHO and PCP-11 than with the force limited Borodontic probe and that the bigger diameter of the Borodontic probe provokes a higher gingival tonus.

REFERENCES

1. Lange, D.E. : Attitudes and behavior with respect to oral hygiene and Periodontal treatment needs in selected groups in west germany. Public Health Aspects of Periodontal disease. Ed.: FRANDSEN, 83-97, A.Quintessenz, Berlin (1984).

2. Lange, D.E.: Die Messung der Zahnfleischtaschen und parodontalen Taschen. Quintessenz 35, 2319-2323 (1984).

3. Tibbetts Jr, L.S.: Use of diagnostic probes for detection of periodontal disease. J Am Dent Ass 78, 549-555 (1969).

4. Lange, D.E. und Meijer, E.: Untersuchungen über individuelle Unterschiede bei parodontalen Taschenmessungen mit einer druck-kalibrierten Sonde. Dtsch Zahnärztl Z 38, 866-869 (1983).

5. Kalkwarf, K.L., Kaldahl, W.B. und Patil, K.D.: Comparison of manuel and pressure-controlled periodontal probing. J Am dent Ass 57, 467-471 (1986).

6. Esmilie, R.D.: The 621 periodontal probe. Int Dent J 31, 287 (1981).

7. Mühlemann, H.R. und Son, S.: gingival sulcus bleeding- a leading symptom in initial gingivitis. Helv odont Acta 15, 107 (1971).

8. Lange, D.E., Plagmann, H.-Ch., Eenboon, A. und Promesberger, A.: Klinische Bewertungsverfahren zur Objektivierung der Mundhygiene. Dtsch Zahnärztl Z 32, 44-47 (1977).

9. Ramfjord, S.P.: Indices for prevalence and incidence of periodontal disease. J Periodont 30, 51-59 (1959).

10. Marthaler, Th. M., Engelberger, B. and Rateitschak, K.H.: Bone loss in Ramfjord´s index: Substitution of selected teeth. Helv Odont Acta 15, 121 (1971).

11. World Health Organization (WHO). Epidemiology, etiology and prevention of periodontal diseases. Tech Rep Ser, No 621, WHO, Geneva (1978).

© 1991 Elsevier Science Publishers B.V.
Recent advances in periodontology Vol. II,
S.I. Gold, M. Midda and S. Mutlu, eds.

TRANSPLANTATION OF UNERUPTED WISDOM TEETH

*HIROKI GAMA, **MASAMITSU KAWANAMI, **HIROSHI KATO and **NOBUKAZU TSUKUDA.

*Takugin Health Insurance Society Clinic, Odori Nishi 3, Chuo-ku, Sapporo.   ** Department of Periodontology and Endodontology, Hokkaido University School of Dentistry, Kita 13, Nishi 7, Kita-ku, Sapporo, Japan.

INTRODUCTION

   There have been few detailed reports about the periodontal healing process after transplantation of unerupted wisdom teeth. This presentation describes clinical findings in three cases of transplanted unerupted wisdom teeth into the socket of mandibular second molars which were extracted because of root resorption or root fracture.

CASE I
   In March, 1989 a 33-year-old female. Root resorption was found at the surface of the distal root of the mandibular left second molar which was adjacent to the unerupted wisdom tooth(Fig.I-1). The wisdom tooth was extracted following the extraction of the second molar. The wisdom tooth was retrofilled with amalgam(Fig.I-2). It was transplanted into the socket of the second molar after being splinted to the elongated acrylic crown of the mandibular left first molar(Fig.I-3). Glass Ionomer Cement was overlayed as a periodontal pack(Fig.I-4). The uncomfortable symptoms had mostly disappeared and slight oppressive pain was felt at the location of transplant after 16 days. After 21 days the periodontal pack was removed and slight percussion pain was found around the transplanted tooth. But there was no subject symptom. The tooth mobility was 1 degree. The probing depth at the distal site was 6mm. The splint was removed 42 days later. The depth was 4mm at the distal site. After 14 months the tooth was well maintained.

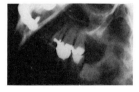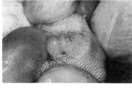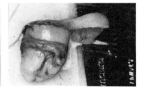

Fig.I-1. At initial visit.
Fig.I-2. Retrofilling with amalgam.
Fig.I-3. The tooth connected to the elongated acrylic crown of the mandibular left first molar.

440

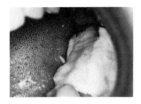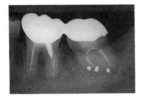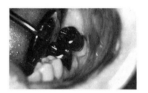

Fig.I-4. Glass Ionomer cement pack.
Fig.I-5,6. 9 monthes after transplantation.

CASE I   Changes in probing depth

12 weeks after transplantation
(3 weeks after transplantation)

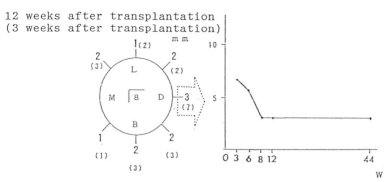

CASE II
    In August 1987, a 24 year old female complained of a slight
pain around the mandibular right second molar.Root canal   treatment   was   performed,however   there was root   resorption at the
surface of the distal root where it was making contact with   the
mandibular right unerupted wisdom tooth(Fig.II-1), such that
inflammation continued. In June, 1989 the wisdom tooth was   extracted for transplantation following the extraction of the
second molar(Fig.II-2). After retrofilling of the Apex with
amalgam, it was transplanted into the socket of the second
molar(Fig.II-3). Occlusal adjustment and temporary splinting with
Glass Ionomer Cement overlaying the gingiva   was   performed.   The
patient complained only of slight pain. Periodontal swelling and
gingival   redness   did not occur after the   transplantation.   The
tooth mobility was 1 degree and the probing depth was less   than
3mm except 6mm at the distal site 21 days later. However after 3
months the probing depth around the whole tooth was 3mm and   the
mobility was less than one degree(Fig.II-4).   After   14   months
the tooth was well maintained(Fig.II-5,6).

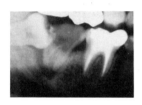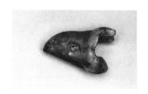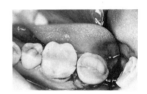

Fig.II-1. At initial visit.
Fig.II-2. Root resorption   at   the   surface   of   the distal   root.
Fig.II-3. Transplantaion   into the socket of   the   second   molar
(mirror view).

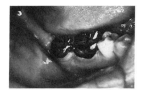 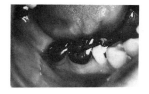 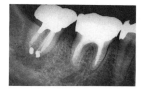

Fig.II-4. At 3 months after transplantation.
Fig.II-5,6. At 14 months after transplantation.

CASE   II   Changes in probing depth

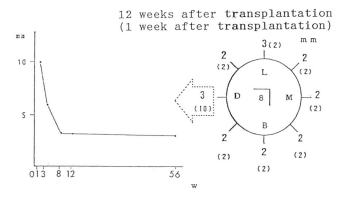

12 weeks after transplantation
(1 week after transplantation)

CASE III
  In February, 1989 a fistula was found at the lingual interdental papillae between the mandibular left first and second molar of a 50-year-old male. Root canal treatment was begun and then on April 7th root canal filling was performed. Fistula appeared at the same place 4 months later. It was shown on radiograph that Guttapercha point #60 went through the fistula to the root Apex(Fig.III-1). Therefore root fracture was suspected.
In September. 1989 the second molar was extracted and root fracture was found from crown to root. The mandibular left unerupted wisdom tooth was transplanted into the socket of the second molar. Only slight pain and swelling were noted after transplantation. The subject symptom disappeared two weeks later.The probing depth was less than 3mm around the whole tooth surface except 7mm at the distal site three weeks later. All of the depths were 3mm and the mobility was 1 degree two months later. The tooth was well maintained after 11 month(Fig.III-2,3).

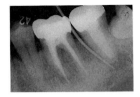 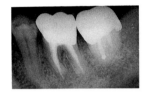 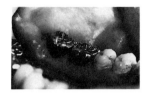

Fig.III-1. Guttapercha point went through the fistula to the root apex.
Fig.III-2,3. 11 months after transplantation.

CASE III Changes in probing depth

8 weeks after transplantation
(3 weeks after transplantation)

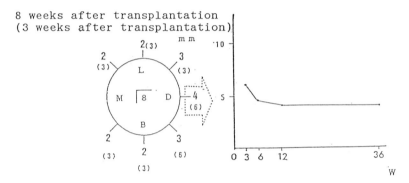

DISCUSSION

If a mandibular second molar accompanied with a horizontally-buried or partially erupted wisdom tooth has poor prognosis because of excessive root resorption or root fracture, both teeth will usually be extracted. In this study the transplantation of the wisdom teeth into the socket of the second molar was per-formed as the periodontal membranes of the wisdom teeth were healthy, which is good for transplantation. As the unerupted wisdom teeth made contact with the distal surface of the second molar, the distal wall of the second molar's socket became defec-tive. The transplanted teeth didn't fit well into the sockets at the distal site which seemed bad for transplantation.
However according to the clinical observation, the probing depth at the distal site became shallow within a few weeks after transplantation. These cases were all clinically well maintained. The type of periodontal attachment to the site or resistance against periodontitis is, however, unknown. Any symptom of root resorption or ankylosis has not been found. Long term observation will be continued.

REFFERENCES

1.Kehoe JC (1986) J American Dental Association 112:224-230
2.Nasjleti CE, Castelli WA, Caffesse RA (1982) Oral Surg. 53:557-566

© 1991 Elsevier Science Publishers B.V.
Recent advances in periodontology Vol. II,
S.I. Gold, M. Midda and S. Mutlu, eds.

CLINICAL STUDY OF BRUXISM

- ANALYSIS OF JAW MOVEMENT IN BRUXISM DURING SLEEP BY LED-PHOTENTIOMATIC
SYSTEM -

YOSHIHIRO KATO, HIROCHIKA NAKAGAWA, TAKATSUNE TAKAMATSU, AKITO INABA, HIROSHI
KATO*, TAKAKI MAKINO, YOSHIAKI SAKAKIBARA, SHIN TANOI, MITSUHIRO MATSUO,
YASUHARU NAKAJIMA and YUSUKE KOWASHI

Dept. of Periodont., School of Dent., Higashi-Nippon-Gakuen Univ., 1757
Kanazawa, Ishikari-Tobetsu (Japan) and *Dept. of Periodont., School of Dent.,
Hokkaido Univ., N-3, W-7 Sapporo (Japan)

INTRODUCTION

Bruxism has been considered to be one of the important factors accelerating the
progression of periodontal lesions. But the detailed mechanism of bruxism has
not yet been established. Bruxism has been examined with electric myogram in the
past. However, we have obtained few informations about jaw movement during
sleep at night. Periodontal destruction by bruxism might be due to not only extension of duration of the muscle activity but also differences of jaw movement
types. Therefore, we developed the nocturnal jaw movement recording system[1].

The purpose of the present investigation was to examine the characteristic of
the jaw movement with bruxism by using our improved system available for recording two directions (lateral and anterior) of the jaw movement.

MATERIAL AND METHODS

Subjects

Three adult volunteers ranging in age from 27 to 32 were selected. Non of the
subjects had any clinically detectable abnormality of the masticatory muscles
or temporomandibular joints. Additionally two of them were conscious of bruxism
(subject nos. 1 and 2), and another was not conscious of it (subject no. 3)(Table
1). Each subject participated in our experiment for two nights and two nights (or
more) of adaptation period was prepared in advance of the experimental period.

Measuring devices

We recorded muscle activity, tooth contact, grinding sounds and jaw movement
during sleep. EMG signals were obtained from bilateral masseter muscles by using
surface electrodes. Tooth contact was picked up with a microvibration pick up (MT
pick up, Nihonkoden, Tokyo) on the forehead (Fig. 1-A). Grinding sounds were recorded with a condenser microphon (MKH816 TU-3, Sennheiser, Germany). Jaw movement in two directions was recorded by using LED - Photentiomatic system. This appliance consisted of two Photentiomatics (MPC-1001, Moririka LTD., Yokohama) con
nected to acrylic plate on upper anterior teeth and two LEDs connected to
acrylic plate on lower anterior teeth (Fig. 1-B). These data were transmitted

with wireless system and synchronously traced on recording paper at chart speed of 5.0mm/sec (Fig. 1-C).

<u>Measurements and analysis</u>

The recorded EMG and jaw movement pattern were classified into grinding, clenching and others. The characteristics of the jaw movement for each type were as folloes: 1) Grinding type. We obtained periodic jaw movement with or without grinding sound in addition to muscle activity and tooth contact (Fig. 2). 2) Clenching type. This type had the period of the muscle activity without jaw movement (Fig. 3). 3) Other type. This type was other jaw movement with muscle activity than grinding and clenching (Fig. 4).

In three volunteers, the duration time of three bruxism types was measured from EMG activity and jaw movement, and calculated the percentage of each type.

Each recorded jaw movement was analysed by following method. The figures were traced onto a transparent film and the pattern of the most frequently appeared (MFA) was selected from each volunteers. When the interval between two EMG events was less than 10 sec, these patterns were considered to be one unit. The proportion of unit included MFA (MFA unit) was evaluated.

RESULTS

The mean percentages of each jaw movement type are shown in table 1. The proportions of grinding and others were higher in nos. 1 and 2 subjects compared to no. 3. On the contrary the proportion of clenching was lower in nos. 1 and 2 subjects compared to no. 3.

The proportion of MFA unit are given in figure 5. The MFA unit constituted about half of total unit numbers.

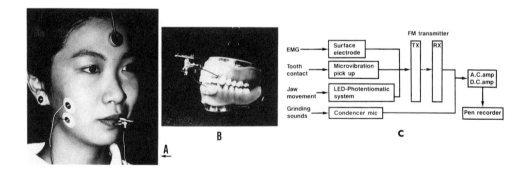

Fig.1-A. This figure illustrates proper placement of the surface electrodes, a reference electrode, a microvibration pick up on the forehead and LEDs (lower teeth) - Photentiomatics (upper teeth) assembly.
Fig. 1-B. Sensor parts of LED-Photentiomatic system.
Fig. 1-C. EMG, tooth contact, grinding sounds and two directions of jaw movement were recorded synchronously during sleep.

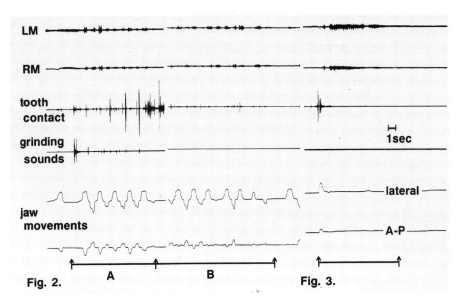

Fig. 2. Grinding type: Periodic EMG activity and jaw movement were observed with (Fig. 2-A) or without (Fig. 2-B) grinding sounds.
Fig. 3. Clenching type: This type has the period of the muscle activity without jaw movement.

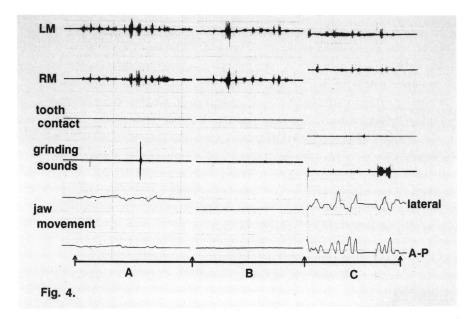

Fig. 4. Other type: Other jaw movement with muscle activity than grinding and clenching. Periodic EMG activity with irregular jaw movement (Fig. 4-A) or no jaw movement (Fig. 4-B). Unclassifiable EMG activity and jaw movement (Fig. 4-C).

Table 1. Conscious bruxism, sleeping time, duration of muscle activity and percentages of each bruxism type; mean and standard deviation

Subject no.	Conscious bruxism	Sleeping time (h)	Duration of muscle activity (min)	TYPE A (%)	TYPE B	TYPE C
1.	+	7.2± 1.2	10.6± 3.3	47.5± 7.3	15.1±12.7	37.5± 5.5
2.	+	6.0± 0.3	10.8± 3.7	52.2±14.6	24.0±10.9	24.4± 3.0
3.	–	7.6± 0.5	8.5± 1.2	17.4± 1.6	70.6± 7.4	12.0± 5.9

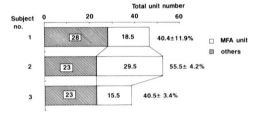

Fig. 5. Proportion of MFA units. Columns represent the total number of unit. The blank portion shows the number of MFA unit. Figures outside the columns indicate percentage of MFA unit (mean ± standard deviation).

DISCUSSION AND CONCLUSION

This paper reports the findings of bruxism patterns in three volunteer using jaw movement recording system developed by us. The subjects were divided into two groups. Two of them were conscious of bruxism, and another was not.

The bruxism pattern were classified into grinding, clenching and others. The result of mean percentage of each bruxism type were similar to our previous study[2]. In both studies, subjects who were conscious of bruxism showed higher proportion of grinding pattern. Although the incidence was significantly low, grinding was observed in subjects without conscious bruxism. Additionally, considerable number of similar jaw movement pattern was observed in each subject. It was indicated that such similar jaw movement increase might be one of the factors accelerating the progression of periodontal lesions in guiding teeth.

It was concluded that the jaw movement pattern observed with EMG activity was capable of making more detailed diagnosis of bruxism.

REFERENCES

1. Takamatsu T, Kato Y, Nakagawa H, Bando S, Fujii T, Nakajima Y, Kowashi Y, Hoshi M, Kato H (1988) In: Ishikawa J, Kawasaki H, Ikeda K, Hasegawa K (eds) Recent Advances in Clinical Periodontology, Excerpta Medica, Amsterdam, pp 495-462

2. Kato Y, Nakagawa H, Takamatsu T, Inaba A, Kato H, Makino T, Kowashi Y (1990) J Japan Ass Periodont 32:May 132

© 1991 Elsevier Science Publishers B.V.
Recent advances in periodontology Vol. II,
S.I. Gold, M. Midda and S. Mutlu, eds.

STUDIES ON THE EFFECTS OF DIFFERENT KINDS OF TOOTHBRUSHES ON BOTH PLAQUE REMOVAL AND TOOTHBRUSHING PRESSURE, IN THE SCRUBBING METHOD OF TOOTHBRUSHING   (REPORT2)

*JOICHIRO SUZUKI, NORIKO SEKI, MASATO FUKUSHIMA, YOSHIHIKO SHOJI, ICHIRO WATANABE, TAKAAKI WATANABE, TAKASHI ARAI and JIRO NAKAMURA

Department of Periodontics and Endodontics, Tsurumi University School of Dental Medicine.   , 2-1-3, Tsurumi, Tsurumi-ku, Yokohama, Japan 230

INTRODUCTION

The purpose of this study was to investigate the effects of different types of toothbrushes on toothbrushing pressure and plaque removal in the scrubbing method.

Two sequential experiments were carried out to evaluate the following factors in this study.

EXP.1. Nylon bristle toothbrushes with different lengths of shanks and different types(tapered and round) of bristle tips.

EXP.2. Nylon bristle toothbrushes differing in hardness and the number of bristles.

MATERIALS AND METHODS

Twelve(EXP.1) and Nine(EXP.2) subjects participated in this study. Plaque score were measured before and after toothbrushing. Then plaque removal rates were calculated. Toothbrushing pressure was determined by Watanabe's method.(Watanabe,T.J.Japan.- Ass.Periodont.,27:779-794,1985.)

Toothbrushes

EXP. 1: Four kinds of toothbrushes which were different in length of shank (30mm, 40mm) and type of bristles tip (round type, tapered type) respectively were used in this study. Referring to the results of our previous reports, the dimension of new toothbrushes were determined as follows; nylon bristles 10mm long and 0.20mm in diameter, brushing surface: 30mm long, bristle: 3rows with 26tufts, and a straight handle. (Fig.1-A)

EXP. 2: Nine kinds of toothbrushes which were different in the hardness of total bristles(7kg,10kg,12kg) and the number of bristles were used in this study. The toothbrushes were designed as follows ; nylon bristle (0.20mm, 0.25mm, 0.30mm in diameter),

rounded ends ,10mm in length, 3rows, 26tufts, straight handle
the brushing surface 25mm long. (Fig.1-B)

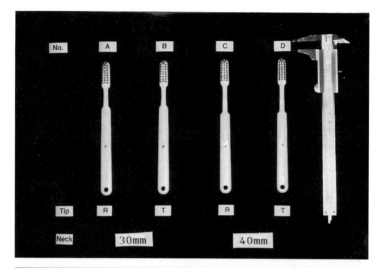

A

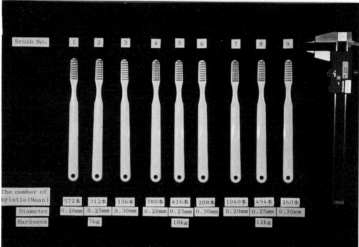

B

Fig.1 A:Toothbrushes(EXP. 1) B:Toothbrushes(EXP. 2)

RESULTS

<u>EXP. 1</u>: The average toothbrushing pressure of the toothbrushes
with a 40mm long shanks(301.6 ± 84.1g/cm^2)was higher than that of
those with a 30mm long shanks(294.7 ± 74.8g/cm^2), and that with a
tapered bristle type(316.7 ± 90.4g/cm^2)was higher than that with a

round type bristles($279.6\pm61.7g/cm^2$). However statistically significant differences were not found among the four toothbrushes in brushing pressure and in plaque removal on total teeth surfaces and on distal surfaces of the most posterior teeth($P<0.05$; two-way ANOVA) .(Fig. 2-A,B)

EXP. 2: There was a tendency that toothbrushes with harder bristles showed higher toothbrushing pressure(7kg: $296.-3\pm74.0g/cm^2$, 10kg: $411.9\pm127.8g/cm^2$, 12kg: $405.7\pm152.7g/cm^2$) . Statistically significant differences were found among the three different hardness($P<0.01$). Statistically differences were not found among the three different numbers of bristles in toothbrushing pressure, among the three different hardness and numbers of bristles in plaque removal. But toothbrushes with harder bristles and with bristles in lager diameter showed a tendency of higher plaque removal. When the elasticity of all the toothbrush bristles is the same, a toothbrush with a smaller number of bristles per tuft is more effective for plaque removal than one with a larger number of bristles. (Fig. 2-C,D)

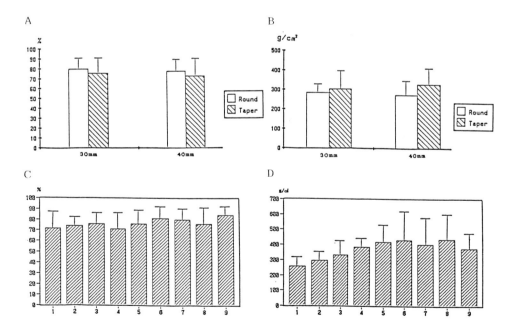

Fig. 2 A:Total Plaque Removal B:Toothbrushing Pressure (EXP. 1)
        C:Total Plaque Removal D:Toothbrushing Pressure (EXP. 2)

CONCLUSION

The better toothbrushes for the scrubbing method would seem to be those which have a 40mm-long shank, rounded bristle tips and harder bristles.

REFERENCES

1. Rodda, J. C. : A comparison of four methods of toothbrushing. New Zeal. Dent. J. , 64; 162-167, 1986.

2. Carrannza: Glickman's Clinical Periodontology, 5th ed. W. B. Saunders, Philadelphia and London, 1979, 736-758.

3. Wilkins, E. M. : Clinical Practice of the Dental Hygienist, 4th. ed. , Lea & Febinger, Philadelphia, 1976, 308-320.

4. McClure, D. B. : A comparison of toothbrushing techniques for the preschool child. J. Dent. child, 33: 205-210, 1966.

5. Ramfjord, S. P. : Indices for prevalence and incidence of periodontal disease. J. Periodonto. , 30: 51-59, 1959.

6. Wade, A. B. : Brushing practice of a group with periodontal disease,edited by John, E. E. , et al. , Henly Kinpton London, 1972, pp. 218-223.

7. Arai, T. : A comparison of plaque removal by different toothbrushes and toothbrushing methods. The bulletin of tokyo medical and dental university. Vol. 24, No. 2 pp. 177-188. june, 1977.

8. WATANABE, T. : A study of toothbrushing pressures by the specifically designed intraoral telemetry system . J. Japan. Ass. Periodont. , 27: 779-794, 1985.

© 1991 Elsevier Science Publishers B.V.
Recent advances in periodontology Vol. II,
S.I. Gold, M. Midda and S. Mutlu, eds.

EFFECTS OF DIFFERENT TOOTHBRUSHING METHODS AND TOOTHBRUSHING PRESSURES ON GINGIVAL SOFT TISSUE

＊MUNENORI SHIONO, KAZUHIKO SUGAYA, TAKASHI ARAI AND JIRO NAKAMURA
Department of Periodontics and Endodontics, Tsurumi University School of
Dental Medicine, 2-1-3 Tsurumi, Tsurumi-ku, Yokohama, Japan 230

INTRODUCTION

The importance of toothbrushing as a therapeutic aid in the control of periodontal disease is an established fact[1]. The effects of toothbrushing on the gingival soft tissue have been reported by many researchers[2,3]. But, the effects of toothbrushing on the gingival surface immediately after brushing weren't reported.

The purpose of this study was to determine the immediate effects of different toothbrushing methods and toothbrushing pressures on gingival soft tissue. The following two investigations were undertaken.

Experiment 1) The number of oral exfoliative cells resulting from different brushing methods was measured and the gingival surface immediately after brushing was observed.

Experiment 2) The same evaluations at different brushing pressures were performed.

MATERIALS & METHODS

Experiment 1) There were 14 subjects(13 males, 1 female), each with both clinically normal dentition and gingiva. Rolling, horizontal and scrubbing methods with a medium bristle brush (PERIO Ⅱ ᴿ M by Sunstar Comp.Japan) were evaluated for the following items. ① The numbers of oral exfoliative cells in rinsing solution before and after brushing (included during brushing) were counted using microscope.② SEM investigation of gingival surface after brushing using a replica technique employing a hydrophilic silicone rubber impression material. The experimental schedule and the sampling and impression methods are shown in Fig.1.

Experiment 2) 10 subjects (9 males,1 female) were used. Toothbrushing at different pressures(routine brushing pressure and high pressure),performed with a rolling and a scrubbing method, were examined as in ① and ②. The experimental block diagram is shown in Fig.2-a. This system could record one set of data from a strain-gage on the toothbrush and another set of data from the pressure-transducer on the tooth surface[4].This is reproducible at the same pressure on all teeth except the upper first molar(Fig.2-b,c,d).

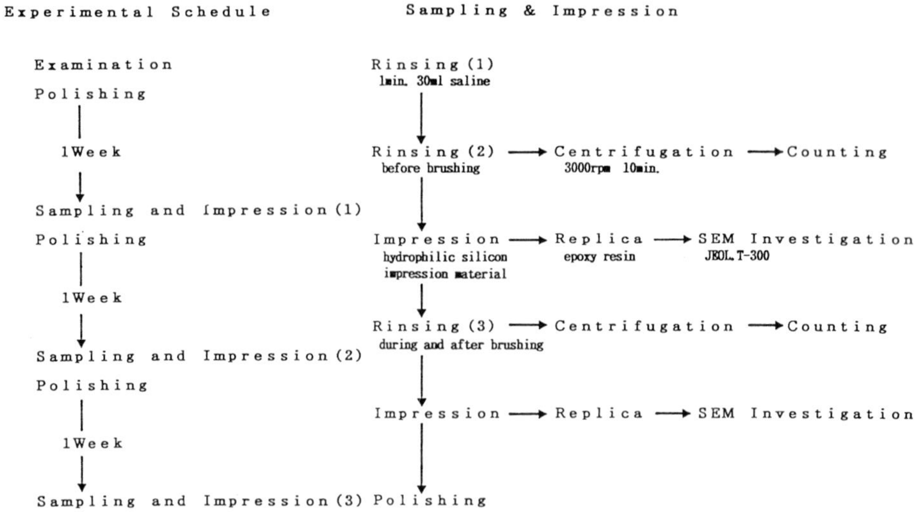
Experimental Schedule
Sampling & Impression
Examination
Polishing
1Week
Sampling and Impression (1)
Polishing
1Week
Sampling and Impression (2)
Polishing
1Week
Sampling and Impression (3)
Rinsing (1)
1min. 30ml saline
Rinsing (2)
before brushing
Centrifugation
3000rpm 10min.
Counting
Impression
hydrophilic silicon impression material
Replica
epoxy resin
SEM Investigation
JEOL T-300
Rinsing (3)
during and after brushing
Centrifugation
Counting
Impression
Replica
SEM Investigation
Polishing
Fig.1

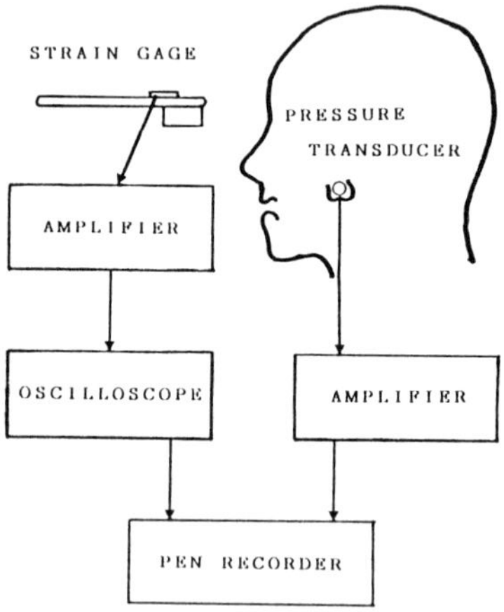
STRAIN GAGE
PRESSURE
TRANSDUCER
AMPLIFIER
OSCILLOSCOPE
AMPLIFIER
PEN RECORDER
Fig.2-a

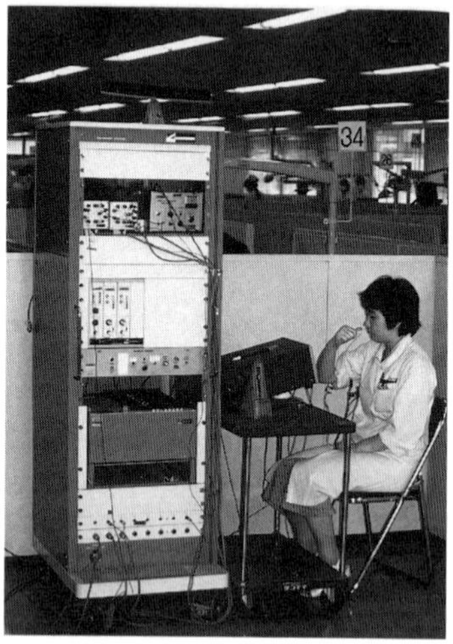
Fig.2-c

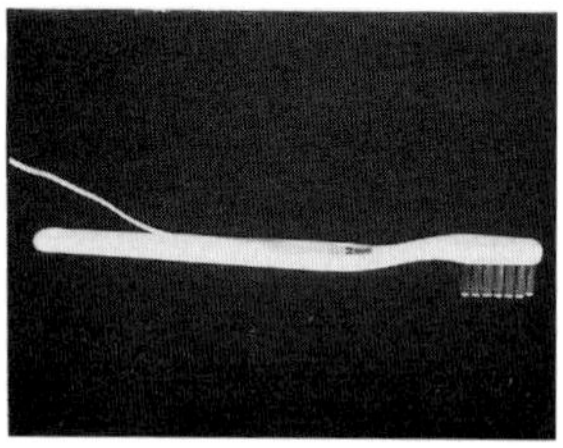
Fig.2-b

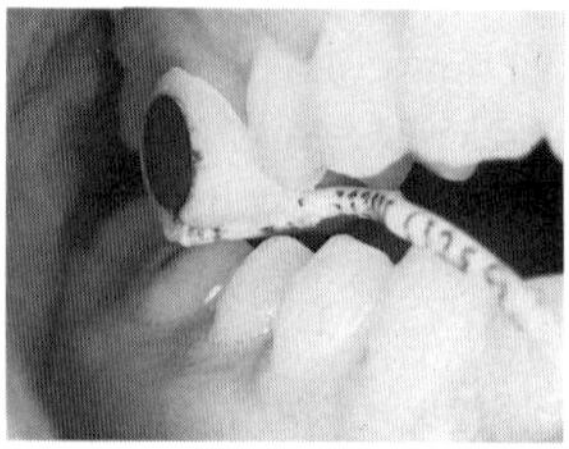
Fig.2-d

RESULTS

Experiment 1) The rolling method showed the highest number of exfoliative cells during brushing ($26.0 \pm 6.3 \times 10^4$ /ml), compared to the horizontal ($20.5 \pm 3.2 \times 10^4$ /ml) and the scrubbing method($12.5 \pm 2.2 \times 10^4$ /ml)(Fig.3-a). Statistical significance was recognized among the three brushing methods ($P < 0.05$). There was a difference in the location of gingival abrasion among brushing methods (Fig.3-b, c, d).

Experiment 2) The number of exfoliative cells using scrubbing method at routine pressure($11.7 \pm 4.5 \times 10^4$ /ml, 1246.1 ± 513.5 g/cm^2) was slightly lower than that at high pressure ($12.1 \pm 5.2 \times 10^4$ /ml, 2036.3 ± 713.5 g/cm^2) (Fig.4-a, b).Statistical significance was recognized between the brushing pressures ($P < 0.05$), but not recognized between the number of exfoliative cells. The number of oral exfoliative cells using rolling method at routine pressure ($18.9 \pm 3.8 \times 10^4$ /ml, 498.3 ± 84.8 g/cm^2) was lower than the high pressure ($23.1 \pm 3.5 \times 10^4$ /ml, 687.6 ± 212.9 g/cm^2)(Fig.5-a ,b). Statistical significance was recognized between the brushing pressures ($P < 0.05$),but not recognized between the number of exfoliative cells.

Oral Exfoliative Epitherial Cells at Different Brushing Methods.

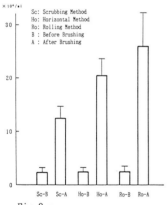

Fig.3-a

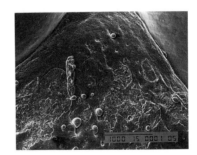

Fig.3-c Horizontal

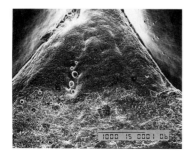

Fig.3-b Scrubbing

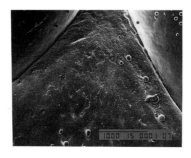

Fig.3-d Rolling

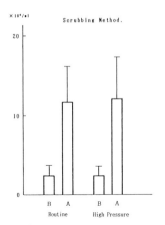

Fig. 4-a

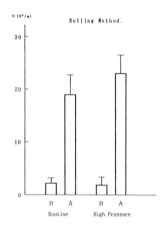

Fig. 5-a

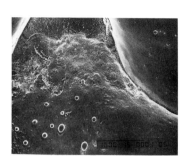

Fig. 4-b High Pressure

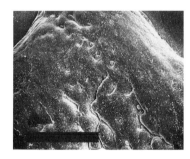

Fig. 5-b High Pressure

CONCLUSIONS

① The number of oral exfoliative cells was significantly influenced by the brushing methods.

② It can be considered that there is no effect of brushing pressures on the number of oral exfoliative cells.

③ SEM observation using the replica technique is very useful for evaluating gingival surfaces without biopsy.

REFERENCE
1. Takashi ARAI and Shiro KINOSHITA (1977):A Comparison of Plaque Removal by Different toothbrushes and Toothbrushing Methods,Bull.Tokyo Med.Dent.Univ. 24:177-188.
2. Shinji OKAWARA (1965):The Effects of Toothbrushing on the Gingival Tissue, Japan.J.Conserv.Dent.,8:305-335.
3. Leena SANDHOLM, Maija-Liisa NIEMI and Jukka AINAMO (1982):Identification of Soft Tissue Brushing Lisions -A Clinical and Scanning Electron Microscopic Study-,J.Clin.Periodontol.,9:387-401.
4. Takaaki WATANABE,Tohru MAKITA,Hisao MATSUURA,Takashi ARAI and Jiro NAKAMURA (1981):A Study of the toothbrushing Pressures -Relationship between Tooth-brushing Speed and Toothbrushing Pressures-,J.Japan.Ass.Periodont.,23:499-508

© 1991 Elsevier Science Publishers B.V.
Recent advances in periodontology Vol. II,
S.I. Gold, M. Midda and S. Mutlu, eds.

EFFECT OF PERIODONTAL TREATMENT ON PERIODONTALLY-INVOLVED ROOT SURFACES
-WHAT SURFACE CHARACTER OF EXPOSED CEMENTUM IS NEEDED FOR NEW ATTACHMENT?-

MASATOSHI UEDA, YOSHIHIRO TERANISHI, NAOKI NAKAGAKI, AKIRA YAMAOKA, MIBU UEMURA*, HIDEAKI NOSHI*, MASAKI KAMBARA*, KOJI KONISHI*
Department of periodontoligy, *Preventive Dentistry, Osaka Dental University, 5-31 Otemae, 1-chome, Chuo-ku, Osaka 540, Japan.

INTRODUCTION

Exposed cementum in the periodontal pocket have many complex conditions, for example, the adhesion of plaque and calculus, the immersion of bacterium, the formation of supercalcified layer. The root treatment for this exposed cementum is most important to obtain new attachment of connective tissue including plaque control in the prognosis of periodontal treatment. We had already reported the surface properties of exposed cementum treated by root planing or citric acid treatment, which influence new attachment. This study was made to investigate the effect of the air power abrasive system (APA system) on the exposed root surface.

MATERIALS AND METHODS

As the experimental teeth, periodontally involved teeth were employed which were diagnosed as the indication of extraction of tooth after inspection and examination and no anamnesis of scaling and root planing. And the periodontally not involved teeth, which were diagnosed conveniently as extraction in the case of impacted tooth and orthodontic treatments, were used as control teeth. The experimentally teeth were divided into the following four groups:
(1) The scaling group, whose exposed root surfaces were removed dental plaque and calculus, as far as possible, with a curette-type scaler(S group).
(2) The group, in which the exposed root surfaces of the scaling group(1) were further treated with APA system for 20 seconds (S+A group).

(3) The group, whose exposed root surfaces were planed to the smooth surface with a curette-type scaler(R group).

(4) The group, in which the exposed root surfaces of root planing group(3) were further treated with APA system for 20 seconds (R+A group).

The qualitative and quantitative analysis of elements on the few um layer of the experimental cementum surface was made by X-ray microanalyzer(XMA : Hitachi S-560 type scanning electron microscope connected with a Kevex-7000 energy-dispersing type X-ray analyzer and a data-analyzing computer with a CRT-display). The chemical analysis of elements on the topmost surface (nm units) of materials was also made by X-ray photoelectron spectroscopy(XPS: Shimazu type 750 connected with data-processing apparatus, Mitsubishi electronic, Multi-16, Software, Espac 200).

The morphological status of exposed cementum in each groups were observed by a scanning electron microscope(SEM).

The contact angle was measured by the new method improved the sessile drop method. 1ul redistilled water was dropped on the root surface, the shape of a drop was photographed with an unique camera, the height and radius of drop image on film was measured and its contact angle was calculated.

RESULTS AND DISCUSSION

The statistical difference between groups couldn't be found in Ca, P and Ca/P by X-ray microanalyzer (Table 1). However, the value of Ca, P and Ca/P in the APA system groups added to S and R groups showed to be close to the intact cementum. Besides, another trace elements, e.g. Mg, Na, Al, Si, Cl, Fe, Cu and Zn, could be detected in all groups.

Table 1 Concentrations of Ca and P of exposed cementum measured with XMA

Groups	Ca (%)	P (%)	Ca/P
S	$24.05 \pm 1.12*$	11.19 ± 0.51	2.15
S+A	23.15 ± 1.10	10.87 ± 0.41	2.13
R	23.73 ± 1.13	11.09 ± 0.53	2.14
R+A	22.32 ± 0.95	10.58 ± 0.39	2.11
IC**	22.43 ± 1.17	10.68 ± 0.55	2.10

* Standard deviation of the mean
** Intact cementum

On the other hand, the relative concentration of the target
element and Ca/P by XPS analysis showed that in the comparison
between S and R groups versus S+A and R+A groups, the increase of
the Ca/P ratio was observed due to an increase of Ca concentration
(Table 2). From these findings it can be estimated that the
application of APA system does not give the difference in the
element compositions, but the Ca/P on the topmost surface in
exposed cementum is different from the surface layer (um deeper
from surface).

Table 2   Relative concentrations of the target elements of
exposed cementum surface measured with XPS analysis

| Groups | Concentration (%) | | | | | Ca/P ratio |
	Ca	P	O	F	N	
S	11.6+0.1*	10.6+0.3	63.5+1.4	2.5+0.7	11.6+1.4	1.1+0.1
S+A	16.6+2.2	12.0+1.8	64.3+0.4	1.8+0.3	5.3+0.4	1.4+0.1
R	10.7+0.7	9.4+0.3	67.8+0.8	1.5+0.5	10.6+0.9	1.1+0.4
R+A	12.7+1.9	9.2+1.6	65.1+1.3	3.0+0.4	10.0+0.9	1.4+0.1
IC**	12.3+2.0	9.0+1.1	64.4+1.2	1.3+0.2	13.1+2.1	1.3+0.1

 * Standard deviation of the mean
 ** Intact cementum

The SEM observation showed that the striae with a curette type
scaler in S and R groups could be observed on the surface of
exposed cementum, but, in APA system groups, this striae became to
be weaker(Fig.1a and b).

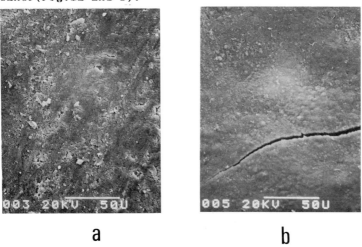

a   b

Fig. 1   The surface of exposed cementum by SEM observation
(a: S and R groups, b: APA system groups)

Contact angle of expose cementum was measured by the improved
method. The contact angle in S group showed to become more
hydrophilic than intact cementum, probably with increase the
surface roughness. In R groups, the contact angle showed higher
value than S group. the application of APA system made the contact
angle to increase to the comparison with only S and R groups, not
beyond the intact cementum(Table 3). It was proved that the
morphological surface became to be more plane and smooth by the
APA system.

Table 3   Contact angles of the
surface of exposed cementum

Groups	Contact angles
S	45.6+0.87*
S+A	50.6+0.95
R	48.2+0.91
R+A	54.0+0.85
IC**	59.9+1.00

 * Standard deviation of the mean
** Intact cementum

These results suggest that the characteristic properties
(hydrophobicity, surface net charge and so on) and chemical
composition of the topmost surface on the exposed cementum is
need for new attachment, especially the interaction between
cementum and periodontal tissue.

REFERENCES
1. Ueda M, Teranishi Y, Yamaoka A, Uemura M, Noshi H, Kambara M,
   Konishi K(1989): Some investigations on the surface features
   of human exposed cementum. J. Japan Ass Periodont 31: 112.
2. Ueda M, Teranishi Y, Yamaoka A, Uemura M, Noshi H, Kambara M,
   Konishi K(1990): Some investigations on the surface features
   of human exposed cementum(Part 2). J Japan Ass Periodont 32:
   59.

© 1991 Elsevier Science Publishers B.V.
Recent advances in periodontology Vol. II,
S.I. Gold, M. Midda and S. Mutlu, eds.

FRICTION SOUND AS AN OBJECTIVE SIGN OF COMPLETION OF ROOT PLANING

MOTOYUKI SUZUKI. KOHJI HASEGAWA
Department of Periodontics, Showa University Dental Scool

INTRODUCTION

Root planing is one of the most important procedures in periodontal treatments. However, there are no objective clinical signs to indicate completion of this procedure.

The purpose of this study was to examine the friction sound produced by curettes and root surfaces during root planing and to test the possibility of utilizing the sound changes as an objective parameter for evaluating completion of this procedure.

MATERIAL AND METHODS

Root planed surfaces were classified as pre-root planed and post-root planed according to their friction sounds during rootplaning. During scaling and root planing with the Gracey curette, the friction sounds were analyzed by the Digital Sonagraph ® 7800 (Kay, Pine Brook, U.S.A.). When friction sound increased, the frequency component showed periodic changes(Fig.1.2).

This state indicated completion of root planing and root surfaces satisfying this criteria were classified as post-root planed.

The study consisted of a clinical and laboratory experiment.

Clinical study.

Seven periodontally diseased teeth were utilized in the clinical trial. Observations of the root surfaces, in situ, were made by scanning electron microscopy(SEM) with replica technique.

Laboratory study.

Twenty-one extracted periodontally diseased teeth were used in the laboratory study. Each surface was examined by the following methods. 1) measuring of root surface roughness by profilometer (Surfcom 700A® Tokyo, Japan) 2) SEM observations 3) determination of number of adherent cells by cultured fibroblast technique.

RESULT

Clinical study.

Post-root planed surfaces were smoother than pre-root planed surface as observed by SEM with the replica technique(Fig.3.4).

Laboratory study.

There were statistic reduction of Ra (root surface roughness, profilometer) between pre- and post-root planed surfaces. Average Ra was 5.8± 2.62 (pre-root planed surfaces) and 2.72± 0.79 (post- root planed surfaces)(Fig.5.). Post-root planed surfaces were smoother than pre-root planed surfaces. The result was similar in the clinical study (Fig.6.7).

Adherent cell counts were increased on post-root planed surfaces.

Average cell count was 14.4 ± 7.1 (pre-root planed surfaces) and 38.5± 7.8 (post-root planed surfaces). These values were statistically significant(Fig.8.9.10).

DISCUSSION

Several studies have shown that endotoxin was increased in exposed cementum and was decreased by root planing. Studies have also indicated the inhibition of cellular growth by endotoxin, in vitro. Fibroblast cells have shown good adherence to root-planed surfaces and furthermore, in the study by Dunlap et al (1981), it was concluded that fibroblast cells showed good growth as well as good adherence to root-planed surface. In this study, fibroblast cells similar showed good growth and good adherence to root-planed surfaces, and these results indicated the possible usefulness of friction sound analysis in the clinical judgement of completion of rootplaning.

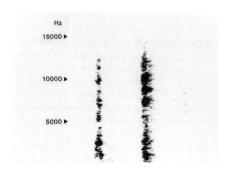

Fig.1.Sonagram of friction
sound pre-planing.

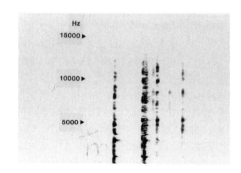

Fig.2.Sonagram of friction
sound post-planing.

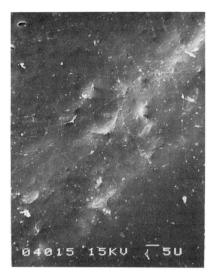

Fig,3.Pre-planed surface
(SEM Replica × 1000)

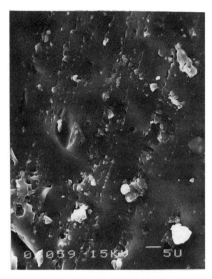

Fig.4.Post-planed surface
(SEM Replica × 1000)

Pre-planed   Post-planed
surface   surface

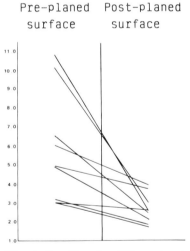

Fig.5.Ra.(by Profilometer)

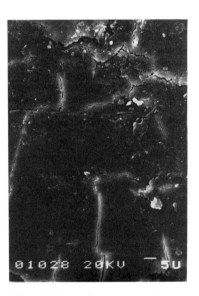

Fig.6.Pre-planed surface
(SEM × 1000)

462

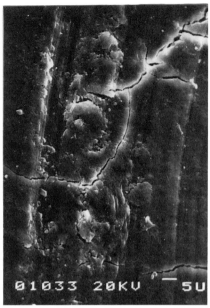

Fig.7.Post-planed surface
(SEM × 1000)

Pre-planed   Post-planed
surface   surface

14.4±7.1   38.5±7.8

Fig.8.Adhereht cell count

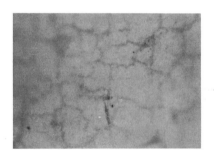

Fig.9.Pre-planed surface
(LM × 100)

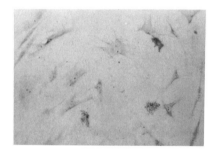

Fig.10.Post-planed surface
fibloblast cell remarkedly
increased   (LM × 100)

1. Aleo,J.J.,et al(1974) J.Periodontol.45:672-675
2. Aleo,J.J.,et al(1975) J.Periodontol.46:639-645
3. Nishimine,D.(1979) J.Periodontol.50:345-349
4. Dunlap,R.M.(1981) J.Periodontol.52:140-142

© 1991 Elsevier Science Publishers B.V.
Recent advances in periodontology Vol. II,
S.I. Gold, M. Midda and S. Mutlu, eds.

EFFECTS OF SUBGINGIVAL WATER JET IRRIGATION ON MODERATE PERIODONTAL POCKETS

NOBUKI MINAMIZAKI,CHISATO SAKURAI,CHIKAKO KURIHARA,TOHRU OHTAKE
AND HAJIME MIYASHITA
Depatment of Periodontics, Showa University Dental School,
2-1-1 Kitasenzoku Ohta-ku Tokyo(Japan)

INTRODUCTION

Many investigations on subgingival plaque control tequnique have been conducted. Subgingival irrigation tequnique is one of it. There are two systems of irrigation tequniques. One is used by syringe and the other is used by irrigator. However, there has been only few studies of subgingival effect of irrigator, except for that of Watts et al[1] , Hagiwara et al[2] .

Hagiwara says that a single distilled water irrigation reduced the total number of subgingival bacteria and the ratio of spirochetas and motile rods until a period of 1 week. We examined that the efficacy of frequently subgigival water jet irrigation on moderate periodontal pockets.

MATERIAL&METHOD

Patient

Nine patients with periodontitis were selected in this study. They were approximately 51 years old with no histry of systemic disease and they had not taken antibiotics for 6 months prior to the start of this study. And they had been no periodontal treatment carried out.

Periodontal pocket

In each of them, at least 2 sites of periodontal pocket $\geq$ 4mm, and radiographic evidence of bone loss, were selected.

Trial design

Fig 1 shows the trial design. Each patient instructed scrub method tooth brushing and interdental cleaning (interdental brush or dental floss). Test site(n=20) received irrigation twice a week for 4 weeks using Water Pik® and Perio Pik® .

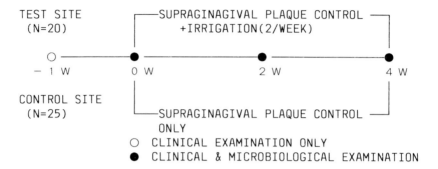

TEST SITE
(N=20)

SUPRAGINAGIVAL PLAQUE CONTROL
+IRRIGATION(2/WEEK)

○ ——————— ● ————————— ● ————————— ●
− 1 W   0 W   2 W   4 W

CONTROL SITE
(N=25)

SUPRAGINAGIVAL PLAQUE CONTROL
ONLY

○ CLINICAL EXAMINATION ONLY
● CLINICAL & MICROBIOLOGICAL EXAMINATION

Fig. 1. Trial design.

The irrigation time was 30 minites for each teeth and distilled water(H_2O) was used as irriqants. The control sites(n=25) received supragingival plaque control only. All pockets were examined, Plaque Index(PLI,Silness&Löe), Gingival Index(GI, Löe&Silness), Probing Pocket Depth(PD) and microbiological findings.

Microbiological findings

Supragingival plaque was removed from the surface to be sampled. The subgingival plaque sample were taken with 3 paperpoints (Johnson&Johonson,Midium) which were inserted into the periodontal pocket until resistance was met and left in place for 30 seconds. The samples were immediately placed into 1.0ml of sterile saline solution. The bacterial sample was suspended by voltexing for 60 seconds and analysed by microscpic studies. The homogenized bacterial suspension was applied to a Petroff-Hauser-counting-chamber(C.A.H.&SON,USA). The sumple was examined by phase contrast microscopy at a magnification of × 1000.Up to 100 cells per samples were counted in randomly selected fields and namely coccoid cells, rods, motile rods, spirochetes were differentiated.

RESULTS
Clinical results

The results from at 0 weeks examination are reported in table 1. No different were found in PLI,GI,and PD between the irrigation sites and the control sites.Thus, after 2 and 4 weeks of supragingival plaque control, the harboring plaque had been reduced from 1.31 to 0.33 for test sites, 1.31 to 0.41 for cotrol sites. There was no significance between the irrigation sites and the control sites. And the mean of GI score sligtly reduced 1.81

to 1.44(P<0.01) for test sites, 1.88 to 1.69(P<0.01) for control sites. There was a significantly improvement GI score(P<0.05) for the irrigation sites.

The mean PD were decreased from 4.95 to 3.87(P<0.01) for the irrigation sites,and from 4.92 to 4.34(P<0.05) for the control sites. The difference between 2 sites regarding mean PD was not statistically significant.

table 1. THE CHANGE OF CLINICAL PARAMETERS

		0W	2W	4W
PLI	TEST	1.31±0.41	0.61±0.37☆	0.33±0.33☆♥
	CONTROL	1.31±0.50	0.48±0.39☆	0.41±0.42☆
GI	TEST	1.88±0.31	1.55±0.44☆	1.44±0.42☆¬
				*
	CONTROL	1.88±0.26	1.45±0.47☆	1.69±0.29☆˩
PD	TEST	4.95±0.94	4.15±0.95☆	3.87±0.99☆♥
	CONTROL	4.92±1.29	4.98±1.55	4.34±2.08★♥

☆Significant difference from week 0(P<0.01)
★Significant difference from week 0(P<0.05)
♥Significant difference from week 2(P<0.01)
* P<0.05

table 2. THE CHANGE OF MICROBIOLOGICAL PARAMETERS

		0W	2W	4W
THE NUMBER OF TOTAL BACTERIA (×10⁷cells/ml)	TEST	8.67±5.57	2.91±2.41☆	0.98±1.41☆♥
	CONTROL	11.09±13.7	10.11±16.7	4.45±6.41☆♥
THE NUMBER OF M&S (×10⁷cells/ml)	TEST	3.59±2.90	0.84±1.14☆	0.19±0.31☆♥¬
				*
	CONTROL	5.00±8.81	5.19±11.3☆	1.75±3.33☆♥˩

☆Significant difference from week 0(P<0.01)
♥Significant difference from week 2(P<0.01)
* P<0.05

Microbiological-findings

There were statistically significant difference in the number of total bacteria and motile rods & spirocheta(M&S) to less than base line(OW) value for both sites. At 4 weeks the number of M&S was significantly improved to the irrrigation sites when compered to the control sites(table 2).

DISCUSSION

The background of this study

Various subgingival irrigaton tequniques have been studied of periodontal disease. However most authers have studied antibiotics or chlorhexidine.

There are only few reports on subgingival washing effect by irrigation tequnique.

There is 2 methods of subgingival irrigation. One is by inserting syringe into the irrigants to slowly lavege in subgingival area, and the other is by use of the irrigator. Recently, subgingival irrigation device system has been introduced. The present study was desiged to evaluated the effect of water jet irrigation on moderate periodontal pockets.

The washing effect of subgingival jet irrigation

Recently several studies have been suggested that various loosely adherent plaque bacteria could be involved in periodontitis.

Fine et al[3] says his paper that limulus activty in loosly adherent plaque consistently higher than in comparable attached plaque sample. And subgingival loosly plaque included motile rods & spirochetes. Our results showed that supragingival plaque control plus water jet irrigation statistically improved M&S counts reduction versus supragingival plaque control only. It was suggested that the reduction of M&S counts was to wash the loosely adherent plaque by water jet irrigation.

Conclusion

It was concluded that water jet irrigation measures in moderate periodontal pockets has beneficial effects on subgingival bacterial flora and improvement of clinical parameters.

REFERENCE

1. Watts E.A.et al(1986) J.Clin.Periodontology 13:666-670
2. Hagiwara et al(1988) Recent advances in clinical periodontology. ELSEVIER SCIENCE PUBLISHERS B.V., Amsterdam, pp 483-486
3. Fine D.H.et al(1978) J.Periodont.Res. 13:17-23

© 1991 Elsevier Science Publishers B.V.
Recent advances in periodontology Vol. II,
S.I. Gold, M. Midda and S. Mutlu, eds.

HISTOLOGICAL STUDY OF MULTINUCLEATED GIANT CELLS IN BONE GRAFTING

KIYOTAKA INUI,YOSHIO MOTEGI,KOHJI HASEGAWA,TETUHIKO TACHIKAWA AND
SYUSAKU YOSHIKI

Department of Periodontics, Department of Oral Pathology, Showa
University Dental School.2-1-1 Kitasenzoku Ohta-ku Tokyo 145 JAPAN

INTRODUCTION

Bone grafting, a future anticipation of new attachment procedures, has been performed in the purpose of promoting active new bone formation in periodontal bone defects. In numerous situations, new bone formation has been observed surrounding and inside the graft materials and on the surface of the facing bone. But concerning the metabolism of these graft materials after implantation, the process is left unknown. Is the graft materials absorbed by osteoclasts or the so-called foreign body giant cells? The purpose of this study was to histochemically determine the characteristics of elicited multinucleated giant cells adhering artificial graft materials.

MATERIAL AND METHODS

Twenty-four rats (SD strain) weighing 150-180g and 24 mice (ddy strain) weighing approximately 25g were used in this study. Isogeneic bone particles (BP) were prepared from femora. The cleaned diaphyses were extracted with absolute ethanol followed by anhydrous ethyl ether. The bones were palverized. Bone particles measuring 80-300μ m were separated by sieving. As artificial graft materials, resorbable ceramic β –tricalcium phosphate (TCP), non-soluble porous hydroxyapatite (pHA) and non-soluble non-porous hydroxyapatite (npHA) were examined, with BP serving as control. Lateral subcutaneous pockets were prepared by blunt dissection over the back area in anesthetized rats and mice. Twenty mg of BP, TCP, pHA or npHA were each embedded in groups of 6 rats and mice. Incisions were sutured at least 2cm from the implantations. After 20 days, specimens were harvested for histologic analysis and enzyme histochemistry. For decalcified light microscopy, specimens were fixed in 4% formalin-calcium with 8% sucrose at 4℃, decalcified in 10% EDTA containing 8% sucrose at 4℃, followed by rinses in cacodylate buffer, pH7.4 and embedding in glycol methaacrylate (JB4,Polysciences) at 4 ℃. Four-micron sections were stained with Mayer's hematoxylin for acid phosphatase activity with (AcP)and without 50mM sodium-tartrate (TRAcP)for 30 minutes at 37 ℃ or for non-specific esterase activity(NSE). The number of stained cells was determined in at least 5 particles per specimen. The intensity of reaction was graded on a scale negative(0) to positive(++). The number of positive cells per circumference of particles was counted. Statistical analysis were done using the Welch t-test (of means).

RESULTS

Implant of pHA and npHA alone showed similar tissue reactions. Each of the particles were surrounded by large and multinucleated giant cells. The interstitial space was composed of connective tissue with small blood vesseles, fibroblast-like cells and mononuclear cells. Implants of BP showed evidence of surface resorption of particles, i.e. resorption bays containing large multinucleated cells. The feature of TCP implants was similar, but interstitial spaces contained more fibrous tissue and mast cells and fewer infiltrative inflammatory cells than in TCP specimens. As the result of TRAcP activity, there was no significant difference in the number of positive cells, both in BP and TCP. But more positive cell adherences were significantly seen in control than in pHA and in npHA(Table.2). AcP activity in mice and rats and the number of positive cells in TCP were similar to thosein BP(Table.1). The number of multinucleated giant cells positive to NSE activity was minimun(Table.3).

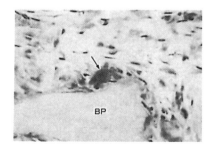 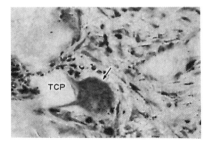

Fig.1
The specimen from BP implant.
Large multinucleated cells (arrow)
surround bone particle.
(mouse,Tartrate resistant acid
phosphatase ×480)

Fig.2
The specimen from TCP implant.
Large multinucleated cells (arrow)
surround TCP particle.
(mouse,Non-specific esterase×480)

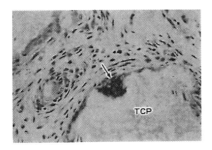

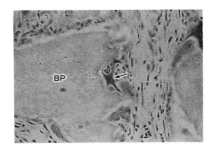

Fig.3
The specimen from TCP implant.
Large multinucleated cells (arrow)
surround TCP particle.
(rat, Tartrate resistant acid
phosphatase × 480)

Fig.4
The specimen from BP implant.
Large multinucleated cells (arrow)
surround bone particle.
(rat, Acid phosphatase × 480)

Table.1
AcP POSITIVE MULTINUCLEATED GIANT CELLS
(MICE)

	+ & ++POSITIVE	++POSITIVE
BP	7.71± 4.47	3.06± 3.36
TCP	9.07± 2.92[NS]	2.01± 1.76[NS]
pHA	2.77± 2.49•••	0.59± 1.41••
npHA	1.71± 1.19•••	0.08± 0.37•••

(POSITIVE CELLS/LENGTH)
[NS] : not significant
•• : $0.001 < p \leq 0.01$
••• : $P \leq 0.001$

Table.2
TRAcP POSITIVE MULTINUCLEATED GIANT CELLS
(MICE)

	+ & ++POSITIVE	++POSITIVE
BP	7.36± 2.50	0.77± 1.41
TCP	7.95± 3.67[NS]	0.69± 1.29[NS]
pHA	1.83± 1.28•••	1.19± 0.59[NS]
npHA	0.69± 1.37•••	0.21± 0.64[NS]

(POSITIVE CELLS/LENGTH)
[NS] : not significant
••• : $P \leq 0.001$

Table.3
NSE POSITIVE MULTINUCLEATED GIANT CELLS
(MICE)

	+ & ++POSITIVE	++POSITIVE
BP	1.15± 1.20	0.14± 0.60
TCP	3.08± 1.92***	0.00± 0.00
pHA	4.06± 2.38***	0.62± 0.98[NS]
npHA	3.23± 1.59***	0.25± 0.61[NS]

(POSITIVE CELLS/LENGTH)
[NS] : not significant
*** : $P \leq 0.001$

DISCUSSION

It is established that macrophages are derived from monocytes of bone marrow origin[1]. Foreign body giant cells are multinucleated cells formed by the fusion of macrophages[2]. Factors such as the composition, size, shape and surface character of the material influence the nature of the foreign body reaction .

Osteoclast which is the multinucleated resorbing cells of bone are formed by the fusion of mononuclear progenitor cells of hematogenous origin[3]. Osteoclast have distinctive features related to their function as the agents of bone resorption. These include cell membrane specialization such as ruffled borders and clear zones of attachment to the bone, and lysozomes with hydrolytic enzymes, especially TRAcP.

Multinucleated giant cells were more frequently seen in TCP rather than in pHA and npHA.The number of TRAcP activity positive cells in TCP were similar to those in BP.

Elicited multinucleated giant cells adhering to graft materials showed enzyme activity similar to those of osteoclasts. It was suggested that artificial graft materials may be absorbed by osteoclasts.

REFERENCES

1. Sutton, J. S. and Weiss, L.(1966) J. Cell. Bio.,28:303-332
2. Mariano, M. and Spector, W. G.(1974) J. Path.,113:1-19
3. Fischman, D. A. and Hay, E. D.(1962) Anat. Rec.,143:329-337

© 1991 Elsevier Science Publishers B.V.
Recent advances in periodontology Vol. II,
S.I. Gold, M. Midda and S. Mutlu, eds.

EXPERIMENTAL STUDY ON PERIODONTAL TISSUE REGENERATION AFTER
BIOACTIVE AND BIOINERT CERAMIC ROOT IMPLANTS

KEN KANNO, TERUYUKI YANAGAWA, TAKASHI YAEGASHI, ATSUSHI KUMAGAI
AND KAZUYUKI UYENO

Department of Periodontology, School of Dentistry, Iwate Medical
University 1-3-27 Chuo-dori, Morioka-shi, Iwate-ken, JAPAN

INTRODUCTION

Recently, bioceramic materials such as artificial roots have
been applicable to periodontal therapy. Generally implanted
roots were maintained mechanically or chemically in created bone
cavities, but there was no definite regeneration in surrounding
periodontal tissues. The present study was designed to evaluate
the periodontal tissue regeneration after ceramic root
implantation into newly extracted root socket with functional
stimulation.

MATERIALS AND METHODS

Implant materials:

Two types of biocompatible implants were used.

(1)APACERAM (PENTAX,Japan): bioactive hydroxylapatite ceramic
root.

(2)BIOCERAM (KYOUCERA,Japan): bioinert single sapphire ceramic
root.

Experimental animals and areas:

Bilateral lower first molars of ten adult beagle dogs were
employed. In addition, bilateral lower second molar areas of
each dog were used as a control.

Methods of implant:

Two types of biocompatible artificial roots, one is a bioactive
hydroxylapatite ceramic root (HAP) and the other a bioinert
bioceram single sapphire root (BCS), were respectively placed
into the mesial root sockets immediately after the mesial root
extraction of bilateral lower first molars of each dog. Some
functional stimulation was added to these artificial roots by
wire-ligature and cementaion with the remnant distal root.

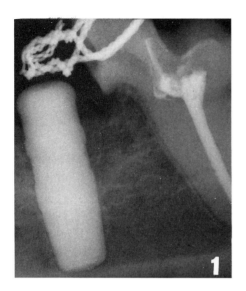

Fig.1

The three-month postoperative radiograph shows good healing at HAP experimental site and no connective tissue layer around the HAP shaft.

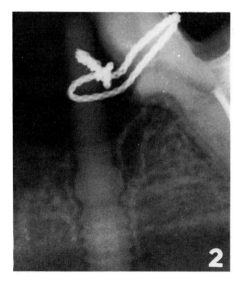

Fig.2

The radiograph taken four months after implantation shows the BCS shaft is surrounded by lamina dura-like appearance at experimental site.

As a control, HAP and BCS artificial roots were implanted into newly created bone cavities at bilateral second molar sites two months after extraction. The bone cavities were made by using PENTAX and KYOCERA-standardized drills and ratchets at the edentulous area.

Experimental periods:

Postoperative tissues were examined macroscopically, radiographically and microscopically up to six months, and some sites over to three years.

RESULTS

Macroscopically, all surgical areas healed by two weeks after the implants at both sites, and were uneventfully maintained during all the experimental periods.

Radiographically, the space between the artificial root and the extraction socket wall near the alveolar crest was filled with newly formed osseous tissues by two months after implantation at both sites. There were occasional signs of osseous adhesion between HAP and the surrounding bones. On the other hand, obvious signs of lamina dura-like appearances were observed at BCS sites.

Microscopically, at HAP sites, severe inflammation and flat, thin fibrous layer were observed between the ceramic root and the surrounding bone one week after implantation. New bone formation was seen along the socket wall two weeks after implantation. Although there were dense fibrous tissue formation and occasional osseous adhesion to the artificial root two months after implantation, no signs of periondontal regeneration could be observed. At BCS sites, dense fibrous tissues, of which arrangement seemed partly to functional orientation, were presented between the artificial root and the bone. However, no apparent signs of periodontal tissue regeneration could be obtained, as the dense fibrous tissue adjacent to the implant shaft revealed no signs of caltification.

The control sites showed almost similar in repair to the experimental sites. However, the osseous repair around the HAP implant was faster at the control site than in the experimental site. The addition of functional stimulation delayed osseous adhesion between the HAP roots and the bones.

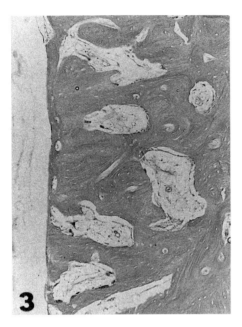 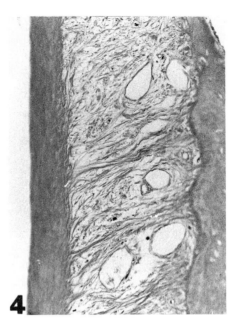

Fig.3

The HAP shaft is integrated with the surrounding bone at the experimental site three months after implantation in this histologic section.(Hematoxyline and Eosin stain)

Fig.4

The arrangement like functional fiber orientation is seen in the connective tissue layer between the BCS shaft and surrounding bone.(Azan-Mallory stain)

CONCLUSION

Amount of periodontal ligament survived on the bone wall of newly extracted root socket was not enough to regenerate the periodontal tissue complex, especially periodontal ligament tissues, even by implantation of two types of ceramic roots into the sockets with functional stimulation.

© 1991 Elsevier Science Publishers B.V.
Recent advances in periodontology Vol. II,
S.I. Gold, M. Midda and S. Mutlu, eds.

EFFECTS OF VARIOUS AGENTS TO REMOVE SMEAR LAYERS ON ROOT PLANED PERIODONTALLY INVOLVED ROOT SURFACES

KOICHI ITO, NAOYUKI SUGANO, JUN-ICHI NISHIKATA, HISASHI UJIIE, KENJI FUJIKAWA AND SEIDAI MURAI

Department of Periodontology, Nihon University School of Dentistry, 1-8-13, Kanda-Surugadai, Chiyoda-ku, Tokyo, 101 (Japan)

INTRODUCTION

The goal of periodontal therapy is the regeneration of periodontium previously destroyed by periodontal disease. The removal of bacterial plaque, calculus and cytotoxic materials from the periodontally involved root surfaces by scaling and root planing is an essential part of periodontal therapy.[1] Characterization of root surfaces after root planing reported that surface smear layers were common.[2-4] There is a possibility that smear layers may contain etiologic factors such as cytotoxic materials and inflammatory agents.[5,6] There is considerable interest in the use of chemical agents to assist in mechanical root instrumentation.

The purpose of this study was to evaluate the effects of various agents to remove smear layers on root planed surfaces using the scanning electron microscope (SEM).

MATERIALS AND METHODS

The proximal surfaces of 21 single-rooted human periodontally involved teeth were scaled and root planed with Gracey scalers (Hu-Friedy Co., Chicago,USA;Nos.5&6) to remove all visible calculus deposits and achieve a smooth, hard, glass-like surface. A specimen was prepared from the proximal surface in size (5 X 5 X 1 mm). The specimens were placed in a beaker containing distilled water and clean for 5 minutes in an ultrasonic cleaner (Vibra Clean 200, MDT Co.,USA; Power high level). Each of six specimens was treated with one of the chemical agents in table 1.

All chemical agents were continuously applied to the specimens by cotton pellets moistened with the agent for 3 minutes. Immediately after the treatment the specimens were immersed in distilled water and gently stirred to stop the chemical reaction. After preparation for this SEM study,all specimens were examined at X 50, X1,000 and X 5,000 with a SEM (JSM-T 100, Japan Electron Optical, Ltd., Tokyo, Japan).

476

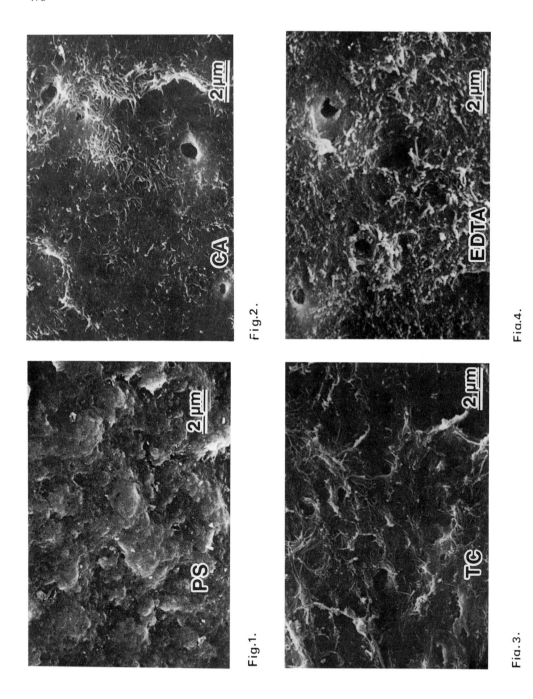

Fig.1.

Fig.2.

Fig. 3.

Fig.4.

Table 1 : Various chemical agents used for specimens

AGENTS		pH
1. Saturated citric acid *	CA	1.0
2. Tetracycline** (100 mg/ml)	TC	1.8
3. Polyacrylic acid ***	PA	2.2
4. Ethylendiaminetetraacetic acid* (15 %)	EDTA	7.2
5. Ampicillin (100 mg/ml)**	AP	10.8
6. Sodium hypochorite# (3 %)	NaOCl	11.8
7. Physiologic saline## (Control)	PS	6.3

* Wako Pure Chemical Industries, Ltd, Osaka, Japan
** Sigma Chemical. Co, St Louis, USA
*** Dentin Conditioner: GC Dental Industrial Corp., Tokyo, Japan
# Koso Chemical Co., Ltd, Tokyo, Japan
Ohtuka Pharmaceuticals, Tokyo, Japan

Figure 1 : Control specimen treated with PS shows some irregular surface with cosiderable debris (smear layers). There is no evidence of exposed collagen fibers and open dentinal tubules (X 5,000).

Figure 2 : SEM of root planed specimen treated with CA displays a relatively flat surface with patent dentinal tubules. Numerous collagen fibers are visible on the surface (X 5,000).

Figure 3 : SEM of root planed surface treated with TC shows numerous exposed collagen fibers and a relatively flat surface with open dentinal tubules (X 5,000).

Figure 4 : SEM of root planed surface treated with EDTA shows numerous exposed collagen fibers and open dentinal tubules. Surface morphology appears to be basically the same as that of surface treated with CA or TC (X 5,000).

RESULTS AND DISCUSSION

Characterization of a dentin surface after root planing reported that surface smear layers were present.[2-4] In this study,teeth were root planed in a clinical situation. After root planing and sectioning procedure, the specimens were washed and debrided in an ultrasonic cleaner. The control specimens treated with PS showed uneven and irregular surface characteristic contained smear layers. There was no evidence of dentinal tubules and exposed collagen fibers on the control specimens (Fig.1).

The smear layers are not removed by rinsing,[3,7,8] the subsequent tissue response may relate to the biological characteristic of the smear layers, possibly contain etiologic factors.[5,6] The smear layers are intimately associated with the tooth surface and virtually removed by demineralizing solution.[7] Acid application not only removes the smear layers and exposes dentinal tubules, but the tubules exhibit widened orifices due to a preferential action on the more highly mineralized peritubular dentin.[7,8] In this study, root planed specimens treated with CA,TC or EDTA had smooth,relatively smear layers-free surfaces with numerous, patent dentinal tubules with a diameter of approximately 0.5 to 1 μm (Figs. 2-4). While PA, AP or NaOCl was relatively ineffective in removing the smear layers and exposing the underlying dentinal surface. The clean surfaces with wider tubular openings appear to offer a more favorable environment for connective tissue attachment.

CONCLUSION

The results suggest that CA, TC or EDTA treatment after root planing may provide an improved substrate for connective tissue attachment.

REFERENCES

1. Wirthlin MR (1981) J Periodontol 52 : 529
2. Jones S, Lozdan J, Boyed A (1972) Br Dent J 132 : 57
3. Lasho DJ, O'Leary TJ, Kafrawy AH (1983) J Periodontol 54 : 210
4. Polson AM, Federick GT, Landenheim S, Hanes PJ (1984)
   J Periodontol 55 : 443
5. Jones WA, O'Leary TJ (1978) J Periodontol 49 : 337
6. Nishimine D, O'Leary TJ (1979) J Periodontol 50 : 345
7. Wilkinson RF, Maybury (1973) J Periodontol 44 : 559
8. Brannstrom M, Johnson G (1974) J Prosthet Dent 31 : 442

© 1991 Elsevier Science Publishers B.V.
Recent advances in periodontology Vol. II,
S.I. Gold, M. Midda and S. Mutlu, eds.

GINGIVAL INFLAMMATION IN PATIENTS TREATED WITH SUBGINGIVAL HIGH-NOBLE AND NON-PRECIOUS NICKEL-CHROMIUM-ALLOY FIXED RESTORATIONS. A COMPARATIVE CLINICAL STUDY.

GABRIELE A. DIEDRICHS, UWE DIEDRICHS and ACHIM SIEPER

Department of Prosthetic Dentistry, Heinrich-Heine-University, Moorenstr. 5, D-4000 Düsseldorf 1 (West-Germany)

INTRODUCTION AND PURPOSE OF THE STUDY

The coronal margin is one of the problematic zones of a fixed restoration. Its quality is determined by whether, and how extensively, the physiological condition of the marginal gingiva is retained.

Economic aspects spured the development of non-precious casting alloys[10]. These efforts in technology of dental materials and their processing tended to reduce costs without functional loss compared to high-gold ceramo-metallic crowns and pontics.

In the Department of Prosthetic Dentistry of Düsseldorf University since 1978 several non-precious nickel-chromium alloys have been applied for fixed restorations.

The purpose of this retrospective clinical study is to evaluate whether the state of the marginal gingiva is affected by subgingival Ni-Cr-alloy fixed restorations compared to the established precious ones in clinical longterm application.

MATERIAL AND METHODS

After an average wearing period of 5.25 years 92 patients with 389 Ni-Cr-alloy crowns and 73 patients with 325 crowns of high-gold alloys were examined. All of them were patients of the Department of Prosthetic Dentistry of Düsseldorf University.

There were five different Ni-Cr-alloys in test (NP2, Ultratek, Wiron 77, Elite and Wiron 88) which had been used for different periods since 1978. The high-noble restorations consisted of Degudent U, Degudent G, Herador H or AM3.

In proof of gingival health of subgingivally crowned teeth Sulcus Bleeding Index according to Mühlemann and Son[4] was assessed and related to the Ramfjord teeth[6] of the same individual. With regard to epidemiologic studies six characteristic teeth represent the individual periodontal state of a patient. In case a tooth was missing or crowned a prescribed substitute tooth was chosen.

Additionally, the coronal margin was probed.

For statistical analysis the X^2-test and the Mann and Whitney U-test as an exact test for randomness in the nonparametric case were applied.

RESULTS

Data of the test samples

In Table1 the data of the test samples are placed together.

TABLE I

DATA OF THE TESTED SAMPLES

Number of crowns, distribution of veneered and non-veneered crowns,
number of patients and average wearing period in months

	n crowns	n veneered	n non-ven.	n patients	average wearing period
Ni-Cr-alloys	389	241	148	92	54
High-nobles	325	267	58	73	72
	714	508	206	165	63

Marginal gingiva and subgingival crowning

In both groups of patients crowned teeth showed a significantly (p<0.05) higher degree of gingival inflammation (SBI $0.62^{+}0.28$) than the non-crowned reference teeth (SBI $0.44^{+}0.23$). No statistical difference between high-gold and non-precious restorations could be found.

In 119 (72%) of in total 165 patients SBI of crowned teeth was higher than the one of the Ramfjord teeth. In 14 (8.5%) cases SBI of the Ramfjord teeth could not be assessed because all teeth in question were crowned.

Marginal gingiva and fit of the coronal margin

The examination of crowns with a contra-angled probe revealed no significant differences between the two types of casting alloys with regard to the proper fit of the coronal margin (minimal marginal gap, accurate margins, no overhangs). The judgement on the marginal fit was classified as "good", "acceptable" in case of a in just one section probable margin and "deficient" if crowns were too short, too extensive or overhanging.

In total 260 (83%) high-gold crowns and 308 (79%) non-precious ones showed clinically perfect margins. While with years the high-gold crowns´ fit was invariantly well, for the non-precious crowns an increasing quality of fit could be stated (Figs. 1 and 2).

There is a slight correlation (p<0.1) between the accuracy of marginal fit and the SBI scores for both types of casting alloys.

The type of casting alloy, however, had no specific influence on the state of the marginal gingiva (Table II). The crownes complained of marginal precision and classified as "acceptable" or "deficient" are summed up as "ill-fitting".

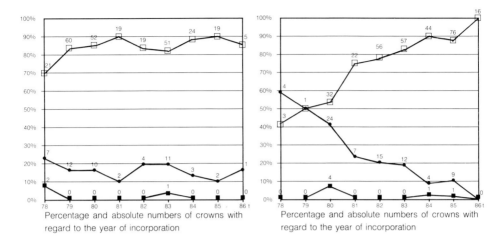

Fig. 1. High-gold crowns' marginal fit
and date of incorporation.

Fig. 2. Ni-Cr crowns' marginal fit
and date of incorporation.

good,   acceptable,   deficient

TABLE II

TYPE OF CASTING ALLOY AND SBI SCORES

Frequency and distribution of SBI scores of teeth with clinically perfect and
ill-fitting Ni-Cr resp. high-gold crowns

| | Ni-Cr-alloys | | | | High-gold alloys | | | |
| | clin. perfect | | ill-fitting | | clin. perfect | | ill-fitting | |
SBI scores	n	%	n	%	n	%	n	%
<0.25	46	89	6	11	60	90	7	10
0.25 – 0.5	81	76	25	24	102	86	16	14
>0.5 – 0.75	112	84	22	16	66	82	15	18
>0.75 – 1.0	57	72	22	28	26	70	11	30
>1.0	12	67	6	33	16	73	6	27
	308		81		270		55	

Marginal gingiva and wearing period

Teeth with longer incorporated crowns showed no significantly increased SBI.
Neither for the group of patients with high-gold restorations nor for the one
with Ni-Cr crowns any significances could be stated. The random distribution
of high-gold and Ni-Cr crowned teeth in the SBI classes concerning the wearing
period was demonstrated.

DISCUSSION

According to other investigations[7][8][9] free gingiva of subgingivally crowned teeth was in a significantly worse condition than the one of non-crowned teeth.

Furthermore, a slight correlation between the accuracy of fit and SBI could be found, thus corroborating in agreement with[2][3][8] that periodontal health is conditioned by the quality of the restorations' margin. Due to improved composition of the alloys and advanced dental techniques Ni-Cr crowns' marginal fit today seems absolutely comparable to that of established precious alloys with fused porcelain veneers. However, the changes of the state of the marginal gingiva can not be simply attributed to ill-fitting coronal margins (for review see[1]).

It has been suggested that periodontal health is affected by some components of casting alloys, i. e. Cu, Be, Ni or Cr[5] . The results of the present study do not support this concept with regard to the tested Ni-Cr-alloys.

CONCLUSION

The results demonstrate that compared to high-noble materials the tested Ni-Cr-alloys per se do not show any specific disadvantages to periodontal health.

REFERENCES

1. Geurtsen W (1990) Dtsch Zahnärztl Z 45:380

2. Kerschbaum Th, Meier F (1978) Dtsch Zahnärztl Z 33:499

3. Lang NP, Kiel RA, Anderhalden K (1983) J Clin Periodont 10:563

4. Mühlemann HR, Son S (1971) Helv Odont Acta 15:107

5. Pierce LH, Goodkind RJ (1989) J Prosth Dent 62:234

6. Ramfjord SP (1959) J Periodont 30:51

7. Sillness J (1970) J Periodont Res 5:225

8. Strub JR, Belser UC (1978) Schweiz Mschr Zahnheilk 88:569

9. Valderhaug J (1978) Zahnärztl Welt/Ref 87:230

10. Weber H (1985) Edelmetallfreie Kronen-, Brücken- und Geschiebeprothetik. Quintessenz Verlag, Berlin

© 1991 Elsevier Science Publishers B.V.
Recent advances in periodontology Vol. II,
S.I. Gold, M. Midda and S. Mutlu, eds.

AN IN VITRO STUDY ON THE BIOCOMPATIBILITY AND INFLUENCE OF GLASS CERAMICS TO OSTEOGENIC CELLS

YOSHITAKA HARA[1], YUKIKO ABE[2], TATSUYA ABE[2], MASAO AONO[2] AND IHACHI KATO[1]

1. Department of Periodontology, School of Dentistry, Nagasaki University, 7-1 Sakamoto-machi, Nagasaki 852, Japan

2. Department of Periodontics and Endodontics, Facultu of Dentistry, Kyushu University, 3-1-1 Maidashi, Higashi-ku, Fukuoka 812, Japan

INTRODUCTION

In recent years, various biofunctional materials have been put to practical use in various fields. But it seems that there are many problems in bonding to bone. Therefore, we tried to make clear the events between materials and cultured cells.

Glass ceramic, which is the one of new biomaterials, have a capacity of direct bond with bone. In the present study, an attempt was made to investigate the biocompatibility and infuluence on the calcification of osteogenic cells, MC3T3-E1.

MATERIALS AND METHODS

Materials used were Glass ceramic (GC) disks of which diameter was 13 mm or granules. MC3T3-E1 derived from new born mouse calvaria was kindly gifted Prof. Kumegawa in Meikai university. Methods were the morphological study under the phase-contrast microscopy, growth curve formation and electron microscopy.

First, cells were inoculated into 24 well multiplates at an appropriate density onto GC and polystyrene coverslips as controls. After 8 days, preparation for electron microscopic study was done. Second, to determine the effect on the calcification, histochemical staining of von-Kossa or alkaline phosphatase (ALP) staining by azo-dye staining method was done.

RESULTS

1) Morphology under the phase-contrast microscopy

MC3T3-E1 cells attached to GC within 24 hours and their numbers increased with time. According to the growth curve, doubling time of cells cultured with GC was shorter than that of controls (Fig. 1). Any cultures reached confluence after 8 days of the cultivation. Phase-contrast microscopy revealed that contact with GC did not bring cellular death nor degeneration.

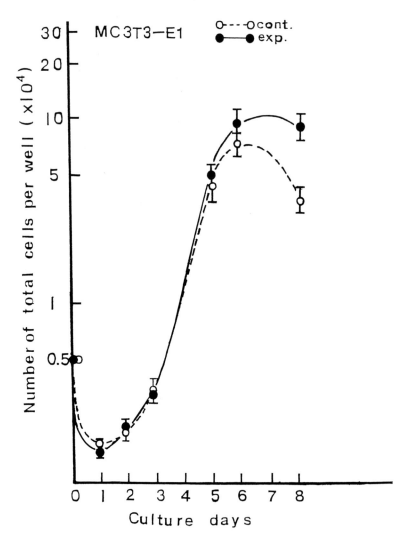

Fig. 1. Growth curve of cells cultured with GC or polystyrene cover slips as controls. Each point showes that mean ± SD. of triplicate cultures. Medium in any cultures was not changed.

2) Ultrastructural study on the interface between MC3T3-E1 and GC.

By transmission electron microscopy, an amorphous structure similar to basal lamina sometimes existed on the wide space between cultured cells and substrates. Cells in cultured with GC prolifferated more three-dimensionally than control cultures (Fig. 2, 3).

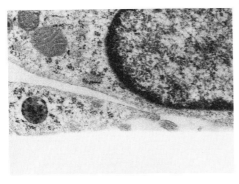

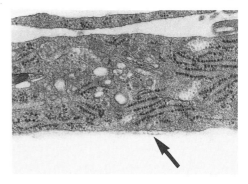

Fig. 2   Fig. 3

Fig. 2. Electron microscopic appearance of control cells cultured with polystyrene cover slips as a control.

Fig. 3. Electron microscopic appearance of cells cultured with GC. Amorphous structure similar to basal lamina (arrow) was observed in part at the interface between cells and GC.

These ultrastructural findings suggest that the biocompatibility of GC was sutisfactory.

3) Effect of GC on the calcification in MC3T3-E1.

Second to clarify the influence of GC on the calcification, histochemical staining were applied.

In cultures with GC, the von-Kossa reaction around some of GC was seen as early as 8th day. On the otherhand, control cells were negative (Fig. 4, 5).

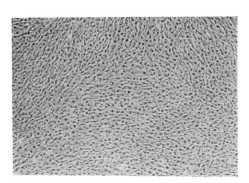

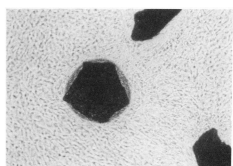

Fig. 4   Fig. 5

Fig. 4. A photomicrograph of MC3T3-E1 at 8th day, stained with von-Kossa's No mineral deposits were found in a control culture.

Fig. 5. A photomicrograph of MC3T3-E1 at 8th day, stained with von-Kossa's method. Positive reactions by silver-nitrate were partly found arround GC.

Reaction of ALP at 8th day was localized on cells which prolliferated three-dimensionally around GC and small polyhedral cells which relatively far apart. Control cells had some scattered positive reaction (Data is not shown).

DISCUSSION

These findings suggest that the biocompatibility of GC is satisfactory.

An amorphous structure similar to basal lamina by the transmission electron microscopy was seemed to be a key factor, of which GC have a direct bond with cells. Further from clinical point of view it seemed to be possible to close the material-tissue interface with osteoblastic cells.

From the histochemical staining, GC facillitated the mineralization of MC3T3-E1 in culture. Further work is in progress to investigate the phenomenon between MC3T3-E1 and GC.

© 1991 Elsevier Science Publishers B.V.
Recent advances in periodontology Vol. II,
S.I. Gold, M. Midda and S. Mutlu, eds.

TWO STEP SURGICAL TREATMENT OF LOCALIZED GINGIVAL RECESSIONS

KAYHAN CIVELEK   JOHN WALTERS   CHARLES SOLT   JOHN HORTON
The Ohio State University,College of Dentistry, Department of Periodontology
305 West 12. Ave. Columbus Ohio 43210 (U.S.A.)

INTRODUCTION

The cause of gingival recession has not been defined yet but can be related to
periodontal disease, developmental defects, trauma and dental procedures.
Different surgical treatments have been advocated for treatment of gingival
recessions, such as laterly sliding flap and coronally positioned flap procedures. Both these techniques require enough width of attached gingiva,where as
localized recessions usually observed with narrow band of attached gingiva.
Bernimoulin(1) described a technique which combined the free gingival graft
and coronally positioned flap procedure. It consisted of gingival graft placed
apical to the recession to increase the width of the attached gingiva. Two
months after grafting procedure a mucoperiosteal flap raised and positioned
coronally. Later Maynard (2) advocated similar procedure for the treatment of
localized gingival recession, and found it to be a predictable procedure for the
buccal aspect of the teeth. Matter (3) presented two year results of the similar
procedure. He was able to obtain significant root coverage. Caffesse (4,5) treated recessions with free gingival graft and compared the two year results with
lateral slidind flap procedure. Recently Liu treated recessionswith similar
technique and used Citric acid to initiate connective tissue attachment. (6)
The purpose of this study is to present one year results of the surgical technique that was used to treat localized gingival recession.

MATERIAL AND METHOD

48 years old female patient presented to The Ohio State University,College of
Dentistry, with a chief complain of "unpleasentt toth appearence. Clinical
examination showed, generally stable periodontal structure with normal sulcus
depth. Radiographic evaluation did not reveal any periodontal breakdown.
Radiographic evaluation of tooth # 22 showed normal interproximal bone-tooth
relation. Sulcus depth, the distance from gingival margin to the C.E.J., and
the width of attached gingiva was measured at the initial periodontal examination and two and twelve months after the procedure. Biometric evaluation
showed 6.0 mm. recession which was the distance between the margin of the gingiva
and the C.E.J. on tooth # 22. The width of attached gingiva was 1mm. and the
sulcus depth noted as 1mm.all around the tooth. All measurements were done
with Michigan probe. A plaque control program was initiated; this program
included scaling, education in oral physiotherapy,and brushing technique.

Grafting procedure

Local anesthesia was obtained using 2%xylocaine with 1:50 000 epinephrine.
With a No 15 Bard-Parker blade a rectangular area of mucosa was dissected to the
apical area of gingival recession. All loose connective tissue and muscle
fibers were dissected to the periostium. The remaining thin layer of soft
tissue formed a rigid base of lamina propria which allowed for immobilization
of the graft. Masticatory mucosa of the palate served as donor site for the
graft. A 2cmX1.5cmX0.5cm autograft was taken from patate. The graft was stored
in a gauze sponge moistened with a normal saline. The graft was secured to
it's bed two simple interrupted sutures, and with figure eight suture from
the periosteum to the tooth. Both surgical sites were packed with periodontal
dressing and prefabricated maxillary occlusal stand was used by the patient
for one week to prevent post op. discomfort. Sutures were removed one week
after the surgery. The patient was seen four weeks after the surgery for
reevaluation.

Coronally positioning

Two months after the initial surgery local anesthesia administered with
 2%xylocaine with 1:50 000 epinephrine at the previously grafted site. Two
 vertical incision bordering the graft was done. They were connected with sulcular incision alomg the gingival margin that extended to the crest of the
 bone. The bone and the cementum was exposed by reflecting a mucoperiosteal
 flap. To facilitate the coronal placement of the mucoperiosteal flap the
 periosteum was severed at the base of the flap using an undermining incision.
The papillae were trimmed with iris scissors to create a normal appearence.
The flap was placed to the level of C.E.J. and sutured by interrupted sutures
at the papillae and in the vertical incisions laterally. Surgical site was
packed with periodontal dressing. The pack and the sutures were removed
 ten days after the surgery.

RESULTS

Clinical healing after both procedures showed normal pattern. One week
after the intial procedure the graft tissue was grayish-white in color. The
desquamated tissue could be removed easily with a cooton swab and slight
hemorrhage noted. The tissue bed adjacent tothe graft was erythamatous,
soft and tender. Donor site normal granulation tissue one week after the
surgery. One month after the surgery clinical healing was completed.
Ten day after the second procedure the soft tissue at the surgical site
was inflamed with an erythematous appearance the wound edges was slightly
rolled and a narrow depression was observed at the surgical site. The gingiva
appearededematous and was soft in consistency.

Biometric evaluation

After two months attached gingiva was 5 mm at the surgical site,sulcus
depth was found tobe 2 mm.and recession measured as 2.5..These results
were stable one year after the surgery.

DISCUSSION

The management of gingival recessions are possible with mucogingival surgeries.
Two step surgical treatment presents an alternative to pedicle grafts and
coronally positioned grafts. We were able to obtain 58.30 % root coverage.
This results were stable after one year. The major gain was in the width
of the attached gingiva. Since the sulcus depth was 1 mm at the initial
exam where the distance from gingival margin to the M.G.J. was also noted
as 1 mm these data was evaluated as lack of attached gingiva but 1mm. of
keratinized gingiva. Sulcus depth increased from 1 mm. to 2 mm. at the end
of one month this change accepted as pathological alteration. Where as Caffesse
was able to reduce the pocket depth after one month. The biometrical evaluation
of the present study show similarity with previous studies. Bernimoulin;
in his original study on 20 sites had an average 2.43 mm of recession
to begin with at the end of one year the average recession was 0.84mm.
Matter later treated 36 recession sites with an average of 2.91cm. with the
similar technique. After one month the average was 0.81. and was stable for
years. He had an average of 65% root coverage. Caffesse was able to have
64.24% root coverage. These studies agree with the present report. Recently
liu tried citric acid to initiate attachment of gingival fibers to the cementum, his results with the rest of the literature for root coverage. He advo
cated the measurement sulcus depth as part of the whole recession. The present
study does not advocate this surgical technique as a the one and the only
surgical technique for recession treatment. Since the cause of the recession
is not clear different recessions may be a good candidate for different treatment
techniques. When surgically treating the exposed roots the adjacent teeth
and the interproximal bone has great importance. One should never attempt
to cover the root surface coronal to the level ao adjacent interproximal bone.
More cases are needed to accept this procedure as a predictable technique.
The nature of the attachment between soft tissue and the cementum can be
the next step in investigating this technique.

REFERENCES

1. J.P. Bernimoulin, B. Luscher and H.R. Muhlemann:Coronally Repositioned
    Periodontal Flap. J. of Clinical Periodontology: 1975,2 1-13

2. J.G. Maynard : Coronal Positioning of a Previously Placed Autogenous
    Gingival Grafts: J. of Periodontology 1977: 48   151-155

3. J. Matter : Free Gingival Graft and Coronally Positioned Flap: J. of
    Clinical Periodontology 1979: 6 437-442

4. R.G.Caffesse and E.A. Guinard: Treatment of Localized Gingival Recessions
    Part II Coronally Repositioned Flap with a Free Gingival Graft: J. of
    Periodontology 1978 49 357-361

5. R.G. Caffesse and E.A. Guinard : Treatment of Localized Gingival Recessi-
    ons Part IV Results after three years: J. of Periodontology: 1980 51
    167-170

6. W.J. Liu and C.W. Solt: Surgical procedure for Treatment of Localized
    Recession in Conjunction with Root sutface Citric Acid Conditioning:
    J. of Periodontology 1980 51 505-509

© 1991 Elsevier Science Publishers B.V.
Recent advances in periodontology Vol. II,
S.I. Gold, M. Midda and S. Mutlu, eds.

EFFECTS OF MECHANICAL STRESS ON BONE RESORPTION

M. MATSUNAGA, T. SETOGUCHI, M. NAKAMURA, M. YOKOTA* and T. SUEDA
Department of Periodontology, School of Dentistry, Kagoshima Univ.
1208-1 Usuki, Kagoshima-city, 890 (Japan)
*Department of Periodontology and Endodontology, Kyusyu Dental College

INTRODUCTION

The mechanisms of alveolar bone resorption observed in periodontal disease are not well clarified. Recently, PGE_2 is thought to be a chemical mediator of the bone resorption[1]. And the increase of PGE_2 synthesis by the bone cells cultured under the stressed condition was previously reported[2,3].

The amount of alveolar bone loss observed on radiograph is larger where occlusal trauma or food impaction can be seen[4,5]. These sites seem to be affected by the mechanical stress as well as the inflammation caused by plaque.

Then we studied the effects of the mechanical stress on the bone resorption, and the relation between the PGE_2 and the activity of the bone resorption promoted by mechanical stress *in vitro*.

MATERIAL AND METHODS

The calvaria of 19 day-old Wistar strain rat fetuses, which were prelabeled by injecting the pregnant rats with ^{45}Ca (2.2 MBq) 24 hours prior to sacrifice, were used for this study. Part of bones were killed by 2 cycles of freeze-thawing ("killed" bone). The bones were placed on the stainless steel mesh to keep them at the gas-liquid interface.

They were precultured for 24 hours to remove exchangeable ^{45}Ca in 2.0 ml chemically defined medium (BGJb medium Fitton Jackson modification) supplemented with bovine serum albumin fraction V (1 mg/ml), ascorbic acid (300 µg/ml) and antibiotics (100 U/ml penicillin, 100 µg/ml streptomycin), at 37 ° C in an atmosphere of 5% CO_2 in air.

The bones were transferred to 2.25ml fresh medium or fresh medium containing indomethacin ($10^{-5}M$), and cultured for 48 hours. One hour after transference, the mechanical stress was applied to some bones. Stainless steel of 3g or 6g weights were used as the mechanical stress. To examine the effect of PGE_2 on this culture system, some bones were cultured in the medium containing PGE_2 ($10^{-5}M$ or $10^{-6}M$). Control bones were cultured in the fresh medium without mechanical stress. After 6 hours, 12 hours, 24 hours and 48 hours, 100 µl medium were collected from each wells. At the end of culture, each bones were decalcified for 6 hours with 1.0 ml of 4N HCl. Then the decalcified bone solutions were neutralized with 1.0 ml of 4N NaOH. The amount of ^{45}Ca in the medium and the solution was counted in a liquid scintillation counter. The bone resorption was expressed as a percent of total ^{45}Ca at each measurement time.

Statistical analysis was performed using Student's t test for unpaired samples.

RESULTS

The percentage of ^{45}Ca release after 48 hours culture from the living bone and the killed bone is showed in Fig.1. ^{45}Ca release of the killed bone was significantly lower than that of the living bone (P<0.001).

The effects of PGE₂ on ^{45}Ca release are showed in Fig.2. The percentage of ^{45}Ca release after 48 hours culture with PGE₂ was significantly higher than that of control group (P<0.001). But there were no statistical differences between $10^{-5}M$ group and $10^{-6}M$ group.

The effects of the mechanical stress on ^{45}Ca release for 48 hours are showed in Fig.3. The stressed group showed more ^{45}Ca release than the unstressed group after 48 hours culture (3g group: P<0.01, 6g group: P<0.05). But there were no statistical differences between 3g group and 6g group.

The effects of indomethacin ($10^{-5}M$) on ^{45}Ca release for 48 hours from mechanically stressed bone are showed in Fig.4. We used only the 3g weight, because there were no statistical differences between 3g weight group and 6g weight group on ^{45}Ca release (Fig.3).

After 48 hours culture, ^{45}Ca release stimulated by the 3g weight group was significantly higher than that of the control group (P<0.001), and the activity was suppressed by indomethacin. But there were no statistical differences between stressed group and suppressed by indomethacin group.

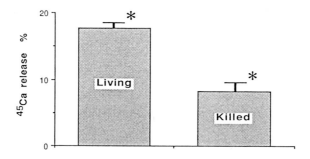

Fig.1 Percentage of ^{45}Ca release from the living bone and the killed bone after 48 hours culture (* P<0.001).

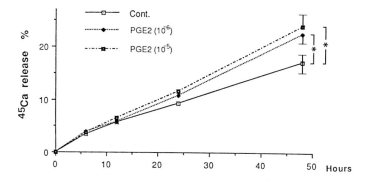

Fig.2 Effects of $PGE_2(10^{-5}M, 10^{-6}M)$ on ^{45}Ca release for 48 hours. (* P<0.001)

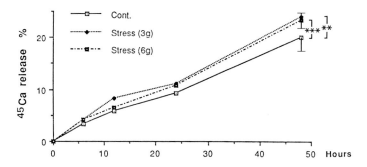

Fig.3 Effects of the mechanical stress on ^{45}Ca release for 48 hours.
(** P<0.01, *** P<0.05)

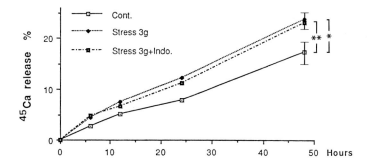

Fig.4 Effects of the mechanical stress (3g) and indomethacin $(10^{-5}M)$ on ^{45}Ca release for 48 hours. (* P<0.001, ** P<0.01)

DISCUSSION

^{45}Ca release was stimulated by PGE$_2$ on this culture system. Similarly ^{45}Ca release was stimulated by the mechanical stress. But indomethacin had no effect on ^{45}Ca release stimulated by mechanical stress. Indomethacin is said to inhibit the synthesis of prostaglandins. These results indicate that ^{45}Ca release stimulated by the mechanical stress with 3g weight is modulated by some factors as well as prostaglandins.

There were no statistical differences between the 3g weight group and the 6g weight group on ^{45}Ca release (Fig.3). This tendency may indicate that the stress used in this study was too heavy. It seems to be important to investigate the influence of the light stress on the bone resorption.

REFERENCES

1. Klein,C.D. and Raisz,G.L.: Prostaglandins: Stimulation of bone resorption in tissue culture. Endocrinology 86:1436-1440,1970.

2. Harrell,A., Dekel,S. and Binderman,I.: Biochemical effect of mechanical stress on cultured bone cells. Calcif. Tissue Res. (Suppl.) 22:202-209, 1977.

3. Somjen,D., Binderman,I., Berger,E. and Harell,A.: Bone remodelling induced by physical stress is prostaglandin E$_2$ mediated. Biochim.Biophys.Acta 627:91-100,1980.

4. Lindhe,J. and Svanberg,G.: Influence of trauma from occlusion on progression of experimental periodontitis in the beagle dog. J.Clin. Periodontol., 1:3-14,1974.

5. Miyagawa,M., Lin,C., Kamatsuki,K., Ohkura,H., Kowashi,Y., Sueda,T. and Kinoshita,S.: Clinical study of the food impaction of patients with periodontal disease - Its frequency, classification and relation to clinical signs. J.Jpn.Ass.Periodontol., 24:201-209,1982.

© 1991 Elsevier Science Publishers B.V.
Recent advances in periodontology Vol. II,
S.I. Gold, M. Midda and S. Mutlu, eds.

PREVALENCE OF PERIODONTAL DISEASE IN MENTALLY AND PHYSICALLY HANDICAPPED PEOPLE
IN NAGASAKI PREFECTURE, JAPAN

YUTAKA OSADA[1], KATSUNORI TANAKA[2], TOMIO WATANABE[2], YOZO INAZAWA[2], KAZUHIRO
TERATANI[2], KAZUHIKO MATSUTANI[2], YOSHITAKA HARA[1] AND IHACHI KATO[1]

[1]Department of Periodontology, Nagasaki University School of Dentistry,
7-1 Sakamoto-machi, Nagasaki, Japan
[2]Nagasaki Dental Health Center, 3-19 Mori-machi, Nagasaki, Japan

INTRODUCTION

There are about 2 million physically and mentally handicapped people in Japan.
Many of them are in need of dental treatment. However, there are not enough
dental services to cope with their special needs. Also, there have been few
epidemiological studies[1-2] done on the periodontal status of handicapped people.

In Nagasaki there are about 60 thousand of these people living either at home
or in one of Nagasaki's 52 institutions. The Nagasaki Dental Association was
entrusted by the prefecture to ensure the maintenance and improvement of the
people's oral health. Therefore, in 1985 the Nagasaki Dental Health Center was
opened and is mainly concerned with the needs of the handicapped.

The purpose of this study was to investigate the prevalence of periodontal
disease and periodontal status in institutionalized handicapped people in
Nagasaki prefecture.

MATERIAL AND METHODS

Subjects

From January 1988 until June 1990, we examined people in 8 institutions which
specialized in the rehabilitation of severly physically and mentally handicapped
people. 174 test subjects (92 male, 82 female all over 17 years old) aged 17-68
(average: 30.9 yrs), were randomly selected for examination in this study.
These subjects suffered from mental retardation (82.8%), epilepsy (27.6%),
physical disability (17.8%), cerebral palsy (13.8%) and Down's syndrome (11.5%)
in this order. Please note that over half of these people suffer from 2 or 3
of these conditions.

Of the 174 subjects, only 107 of them were able to take an IQ (intelligence
quotient) test. 79 people (73.8%) scored below 35, while 28 people (26.2%)
scored above 36. So over half of the subjects were severely mentally deficient.

Clinical examination

On each of the 6 representative teeth (# 16, 21, 24, 36, 41 and 44) in all of
these subjects, we examined the mesio-buccal sites and measured Probing Pocket
Depth (P P D), Gingival Index (G I Löe & Silness[3]), Plaque Index (Pl I
Silness & Löe[4]), and Calculus Index (C I Green & Vermillion[5]).

496

Also, we took dental X-rays to check for bone loss (vertical bone loss of 2mm or more from the cement-enamel junction), and together with knowing the attachment level, we could diagnose health, gingivitis, periodontitis or gingival hyperplasia.

We also checked whether or not the subjects we taking antiepileptics.

The examiner is one periodontist who was responsible for examining all of the subjects.

RESULT

The rate of prevalence of periodontal disease by age

We can clearly state that almost all of institutionalized handicapped people suffer from periodontal disease. The prevalence of gingivitis decreased with age, while the prevalence of periodontitis increased. For the young adult group, the prevalence of periodontitis was much higher than healthy people of this age (Fig.1).

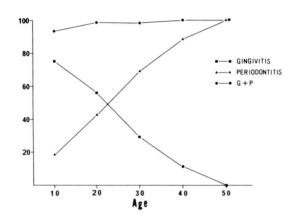

Fig.1.   Prevalence of periodontal disease by age (%)

The rate of prevalence of periodontal disease by IQ level

We divided the subjects into 2 groups: those below 35 and those above 36. Those with a lower IQ group had a greater occurence of periodontitis, while those with a higher IQ group suffered mainly from gingivitis (Fig.2).

The distribution of the maximum PPD of each subject

About 24% had shallow pocket depth, while the remaining 76% had at least 1 of 6 representative teeth with a deep pocket depth of over 4mm (Fig.3).

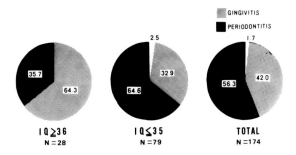

Fig.2.   Prevalence of periodontal disease by IQ level (%)

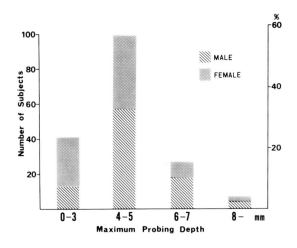

Fig.3.   Distribution of maximum probing depth of each subject

The mean and SD of the PPD, PlI, GI and CI by sex and IQ level

   Compared with healthy people, all of the subjects had high scores. Divided
into sex, the male had much higher scores than the females. And divided by IQ
level, the lower IQ group had much higher scores than the higher IQ group
(Table 1).

Gingival hyperplasia

   Of 42 people who were taking antiepileptics, 16 had gingival hyperplasia (38%).
Most of those with gingival hyperplasia, had such misalignments and malocclusion
as crowding, diastema and open bite.

498

Table 1   Means and S.D. of clinical parameters by sex and IQ level

	n	PPD (mm)	PlI	GI	CI
Total	174	3.20 ± 1.26	1.87 ± 0.59	1.55 ± 0.55	1.54 ± 0.82
Male	92	3.38 ± 1.27	1.98 ± 0.57	1.65 ± 0.54	1.73 ± 0.72
Female	82	3.00 ± 1.21	1.74 ± 0.60	1.44 ± 0.55	1.33 ± 0.87
IQ ≦35	79	3.35 ± 1.32	1.93 ± 0.58	1.59 ± 0.54	1.59 ± 0.81
IQ ≧36	28	2.75 ± 1.03	1.67 ± 0.63	1.31 ± 0.56	1.34 ± 0.89

DISCUSSION AND CONCLUSION
1. From this study, the periodontal status of instituionalized handicapped
people was extremely bad. They had poor oral hygiene, severe gingival inflammation, and deeper pocket than healthy people.
2. We can state that almost all of the subjects suffer from periodontal disease.
For the 10-30 year old group, the rate of periodontitis was higher than healthy
people of the same age. Therefore it is necessary to have some sort of prevention and treatment of the periodontal disease in these young people especially.
3. Because there was a marked difference in the periodontal status between
those of high and low IQ's, it is a necessity to instruct these people about
oral health and hygiene, and help them in ways suited to their special needs.
4. Because, now, within the prefecture there is very little chance for these
handicapped people to receive dental care, we must think of Normalization[6].
This means that we should help make it possible for these handicapped people to
have the chance to enjoy, together with everyone else, as normal a life as
they can. Finally and most importantly, through the maintenance and improvement
of the oral health of these handicapped people, dentists must help them find
ways of doing for themselves to become more self reliant and therefore more
able to lead a normal life.

REFERENCES
1. Suzuki Y, Maita E, Horiuchi H, Suzuki R (1984) J.Jap.Ass.Periodont.26:749-756
2. Kato H, Itatsu K, Nomura M, Tsunakawa K, Sasaki T, Nishio N, Ishikawa S,
    Mizumoto S, Iino M, Takamatsu T (1981) J.Jap.Ass.Periodont. 23:378-385
3. Löe H, Silness J (1963) Acta.Odontol.Scand. 21:533-551
4. Silness J, Löe H (1964) Acta.Odontol.Scand. 22:121-135
5. Green JC, Vermillion JR (1960) J.A.D.A. 61:172
6. Nirje B (1969) In: Kigel R, Wolfensberger W (eds) The Normalization princi-
    ple and its Human Management Implication. In Changing Patterns in Residen-
    tial Services for the Mentally Retarded. Washington D.C. President's
    Committee on Mental Retardation

© 1991 Elsevier Science Publishers B.V.
Recent advances in periodontology Vol. II,
S.I. Gold, M. Midda and S. Mutlu, eds.

THE CLINICAL EFFECTS OF A DENTIFRICE CONTAINING THE SEMICONDUC-
TOR, POWDERED TiO$_2$

KOJI TANAKA, KOICHI ITO, NORITSUGU MAKINO, HIDEHIKO KIKUCHI,
HIDEYASU AKUTAGAWA AND SEIDAI MURAI
Dept. of Periodont., Nihon Univ., School of Dent., 1-8-13 Kanda-
Surugadai, Chiyodaku, Tokyo, Japan

INTRODUCTION

Recently, chemical plaque control has drawn great attention as
an aid of conventional tooth brushing. Chrolhexidene (CH) is the
only chemical agent which is admitted the inhibitory effect of
plaque formation unanimously. Unfortunately, CH has unacceptable
side effects such as tooth staining, burning sensation, etc.
Recently unique chemical agent, semiconductor, powdered TiO$_2$ was
introduced in Japan. The semiconductor, powdered TiO$_2$ is reproted
to have bactericidal effects under irradiation with fluorecent
lamp in vitro[1-4].

The purpose of this study was to examine the effects of a
dentifrice containing the semiconductor, powdered TiO$_2$ on plaque
formation and gingivitis in human volunteers.

MATERIALS AND METHODS
Materials

Subjects. The subjects were systemically healthy 30 dental
students aged 23-29. They had at least 24 sounded teeth and do
not have any restorations on buccal (facial), lingual (palatal)
and interproximal surfaces of their teeth. Their probing sulcus
depth were less than 3mm and the teeth which showed gingival
recession 2mm or more from cement-enamel junction and third
molars were excluded from this study.

Dentifrices. The test and placebo dentifrices were supplied by
Shiken Co.,Ltd. (Osaka,Japan). The test dentifrice contained 5%
powdered TiO$_2$. The placebo dentifrice was identical except for
exclusion on TiO$_2$.

Methods. This study was conducted as double blind, cross over
design. After 2-week prestudy period, the 10-week experimental

period were divided into two 4-week periods, separated by a 2-week interval. (Fig.1) The first day of prestudy period, the oral hygiene status and the gingival conditon were assessed according to the criteria of PSS (Quigley and Hein) and GI (Loe and Silness). Following the examination, all participants were subjected to professional tooth cleaning with scaling and polishing. All of participants were asked to brush their teeth without any dentifrice as usual manner. At the end of prestudy period, clinical indices were recorded and teeh were professinally cleaned. Then each student was assigned test or placebo detnfrice and instructed to brush their teeh near fluorescent lamp more than 2 times a day. At the end of experimental period 1, interim period and experimental period 2, clincal examination and professional tooh cleaning were repeated.

Mean values for PSS and GI following 4 week brushing with test and placebo dentifrice were caluculated. Statistical analysis of the data was performed Student t-test for paired comparison.

RESULTS AND DISCUSSION

Table.1, 2 present the results of this study. The indices of PSS following 4 week use of test dentifrice were slighly lower than that of control dentirice. This tendency was pronounced at buccal surface and anterior teeth. However, all differences between test and placebo dentirice are not statistically significant. Brushing with test dentifirice slightly improved gingival conditon when compared to placebo dentifrice. This improvement was not also statistically significant. Gingival inflammation is usually concomitant with plaque formation. In this study, the

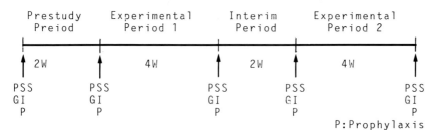

Fig.1 Experimental Design

amount of plaque reduction after using test dentifrice may slightly affect on gingival condition.

Powdered semiconductor irradiated with visible light possess the ability to dicompose organic substances[1] and bactercidal effects[2]. It has been postulated that the bactericidal effect depends on a redox reaction between semiconductor and coenzyme A in which the latter is oxidized intracellulary in the microbial cells[2]. Several studies demonstrated that the powdered TiO_2 itself, or dentifrice containing the powdered TiO_2 has bactericidal effect on Streptococcus munants, Bacteroides gingivalis or other oral bacteria[3,4]. However this study failed to show the inhibitory effect of a dentifrice containing the powdered TiO_2 on plaque formation and gingivitis in human. In vitro study, which showed the bactericidal effects of semiconductor, the light was placed short distance from an incubator. In the oral cavity, especially for posterior teeth, it is difficalt to obtain enough light which bring about semiconductor's bactericidal effects on plaque bacteria. The devices which can access enough light to the oral cavity may be needed when using a dentifrice containing powdered TiO_2 as an aid of conventional tooth brushing for expecting plaque reduction. The dentifrice used in this study contained 5% TiO_2. Was the amount of TiO_2 contained in dentifrice used for one time brushing enough to exert bactericidal effect in human? The mean time which subjects brush their teeth is almost 3 minutes. Is this duration enough to reduce plaque formation?

Further study is needed to elucidate the effect of dentifrice containing the powdered TiO_2 in vivo.

TABLE 1.
THE MEAN PSS AFTER USING TEST AND PLACEBO DENTIFRICE

	Test		Placebo
Total	0.61 ± 0.27	-NS-	0.62 ± 0.25
Maxilla	0.59 ± 0.33	-NS-	0.62 ± 0.26
Mandible	0.63 ± 0.29	-NS-	0.64 ± 0.26
Anterior	0.41 ± 0.26	-NS-	0.46 ± 0.26
Posterior	0.76 ± 0.33	-NS-	0.76 ± 0.21
Buccal(Facial)	0.50 ± 0.21	-NS-	0.58 ± 0.27
Lingual(Palatal)	0.63 ± 0.27	-NS-	0.64 ± 0.19

Mean $\pm$ SD
NS: No significant difference $P < 0.05$

TABLE 2.
THE MEAN GINGIVAL INDEX AFTER USING TEST AND PLACEBO DENTIFIRICE

	Test		Placebo
Total	0.48 ± 0.18	-NS-	0.51 ± 0.19
Maxilla	0.49 ± 0.20	-NS-	0.49 ± 0.17
Mandible	0.47 ± 0.19	-NS-	0.52 ± 0.21
Anterior	0.39 ± 0.20	-NS-	0.44 ± 0.25
Posterior	0.54 ± 0.19	-NS-	0.57 ± 0.17
Buccal(Facial)	0.25 ± 0.18	-NS-	0.28 ± 0.19
Lingual(Palatal)	0.29 ± 0.23	-NS-	0.25 ± 0.20
Interproximal	0.68 ± 0.21	-NS-	0.76 ± 0.21

Mean ± SD
NS:No significant difference $P < 0.05$

CONCLUSION

The use of dentifrice containing powdered TiO_2 as an aid of conventional tooth brushing showed the tendencies to reduce plaque formation and to improve gingival condition when compared to placebo dentifrice. However, these differences are not statistically significants.

ACKNOWLEDGEMENT

The authors wish to thank Shiken Co.,Ltd. for supplying the test and control dentifrices.

REFERENCES

1) Freund T, Gomes T (1969) Catal Rev 3: 1

2) Matsunaga T (1985) J Antibact Antifungi Agents 13: 211-220

3) Onoda K, Watanabe J, Nakagawa Y, Izumi I (1988)
   Denkikagaku 56: 1108-1109

4) Isogai E, Miura H, Isogai H, Wakizaka H, Ueda I, Ito N
   (1988) J Dent Health 38: 588-589

© 1991 Elsevier Science Publishers B.V.
Recent advances in periodontology Vol. II,
S.I. Gold, M. Midda and S. Mutlu, eds.

7 YEARS OF OSTEOINTEGRATED IMPLANTOLOGY EXPERIENCE OF THE UNIVERSITY OF PADUA (ITALY)

G.A. FAVERO   M.D. D.D.S. PH. D.
G.P. CORDIOLI   M.D. D.D.S. PH. D.
A. BELTRAME   M.D. D.D.S. PH. D.

UNIVERSITA' DI PADOVA

CORSO DI LAUREA IN ODONTOIATRIA E PROTESI DENTARIA

CORSO DI PERFEZIONAMENTO IN IMPLANTOLOGIA ORALE ED EXTRAORALE

INTRODUCTION

The concept of osseointegration proposed by Branemark has profoundly changed the clinical implantology approach towards the edentulous patient. [1-3-4-8] The success of the biological principles of osseointegration [6] (Albrektsson 1986) for bone-bond prosthesis has given us the possibility to be able to compare and discuss them on a common basis.

Since 1984, the University of Padova has become an international pioneering center "for osseointegration", and has been able to compare its implantology follow-up [9] with that of Swedish and foreign universities, achieving the same long-term success. [2-7]

The effective scientific value and the long period of clinical application of the Branemark system [1-2-5] (Branemark 1977, Adell 1981, Van Steemberghe 1987) has addressed our choice principally on this implant technique, though without neglecting, with the application of the same modified software, the use of other technique of osseointegration such as IMZ, STRYKER, BONEFIT ITI, PITT EASY (TPS), etc.

MATERIALS AND METHODS

The present work take into consideration all the implants inserted between 1984 and 1990 at our University Clinic in Padova, with the following results.

504

TABLE I

BONEFIT ITI

YEAR	OVERDENTURE	UPPER	LOWER	SINGLE TOOTH	IN	OUT
1989		3	2	5	17	–
1990	1	2	4	6	21	–

TABLE II

STRYKER

YEAR	TOTAL EDENTULISM		OVER	UPPER	LOWER	IN	OUT
	UP	LOW					
1989	1	1		1		15	–
1990	1	2	1	3	6	38	–

TABLE III

IMZ

YEAR	OVER	UPPER	LOWER	IN	OUT
1987	1	2	1	10	–
1988	4	1	6	34	3
1989	8	4	4	35	2
1990	4	2	7	31	1

TABLE IV

PITT EASY

YEAR	UPPER	LOWER	OVER	UPPER	LOWER	SINGLE TOOTH	TOOTH CONNECTION	IN	OUT
1989	1	1	2	3	9	2	5	48	1
1990		2		3	7		7	48	1

TABLE V

BRANEMARK

YEAR	UPPER	LOWER	OVER	UPPER	LOWER	SINGLE TOOTH	TOOTH CONNECTION	IN	OUT
1984	1	1		1				14	–
1985	3	3		3				45	2
1986	2	6	2	9	14		1	125	3
1987	9	16	1	11	15		6	217	5
1988	19	24	16	22	25	14	11	375	12
1989	16	27	24	21	33	29	14	427	14
1990	12	22	19	20	24	42	12	395	10

FAILURE 2,9%

TABLE VI

TOTAL IMPLANT CASE–REPORT

UNIVERSITY OF PADOVA

BETWEEN 1984 TO 1990

(G.A. FAVERO, G.P. CORDIOLI, A. BELTRAME)

Total of Inserted Implant	1905
Removed	53
Sleeping	6
Protesizzati	1693
Extraoral and Bone–Bond	21
Total Failure Percentage	2,8%

TABLE VII

COMPLICATIONS IMZ

ABUTMENT SCREW FRACTURE	7
FRAMEWORK FRACTURE	2
WOUND DEHISCENCE DURING HEALING PHASE OVER IMPLANT COVER SCREW WITHOUT CLINICAL CONSEQUENCES	35
FISTULA	=

TABLE VIII

COMPLICATIONS PITT EASY

WOUND DEHISCENCE DURING HEALING PHASE OVER IMPLANT COVER SCREW WITHOUT CLINICAL CONSEQUENCES	27
RAPID MARGINAL BONE LOSS AFTER ABUTMENT – CONNECTION	3
ABSCESS	2

TABLE IX

COMPLICATIONS BRANEMARK

FIXTURE OUT	46	(2,9 % UNSUCCESSFUL)
ABUTMENT SCREW FRACTURE	2	
GOLD SCREW FRACTURE	12	
FRAMEWORK FRACTURE	8	
OCCLUSAL MATERIAL FRACT	19	
HEMATOMA (ABNORMAL)	2	
ABSCESS	6	
GINGIVITIS SEVERE	4	
FISTULA	6	
RAPID MARGINAL BONE LOSS AFTER ABUTMENT – CONNECTION	2	
BRUXISMUS POKET FORMATION	6	

CONCLUSION

Our period of observation for Branemark's implant system is sufficient, in scientific terms according to the criteria given by Albrektsson, to be able to give one an initial evaluation of the obtained results.

The percentage of failures, mainly occurring in the initial phases of treatment, is nevertheless encouraging, since it has been seen that the possibility of loss of the osseointegration occurs principally in the immediate post-operatory period and durign the first six months after the implant of the prosthesis 4-6 also in the Swedish and in multi-center 7 case-reports (Branemark 1985, Albrektsson 1987).

It is to be noted that the major loss of fixture occured with a length of 7 mm. This has subsequently led the researchers to use longer fixtures providing that the anatomical conditions allow this.

We have also tried other techniques which have so far shown a good success rate, even with a shorter experimental time. We hope that within a few years that it will be possible to compare and to choose between different techniques with a good long term prognosis and at a lower cost, in order to provide a wider diffusion of implant techniques in the population.

REFERENCES

1. Branemark P.I., Hansson B.O., Adell R., Breine U., Lindsrtom J., Hallen O.: Osseointegrated implants in the treatment of the edentulous jaw. Scand. J. Plast. Reconstr. Surg. 11, suppl. 16, 1977.

2. Adell R., Lekholm U., Rockler B., Branemark P.I.: A 15 year study of osseo integrated implants in the treatment of the edentulous jaw. Int. J. Oral. Surg. 10, 387, 1981.

3. Zarb B., Schmitt A., Baker G.: Tissue integreted prostheses, osseointegration research in Toronto. Int. J. Period. Restor. Dent. 1, 1, 1987.

4. Branemark P.I., Zarb G., Albrektsson T.: Tissue integrated prostheses. Osseointegration in clinical dentistry. Quintessence Co, Chicago 1985.

5. Verbist D., Van Steemberghe D., Coppes L.: The applicability of the osseointegration principle in edentulous people. J. Head Neck Phatol 1, 128, 1982.

6. Albrektsson T., Zarb G., Worthington P., Eriksson A.R.: The long term efficacy of currently used dental implants, a review and proposed criteria of success. Int. J. Oral Maxillof. Implants. 1, 11, 1986.

7. Albrektsson T., Bergaman B., Folmer T., Henry P., Higuchi P., Klineberg I., Laney W.R., Lekholm U., Oikarinen V., Van Steenberghe D., Triplett L., Worthington P., Zarb G.: A Multicenter study of osseointegrated implants, submitted 1987.

8. Favero G.A., Cordioli G.P.: Alternative alle edentulie totali intrattabili: presentazione di un caso clinico. Giornale di Stomatologia e Ortognatodonzia vol. V n. 4, 208, 1986.

9. Favero G.A., Cordioli G.P.: Indagine retrospettiva su 271 impianti dentali ad osteointegrazione secondo Branemark. Giornale di Stomatologia e Ortognatodonzia vol. V n. 4, 109, 1987.

© 1991 Elsevier Science Publishers B.V.
Recent advances in periodontology Vol. II,
S.I. Gold, M. Midda and S. Mutlu, eds.

AN IMPLANTOLOGICAL APPROACH TO THE HEREDITARY HYPODONTIA CASES

ALTAN GÜLHAN, IŞIN ULUKAPI, GAMZE AREN, ELİF ERBAY

INTRODUCTION

The congenital absence of teeth has occured in human species since Paleolithic times (1). Numerical alterations of dentition have strong genetic components. While the absence of certain teeth may be polygenic in nature, generalized hypodontia is probably an autosomal dominant trait. The number of teeth absent and the specific teeth are usually quite variable within families. Parents who have missing only one or two teeth, may have children with several to most of their teeth undeveloped. Conversely, nearly edentulous individuals may have of spring with a near normal complement of teeth. This variability of expression introduces uncertainly in the prognosis for particular families. Awareness of the predilection for future generations to be affected is important, since the best treatment for the congenital absence of permanent teeth is to retain the deciduous teeth (2).

In permanent dentition, this abnormality is relatively common with a prevalence of 3.5% to 6.5%, excluding agenesis of the third molars. It occurs more frequently in girls at ratio of 3:2. Agenesis of only the third molars has a prevalance between 9% and 37%. In the deciduos dentition hypodontia occurs less often (0.1%–0.9%) and has no significant sex distributions. The missing deciduous teeth are most often limited to the upper arch (incisors and first deciduous molars). Oligodontia (severe hypodontia) has a population prevalance of 0.3% in the permanent dentition (1).

Numerious articles have appeared in the literature relating the cause of hypodontia to either environmental factors such as irradiation, tumors, rubella and thalidomide or to hereditary genetic dominant factors, or to both and it is also often seen in connection with a number of syndromes like anhidrotic ectodermal dysplasia, chondroectodermal dysplasia, PHC syndrome, aniridia, glaucome, incontinentia pigmenti, Down syndrome, chelio–gnatho–palatochisis (4, 5,6).

Hypodontia does not affect lip position of facial esthetics. According to the literature occurance of missing third molars is rarely found to be an isolated phenomenon (7,8).

The purpose of this study was to show the importance of examining all family members in hypodontia cases. Because after orthodontic and pedodontic treatment these patients should also be investigated for dental implant indications.

MATERIAL AND METHODS

In this study the cases consisted of 6 patients aged 5 to 30 years from Istanbul University Faculty of Dentistry-Pedodontics and Orthodontics clinics in 1989-1990. Selection criteria were availability of panoromic radiographs and dental casts. The diagnosis of missing teeth was made after clinical observation and radiographic examination. In this study 4 cases were boys and 2 cases were girls. In all cases there were no significant medical history but hereditardy histories were significant.

CASE I(2 brothers, parents are relatives)

a) 5 years old. boy, missing teeth:

```
              II    |    II
              2     |    2
          ----------+----------
       5  II  I  |  I  II  5
          2  1   |  1  2
```

Conservatory and orthodontic treatment of this patient is continuing.

b) 9 years old, boy, missing teeth:

```
            2     |
       -----------+-----------
        5         |        5
```

Conservatory treatment is done.

CASE II(2 brothers, parents are relatives)

a) 13 years old, boy, missing teeth:

```
       7  5  4  3  2  |  2  4  5  7
       --------------+--------------
       7  5  4     2  |  2  4  5  7
```

Conservatory treatment is done and prosthetic treatment is continuing. (Because of the loss of vertical dimension we made overdenture this patient.)

b) 9 years old, boy, missing teeth:

```
       7     4  |  4  5     7
       ---------+---------
          5     |  5
```

CASE III (Mother and daughter, mothers parents are relatives)

a) 11 years old, girl, missing teeth

```
    7  6  5  4  3  2  |  2  3  4  5
    ------------------+------------------
    7     5           |              7
```

Orthodontic treatment is continuing.

b) 30 years old, female missing tooth: primary 5

There are a lot of missing teeth but we can say only surely that upper right 5 is missing, because the patient had perhaps extractions before. Prosthetic treatment is continuing.

All cases are motivated for oral hgyiene.

DISCUSSION

Congenital absence of a tooth may be unilateral or bilateral (9). In our cases we mostly observed bilateral absence of teeth.

Absence of theese teeth can often result in serious orthodontic problems(7). T.M.Joint disfunction and, periodontal, esthetic, and masticatory problems. Treatments of such cases must solve these problems and in younger patients prepare the teeth and the jaws for a later remaining rehabilitation (10,11).

In hypodontia cases the morphologic abnormalities of teeth are often seen, and because of this phenomenon orthodontic treatments can be problematic (for fixing of the brakets-like in case 2-a) Therefore prosthetic treatment is preferred.

Prosthetic treatments in such cases can be bridges or removable partial dentures (12). But particularly bridges such as Maryland bridges can be problematic for younger patients with uncomplete jaw development. In hypodontia cases residual ridges of the patients were often very smooth and problematic for removable partial dentures. In adults the problems of missing teeth can also be solved with an osteointegrated fixture. There are multiple advantages of these fixtures (13,14,15). First there is the obvious psychologic benefit for most patients in having a fixed partial denture instead of a removable partial denture. There may be periodontal advantages such as easier plaque control   and a limited tooth mobility (16).

There may be the question of timing and indications in younger patients. What can we do with younger patients, when is the earlier possibility of an osteointegrated fixture?

We think this problem needs further investigations.

REFERENCES

1. Dermaut LR, Goeffers KR, De Smit AA (1986) Am J Orthod Dentofac Orthop 90:204-210.

2. Jorgenson RJ, Levin LS, Mc Kusik VA (1974) The Dental Clinics of North America 587-588.

3. Finn SB (1973) Clinical Pedodontics W.B.Saunders Co, Philadelphia, pp 616-617.

4. Sofaer JA (1989) Br Dent J 167:209-212.

5. Jones JH, Mason DK (1980) Oral Manifestations of Systemic Disease W.B. Saunders Co, London, pp 506-507.

6. Cohen MM (1961) Pediatric Dentistry CV Mosby Co, ST Luis, pp 128-129.

7. Jarvinen S (1984) ASDC 51:374-375.

8. Ranta R (1985) ASDC 52:125-127.

9. Andlaw RJ, Pock WD, Downer GC (1982) A manuel of Pedodontics. Churchill Livingstone Edinburgh, pp 138-139.

512

10. Abadi BJ, Kimmel NA, Falace DA (1982) ASDC 49:123-126.

11. Barghi N, Aquilar T, Martinez C, Woodall WS, Maaskant A (1987) J Prosthet Dent 57:617-620.

12. Groper JN (1983) ASDC 50:369-371.

13. Behneke N, Tetsch P (1985) Fortschr Zahnarztl Implantol I 266-271.

14. Brinkmann E (1976) Dtsch Zahnarztl 2 31:557-559.

15. Buenviaje TM, Rapp R (1984) ASDC 51:42-46.

16. Van Steenbergh D (1989) J Prosthet Dent 61:217-222.

INDEX OF AUTHORS

514